ALZHEIMER'S DISEASE

Janny Lee

ALLIED
HEALTH
PRESS

Alzheimer's Disease

Author: **Janny Lee**

Allied Health Press
4164 Lakeshore Road
Burlington ON L7L 1A4
Canada
www.alliedhealthpress.com
Email: orders@arclereducation.com

ISBN: 978-1-77956-259-3

ABOUT THE AUTHOR

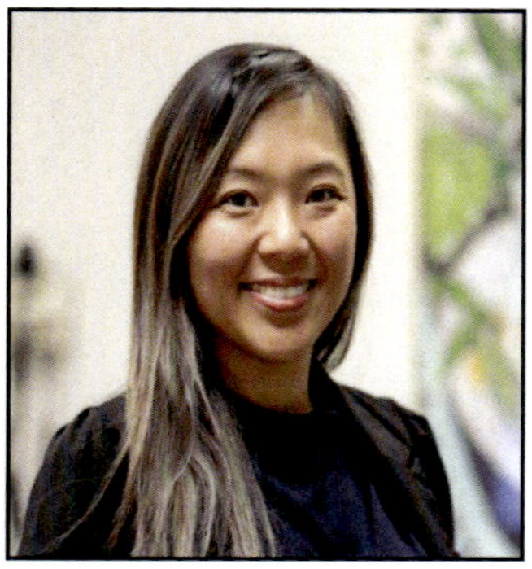

Janny Lee is a dedicated Registered Nurse with a multifaceted background spanning intensive care, community, and emergency care. Currently, Janny is a Clinical Nurse Specialist in Geriatrics in Toronto, Canada, where she is involved in age-friendly initiatives and improving care for older adults. In addition, Janny is an Adjunct lecturer and health tech consultant, offering strategic advisory and clinical transformation. Janny's academic journey is a testament to her commitment to lifelong learning. She earned her Bachelor's in Nursing from the University of New Brunswick, a Master's in Nursing from Athabasca University, and a Master's in Business Administration from the Frankfurt School of Finance and Management. Her dedication to staying abreast of the latest advancements in geriatrics is evident in her active engagement in continuing education. Janny's unwavering dedication to patient care and his diverse experiences and academic achievements exemplify her commitment to excellence in healthcare delivery. She is driven by a profound sense of compassion and empathy, striving to positively impact the lives of those she serves.

Word Roots, Prefixes, and Suffixes by Chapter

Chapter 1 Alzheimer's Disease Basics

corpor: body

myocardi: myocardium (heart muscle)

pneum, pulmon: Lungs, Air

presbyo -: old age

-dynia: pain

-iatry: (specialty, treatment)

Chapter 2 Dementia Due to Alzheimer's Disease (AD)

neuro-: relating to the nervous system or the brain

-cognitive: referring to mental processes

fronto-: frons, frontal lobe of the brain

temporal-: temporalis, temporal lobe of the brain

cardio-: heart

psycho-: psykho, mind or soul

Chapter 3 The Prevalence of Alzheimer's Disease

cerebr-: the brain

cyt-: cell

epi-: over, above, on top

fron-: pertaining to the forehead

hypo-: below

inter-: between, among

intra-: within

Chapter 4 Epidemiology of Alzheimer's Disease

Al-: Relating to Alzheimer's Alzheimerian

Neuro-: Relating to the nervous system Neurodegeneration

-itis: Inflammation of Alzheimeritis

-pathy: Disease or disorder Alzheimeropathy

-genic: Causing Neurogenic

Chapter 5 Diagnosis of Alzheimer's Disease

-osis: Condition or state Neurosis

-logy: Study of Alzheimerology

-plasia: Formation or development Neuroplasia

-ectomy: Surgical removal or excision Neuroectomy

Chapter 6 Alzheimer's Disease Prescription Drug Treatment

acoust/o: hearing, sound

-acusis: hearing

-algia: pain

caps/o, capsul/o: capsule, container

cardi/o: heart

carp/o: wrist bones (carpals)

Chapter 7 Nondrug Treatment for Alzheimer's Disease

-cathisia, -kathisia: sitting

caus/o: burn; burning

cauter/o: heat; burn

cav/o, cavit/o: hollow, cavity

cephal/o: head

Chapter 8 Living with and Caring for Patients with Alzheimer's Disease

cheil/o: lip

gastr/o: stomach

sacchar/o: sugar

seps/o: infection

acro: extremities

Chapter 9 Epidemiologic and Biologic Markers for Alzheimer's Disease

cephal-: head

corp-: body

cardi-: heart

hem-: blood

sex-: six

Chapter 10 Risk Assessment and Prevention of Alzheimer's Disease

-fer-: bear, carry, produce: fertilization

vas-: vessel: vascular tissue

bacteri-: pertaining to bacteria

intra-: within

itis-: inflammation

Table of Contents

List of Figures xiii
List of Tables xv
Preface xvii

1 Alzheimer's Disease Basics 1

Introduction 2
1.1. Overview Of Alzheimer's Disease 4
1.1.1. How Does Alzheimer's Disease Affect the Brain? 4
1.1.2. Stages of Alzheimer's Disease 4
1.1.3. How Long Can a Person Live with Alzheimer's Disease? 5
1.1.4. Brain Changes of Alzheimer's Disease 5
1.1.5. Timing of Brain Changes 6
1.1.6. Brain Changes as Biomarkers 6
1.2. Causes of Alzheimer's Disease 6
1.2.1. Aging and Alzheimer's Risk 7
1.2.2. Genetics of Alzheimer's Disease 7
1.2.3. Hypotheses 12
1.2.4. Health, Environmental, and Lifestyle Factors that May Contribute to Alzheimer's 13
1.3. Signs And Symptoms of Alzheimer's Disease 13
1.4. Diagnosis of Alzheimer's Disease 15
1.4.1. Early Symptoms of Alzheimer's Dementia 15
1.4.2. Diagnosing Alzheimer's Dementia 16
1.4.3. Ruling out Other Conditions 16
1.4.4. Testing Memory Loss and Other Symptoms 16
1.4.5. Laboratory Tests 17
1.4.6. Brain Imaging Tests 17
1.4.7. Future of Diagnosis 17
1.4.8. Benefit of an Early Diagnosis 18
1.5. Treatment of Alzheimer's Disease 18
1.5.1. Treatment for Mild to Moderate Alzheimer's 19
1.5.2. Treatment for Moderate to Severe Alzheimer's 19
1.5.3. Dosage and Side Effects of Alzheimer's Medications 20
1.5.4. Managing Behavioral Symptoms of Alzheimer's Disease 20
1.5.5. Medicines to Be Used with Caution in People with Alzheimer's Disease 20
1.5.6. The Future of Alzheimer's Disease Treatments 21
1.6. Prevention of Alzheimer's Disease 21
1.6.1. Medication 21
1.6.2. Lifestyle 22
1.7. Management of Alzheimer's Disease 23
1.7.1. Pharmaceutical 23
1.7.2. Psychosocial 24
1.7.3. Caregiving 24
1.7.4. Diet 25
1.8. Biochemistry of Alzheimer's Disease 25
1.8.1. Neuropathology 25
1.8.2. Biochemical Characteristics 26
1.8.3. Disease Mechanisms 26
Summary 34
References 35

2 Dementia Due to Alzheimer's Disease (AD) 37

Introduction 38

2.1. Dementia 40

2.1.1. Signs and Symptoms 41

2.1.2. Subtypes of Dementia 41

2.1.3. Clinical Evaluation 44

2.1.4. Assessment Scales 44

2.2. Stages of Dementia 46

2.3. Alzheimer's Disease Progression 50

2.3.1. Preclinical Alzheimer's Disease 50

2.3.2. Mild Cognitive Impairment (MCI) Due to Alzheimer's Disease 51

2.3.3. Mild Dementia Due to Alzheimer's Disease 51

2.3.4. Moderate Dementia Due to Alzheimer's Disease 52

2.3.5. Severe Dementia due to Alzheimer's Disease 52

2.3.6. Rate of Progression Through Alzheimer's Disease Stages 53

2.4. The Diagnosis of Dementia Due to Alzheimer's Disease 53

2.4.1. Criteria for All-Cause Dementia: Core Clinical Criteria 54

2.4.2. Proposed Classification Criteria for AD Dementia 55

2.4.3. Probable AD Dementia: Core Clinical Criteria 55

2.4.4. Possible AD Dementia: Core Clinical Criteria 56

2.4.5. Probable AD Dementia with Evidence of the AD Pathophysiological Process 57

2.4.6. Possible AD Dementia with Evidence of the AD Pathophysiological Process 57

2.4.7. Considerations Related to the Incorporation of Biomarkers into AD Dementia Criteria 58

2.4.8. Pathophysiologically Proved AD Dementia 58

2.5. Dementia Caregiving 58

2.5.1. Family Caregivers 59

2.5.2. Caregiver Burden and Respite Care 60

2.5.3. Environmental Design 60

2.5.4. Communicating 61

2.5.5. Memory Strategies 62

2.5.6. Psychological and Psychosocial Therapies 62

2.5.7. Nursing 62

2.5.8. Incontinence Care 63

Summary 67

References 68

3 The Prevalence of Alzheimer's Disease 71

Introduction 71

3.1. Prevalence of Ad in the United States 73

3.1.1. Prevalence Estimates 74

3.1.2. Mild Cognitive Impairment (MCI) Due to Alzheimer's Disease 76

3.1.3. Underdiagnosis of Alzheimer's and Other Dementias in the Primary Care Setting 78

3.2. Worldwide Prevalence Rates of Ad and Dementia 79

3.2.1. European Studies 80

3.2.2. North American Studies 80

3.2.3. Latin American Studies 80

3.2.4. Asian Studies 81

3.2.5. African Studies 82

3.2.6. Middle East 83

3.3. Methodological Issues in Prevalence Studies 84

3.3.1. Selection Into the Analysis Sample 85

3.3.2. Measurement Validity and Reliability 87

3.3.3. Alternative Timescales and Specification of Longitudinal Models 89

3.3.4. Time-Varying Exposure/ Time-Varying Confounding 90

3.3.5. High-Dimensional Data 91

3.4. Prevalence Rates by Sex 92

3.5. Prevalence by Race Or Ethnicity 93

3.5.1. Ethnic Comparisons Within the United States 93

3.5.2. South America 95

3.5.3. Africa 95

3.5.4. Asia 96

3.5.5. Europe 96

3.5.6. Israel 97

3.5.7. Native Indians 97
3.6. Looking To The Future 98
3.6.1. Continued Population Aging 98
3.6.2. Growth of the Age 85 and Older Population 99
3.6.3. Increased Diversity of Older Adults 99
Summary 103
References 103

4 Epidemiology of Alzheimer's Disease 107

Introduction 108
4.1. Epidemiology of Alzheimer's Disease: Occurrence, Determinants, And Strategies 110
4.1.1. Global Aging 110
4.1.2. Dementia and Alzheimer's Disease 111
4.1.3. Occurrence of Alzheimer's Disease 111
4.1.4. Prevalence 112
4.1.5. Incidence 113
4.1.6. Prognosis and Impact 115
4.1.7. Risk and Protective Factors 115
4.2. Epidemiology of Alzheimer's Disease Modifiable Risk Factors And Prevention 124
4.2.1. Descriptive Epidemiology of Alzheimer's Disease 125
4.2.2. Putative Modifiable Risk Factors and Prevention for Late-Onset Alzheimer's Disease 125
4.2.3. Pre-Existing Diseases 129
4.2.4. Lifestyles 131
4.3. Analytic Epidemiology of Alzheimer's Disease 134
4.3.1. Antecedent Risk Factors that Increase the Risk of Alzheimer's Disease 135
4.3.2. Protective Factors that Reduce Risk of Alzheimer's Disease 138
4.3.3. Genetic Epidemiology 141
Summary 146
References 146

5 Diagnosis of Alzheimer's Disease 149

Introduction 150
5.1. Importance of the Diagnosis of Alzheimer's Disease 152
5.1.1. How Is Alzheimer's Disease Diagnosed? 152
5.1.2. Specialists for Diagnosis 154
5.1.3. What Other Health Problems Can Cause Memory Trouble? 154
5.1.4. Brain Scan Needed to Diagnose Alzheimer's Disease 155
5.2. Alzheimer's Disease Biomarkers 156
5.2.1. Biomarkers in Alzheimer's Disease: Role in Early and Differential Diagnosis and Recognition of Atypical Variants 157
5.2.2. The Clinical Phenotypes of OAD 158
5.2.3. Biomarker Profiles for Typical and Atypical Phenotypes of AD 161
5.2.4. PET Markers 163
5.2.5. MRI Markers 164
5.2.6. CSF Biomarkers 164
5.2.7. Blood-Based Biomarkers (BBBMs) 165
5.2.8. Biomarkers Should be Complementary to Clinical Assessment for AD Diagnosis 166
5.2.9. Biomarkers to Support Clinical Decision Making 168
5.2.10. Who Should Attend Alzheimer's Disease Testing and Diagnosis? 169
5.3. Diagnosis and Management of Alzheimer's Disease 170
5.3.1. Clinical Assessment of Dementia 171
5.3.2. Assessment of Dementia 182
5.3.3. Assessment Instruments for Dementia 184
Summary 187
References 187

6 Alzheimer's Disease Prescription Drug Treatment 195

Introduction 196

6.1. Neurodegenerative Pathways Implicated in AD 198

6.1.1. Amyloid Cascade Hypothesis 198

6.1.2. Tau Hypothesis 198

6.1.3. Cholinergic Hypothesis 199

6.1.4. Excitotoxicity 199

6.1.5. Other Important Etiological Mechanisms 199

6.2. Drug Therapy 200

6.2.1. Approved Drug Treatments 200

6.3. Potential Future Drug Treatments 201

6.3.1. Anti-Amyloid Therapy 201

6.3.2. Immunization 202

6.3.3. Monoclonal Antibodies 202

6.3.4. Tau-Targeted Therapy 203

6.4. Future Directions 203

6.4.1. Early Diagnosis 203

6.4.2. Better Trial Design 204

6.5. An Update on the Novel and Approved Drugs for Alzheimer's Disease 204

6.5.1. FDA Approved Drugs for AD and Their MOA 207

6.5.2. Potential Therapeutic Approach for the Treatment of AD 209

6.5.3. Clinical Trials of Novel Drugs for AD 217

6.5.4. Significance of Research 220

Summary 222

References 222

7 Nondrug Treatment for Alzheimer's Disease 229

Introduction 230

7.1. Need For Non-Drug Treatment for Alzheimer's Disease 232

7.2. Non-Pharmacological Treatment of Alzheimer's 234

7.2.1. Cognitive Training 237

7.2.2. Snoezelen Therapy 238

7.2.3. Reminiscence Therapy 239

7.2.4. Validation Therapy 239

7.2.5. Doll Therapy 243

7.2.6. Ervin Böhm's Psychobiographic Model 245

7.3. Cognitive-Oriented Interventions 246

7.3.1. Cognitive Stimulation 248

7.3.2. Individualized Cognitive Rehabilitation 249

7.3.3. Assessments of Outcomes 250

7.3.4. Limitations 251

7.4. Physical Exercise Interventions 251

7.4.1. Different Types of Physical Exercise Interventions 253

7.4.2. Intensity and Duration of Intervention 254

7.5. Brain Stimulation 254

7.5.1. Deep Brain Stimulation (DBS) 256

7.5.2. Transcranial Direct Current Stimulation (tDCS) 256

7.5.3. Repetitive Transcranial Magnetic Stimulation (rTMS) 256

7.5.4. Transcranial Pulse Stimulation (TPS) 256

7.5.5. Intermittent Theta Burst Stimulation (iTBS) 257

7.6. Nutrition Supplementations 257

Summary 262

References 262

8 Living with and Caring for Patients with Alzheimer's Disease 269

Introduction 270

8.1. Realities of Caring for Someone with Dementia 272

8.1.1. Being a Caregiver for Someone with Alzheimer's 272

8.1.2. Helping Friends and Family Understand 272

8.1.3. Helping Children Understand 273

8.1.4. Advance Care Planning 274

8.2. Everyday Care for a Person With Alzheimer's Disease 275
8.2.1. Bathing 276
8.2.2. Dressing 278
8.2.3. Grooming 278
8.2.4. Healthy Eating and Mealtimes 279
8.2.5. Exercise and Physical Activity 281
8.3. Medical Problems and Going to The Doctor 282
8.3.1. Common Medical Problems 282
8.3.2. Visiting the Doctor 282
8.4. Keeping w Person with Alzheimer's Safe 284
8.4.1. Home Safety 284
8.4.2. Medication Safety 285
8.4.3. Driving Safety 286
8.5. Adapting Activities for People with Alzheimer's Disease 286
8.5.1. At Home 287
8.5.2. Going Out 287
8.5.3. Eating Out 288
8.5.4. Traveling 288
8.5.5. Managing Finances 288
8.5.6. Spiritual Activities 289
8.5.7. Holidays 289
8.5.8. Visitors 289
8.6. Caregiver Support and Self-Care 290
8.6.1. Getting Help from Friends and Family 290
8.6.2. Your Emotional Health 291
8.6.3. Finding Help with At-Home Caregiving 292
8.6.4. Choosing a Long-Term Care Facility 295
8.6.5. Paying for Care 298
8.6.6. Tips for Finding and Hiring In-Home Care Services 300
8.7. Caring for a Person with Late-Stage Alzheimer's 301
8.7.1. When the Person with Alzheimer's Can't Move 301
8.7.2. How to Make Sure the Person Eats Well 302
8.7.3. What to Do About Swallowing Problems 302
8.7.4. Body Jerking 303
8.7.5. Skin Problems 303
Summary 306
References 307

9 Epidemiologic and Biologic Markers for Alzheimer's Disease 309

Introduction 309
9.1. Epidemiology Of Alzheimer's Disease 311
9.1.1. Incidence and Distribution 311
9.1.2. Epidemiological Factors 311
9.2. Blood-Based Biomarkers for Alzheimer's Disease 312
9.2.1. Blood-Based Biomarkers in Sporadic Alzheimer's Disease 313
9.2.2. Blood-Based Biomarkers in Genetically Determined Alzheimer's Disease 317
9.2.3. Factors Associated with Heterogeneity 319
9.2.4. The Road Towards Clinical Implementation 320
9.3. Alzheimer's Disease Biomarker Profiling in a Memory Clinic Cohort Without Common Comorbidities 322
9.3.1. GEDOC Memory Clinic Subcohort 324
9.3.2. Human Brain Tissue 325
9.3.3. CSF Sampling 325
9.3.4. CSF Biomarker Measurements 325
9.3.5. Immunofluorescence Staining 326
9.3.6. Image Biomarkers: PiB PET, FDG PET, and MRI 327
9.3.7. CSF Study Population Characteristics 328
9.3.8. CSF Levels of the Biomarkers Stratified by Diagnostic Groups and b-Amyloid Pathology Status 329
9.3.9. CSF Biomarker Correlations to Age, Sex and One Another 330
9.3.10. Associations Between Mechanistic Biomarkers and Key Elements of Alzheimer's Disease Pathogenesis 331
9.3.11. Stratification of Biomarkers Into Composite Scores 332
9.3.12. Patient Clustering by Biological Mechanisms 333

9.3.13. Immunofluorescence Staining of TRX-1 and AGT in the Human Brain 335
9.3.14. CSF Biomarkers as Evidence of the Pathological Process 337
9.3.15. Sensitivity and Specificity of CSF Biomarkers for Alzheimer's Disease 337
9.3.16. CSF Biomarkers in the Prodromal Stage (Pre-Dementia) of Alzheimer's Disease 338
9.3.17. The Prognostic Value of CSF Biomarkers 338
9.3.18. CSF Biomarkers for the Differential Diagnosis Between Alzheimer's Disease and Other Dementias 339
Summary **342**
References **342**

10 Risk Assessment and Prevention of Alzheimer's Disease 347

Introduction **348**
10.1. Risk Factors for Alzheimer's Disease **350**
10.1.1. Psychosocial Factors 350
10.1.2. Lifestyles 352
10.2. Fall Risk Assessment Among Older Adults with Mild Alzheimer's Disease **354**
10.2.1. Physiological and Cognitive Implications in Alzheimer's Disease 355
10.2.2. Age, Falls, and Alzheimer's Disease 356
10.2.3. The Effects of Education on Falls in Individuals with Alzheimer's Disease 356
10.2.4. Functional Mobility and Fall in Individuals with Alzheimer's Disease 356
10.2.5. The Effects of Gait Aid Usage on Falls in Individuals with Alzheimer's Disease 357
10.3. The Prevention of Alzheimer's Disease **358**
10.3.1. Pharmacologic Approaches to Prevention 360
10.3.2. Lifestyle Modification Interventions 361
10.3.3. Precision Medicine Approaches to Prevention 362
10.3.4. Example of a Personalized Medicine Approach to Dementia Prevention 364
10.4. Challenges For Alzheimer's Disease Therapy **365**
10.4.1. Molecular Pathogenesis of AD 367
10.4.2. Novel Pathophysiological Mechanisms in AD 369
10.4.3. Challenges for AD Therapy 371
Summary **376**
References **377**

Index 381

LIST OF FIGURES

Figure 1.1. Processing of the amyloid precursor protein

Figure 3.1. Deaths per million persons in 2012 due to dementias including Alzheimer's disease 0–4 5–8 9–10 11–13 14–17 18–24 25–45 46–114 115–375 376–1266

Figure 3.2. Hot spot distribution of dementia prevalence in Korea

Figure 4.1. Age-specific prevalence of Alzheimer's disease (per 100 population) across continents and countries.

Figure 4.2. Age-specific incidence of Alzheimer's disease (per 1,000 person years) across continents and countries.

Figure 4.3. Risk factors for Alzheimer's disease

Figure 4.4. Risk of Alzheimer's disease and slowing its progression

Figure 5.1. Clinical analysis

Figure 5.2. Summary of anticipated biomarker results for the different clinical phenotypes of AD

Figure 5.3. FDG-PET for the clinical phenotypes of AD

Figure 5.4. The role of AD biomarkers in the clinical setting

Figure 6.1. AD-pathogenesis

Figure 6.2. The chemical structures of approved drugs for symptomatic treatment of AD

Figure 6.3. The chemical structures of different chaperone molecules: Mizoribine 16, EC3016 17, Avrainvillamide 18, Epolaztaene 19, MKT-077 20, YM-01 21, JG-98 22, Radicicol 23, Geldanamycin 24, 17-AAG 25, Pochoxime C (OS47720) 26, R55 27, and OT1001 28

Figure 7.1. Alzheimer's dementia

Figure 7.2. Identifying and addressing potential contributors to cognitive decline with a personalized, multi-therapeutic approach is supportive of cognitive health. Image depicts the various core strategies for the reversal of AD and MCI and for optimizing brain health

Figure 8.1. Grandson and grandmother potting plant together

Figure 8.2. Advance care planning

Figure 8.3. Caring

Figure 8.4. Preventing

Figure 8.5. Eating a healthy diet important in Alzheimer's disease

Figure 8.6. Yoga

Figure 8.7. Care in the last stages of Alzheimer's

Figure 9.1. Biomarkers and changes in spatiotemporal pattern of Aβ and NFT deposit during disease cascade. Abnormality in CSF Aβ42 and Aβ-PET ('A' abnormality) are biomarkers in pre-clinical stage, followed by abnormality in CSF p-tau or tau-PET and 'N' abnormality (increased CSF T-tau and hippocampal atrophy)

Figure 9.2. Roadmap for the five phases in the development of blood-based biomarkers for the diagnosis of Alzheimer's disease

Figure 9.3. Scatter plots depicting biomarker levels across clinical groups (A–K). Biomarker concentrations are on the y-axis. The median is shown as a horizontal line. P-values were calculated by ANCOVA, adjusting for age

Figure 9.4. Correlation matrix of the analyzed biomarkers

Figure 9.5. Scatter plots of CSF biomarker composite scores in SCD, MCI and AD

Figure 9.6. Multivariate clustering of patients

Figure 9.7. Immunofluorescence co-staining of p-tau with thioredoxin-1 (TRX-1) or angiotensinogen (AGT) in human hippocampal sections

Figure 10.1. Potential risk factors for Alzheimer's disease

Figure 10.2. Implications for preventing Alzheimer's disease and slowing its progression

Figure 10.3. Model of a dementia prevention initiative

LIST OF TABLES

Table 2.1. Diagnosis of mild cognitive impairment (MCI) and mild dementia

Table 2.2. Examples of cognitive assessment tools

Table 2.3. Cognitive assessment tools

Table 3.1. Subgroup analysis of the prevalence of mild cognitive impairment

Table 3.2. Worldwide estimate for the absolute number of cases of dementia according to the Delphi consensus study

Table 3.3. Risk-of-bias assessment of RCTs using the ROB-2 tool. traffic light plot of study-by-study bias assessment. Weighted summary plot of the overall type of bias encountered in all studies performance (i.e., providing a precise estimate of the effect of interest) in dementia research

Table 3.4. Bias

Table 4.1. Factors that modify the risk of Alzheimer's disease

Table 4.2. Common susceptibility genes and their related SNPs in AD and IS

Table 5.1. Clinical features of the different phenotypes of AD

Table 5.2. Summary for diagnosing Alzheimer's disease

Table 5.3. Blood biomarkers and VCID

Table 6.1. Summary of clinical trials conducted for anti-Alzheimer's medicinal plants

Table 6.2. Disease modifying agents for the treatment of Alzheimer's disease in clinical trials

Table 7.1. Reversing AD-associated cognitive health requires addressing potential contributors to cognitive decline with a personalized, multi-therapeutic approach. Each of the strategies mentioned in the table has the ability to improve cognition and brain health, and when practiced together, they create a powerful synergy with sustained improvement

Table 7.2. Criteria for a perfect AD drug

Table 7.3. A selection of conditions in which DBS is being actively researched as a viable treatment option

Table 7.4. A summary of clinical studies examining vegetarian diet impact on ADRD

Table 9.1. Summary of the CSF study population characteristics

Table 9.2. Linear regression models

Table 9.3. Demographic, cognition and biomarker comparisons between clusters
Table 10.1. The effects of diets and life situations negatively influencing the Alzheimer's disease
Table 10.2. Possible mechanisms of the effects of physical activity and exercise interventions on cognitive decline and dementia prevention

PREFACE

Alzheimer's disease (AD) is the primary cause of cognitive decline. This is a neurodegenerative condition that typically impacts individuals who are 65 years or older. It affects various cognitive functions such as language, memory, comprehension, attention, judgment, and reasoning. Dementia is a broad term that encompasses a decrease in cognitive function that is significant enough to disrupt everyday activities. The most common form of dementia is Alzheimer's disease (AD), which accounts for at least two-thirds of all cases of dementia in people aged 65 and older respectively. The neurodegenerative condition known as Alzheimer's disease is characterized by a gradual and subtle decline in behavioral and cognitive abilities, including memory, comprehension, language, attention, reasoning, and judgment. Alzheimer's disease is a leading cause of dementia in the United States. Among the leading causes of death in the United States, it is the sixth most common cause of death. Less than 10% of patients experience the atypical occurrence of early-onset Alzheimer's disease, which is defined as the disease's onset occurring before the age of 65. Although there is no cure for Alzheimer's disease, there are treatments that have the potential to alleviate certain symptoms of the disease.

In Alzheimer's disease, the manifestation of symptoms is dependent on the particular stage of the disease that the patient is currently experiencing. The progression of Alzheimer's disease can be broken down into three distinct stages: preclinical, also known as presymptomatic, mild, and dementia. These stages are determined by cognitive decline. Contrary to the DSM-5 classification of Alzheimer's disease, the stages in question are not the same. The primary and most common initial symptom is sporadic impairment of short-term memory, while long-term memory is relatively unaffected by the condition. It is possible to observe this symptom in the majority of patients, even if it is not the initial symptom that an individual reports experiencing. As a consequence of having a short-term memory impairment, individuals may experience deficits in problem-solving, judgment, executive functioning, motivation, and organization. These deficits can lead to difficulties with multitasking and abstract thinking. There is a spectrum of impairment in executive functioning during the initial phases, ranging from slight to substantial. This impairment falls somewhere in the middle. Additionally, a decline in visuospatial skills occurs concurrently with the development of a language disorder. It is common to observe neuropsychiatric symptoms during the middle to late stages of the disease. These symptoms include apathy, social withdrawal, disinhibition, agitation, psychosis, and wandering. Patients who suffer from this condition may experience difficulties in performing previously acquired motor skills (a condition known as dyspraxia), a loss of sense of smell, and disruptions in their normal sleep patterns. Additionally, they may develop extrapyramidal motor symptoms such as dystonia, akathisia, and Parkinsonian symptoms, which typically appear in the later stages of the disease. These symptoms are most commonly seen in people who have Parkinson's disease. After that, there is a progression that leads to the development of primitive reflexes, the loss of control over bodily functions, and total dependence on healthcare providers.

The book titled "Alzheimer's Disease" provides a comprehensive analysis of the assessment and treatment of Alzheimer's disease, while highlighting the importance of the interprofessional team in enhancing the quality of care for patients suffering from this condition. It provides a comprehensive understanding of the condition, from its underlying biology and pathological mechanisms to its impact on individuals, families, and society. It aims to explore the latest research findings, diagnostic approaches, and treatment strategies, including pharmacological and non-pharmacological interventions. By delving into the complexities of Alzheimer's, the book seeks to increase awareness, reduce stigma, and offer hope to patients and caregivers. It also examines the challenges faced by healthcare systems and policymakers in addressing the growing burden of Alzheimer's disease. Written in an accessible manner, the book is intended for a wide readership, including healthcare professionals, researchers, caregivers, patients, and anyone interested in gaining a deeper understanding of this devastating neurological disorder.

Chapter 1

ALZHEIMER'S DISEASE BASICS

Contents

Introduction 2
1.1. Overview of Alzheimer's Disease 4
1.2. Causes of Alzheimer's Disease 6
1.3. Signs And Symptoms of Alzheimer's Disease 13
1.4. Diagnosis of Alzheimer's Disease 15
1.5. Treatment of Alzheimer's Disease 18
1.6. Prevention of Alzheimer's Disease 21
1.7. Management of Alzheimer's Disease 23
1.8. Biochemistry of Alzheimer's Disease 25
Summary 34
References 35

INTRODUCTION

Alzheimer's disease (AD) accounts for 60–70% of cases of dementia. It is a neurodegenerative disease that typically begins slowly and gets worse over time. The most typical initial symptom is trouble recalling recent events. As the illness progresses, behavioral problems, mood swings, disorientation (including getting lost easily), loss of motivation, self-neglect, and language difficulties can all be symptoms. When a person's health deteriorates, they frequently distance themselves from friends and family. Body functions gradually disappear, which finally results in death. Three to twelve years is the average life expectancy after diagnosis, though the rate of progression can vary. It is unclear what causes Alzheimer's disease. Its development is linked to numerous environmental and genetic risk factors. One of the strongest genetic risk factors comes from an apolipoprotein E allele. A history of head injuries, clinical depression, and high blood pressure are additional risk factors. The development of amyloid plaques, neurofibrillary tangles, and loss of neuronal connections in the brain are primarily linked to the progression of protein misfolding disease. Based on the patient's medical history, cognitive testing, and blood and imaging tests to rule out other potential causes, a probable diagnosis is made. Early signs are frequently confused with typical cognitive aging. A definitive diagnosis can only be made by examining brain tissue, which is only possible after death.

While some treatments may momentarily lessen symptoms, none can halt or reverse its progression. In general, a balanced diet, regular exercise, and social interaction all promote healthy aging and may lower the risk of cognitive decline and Alzheimer's disease. Affected individuals depend more and more on other people for help, which frequently puts a strain on those who provide care. There may be social, psychological, physical, and financial pressures. Physical activity regimens have the potential to enhance daily tasks and yield better results. Antipsychotics are sometimes used to treat behavioral issues or psychosis brought on by dementia, but doing so increases the risk of premature death. Globally, there were about 50 million cases of Alzheimer's disease as of 2020. Although up to 10% of cases have an early onset and affect people in their 30s to mid-60s, cases usually start in those over 65. About 6% of adults 65 and older are affected, with women being affected more frequently than men. The illness bears Alois Alzheimer's name, a German pathologist and psychiatrist who initially reported it in 1906. Alzheimer's financial burden on society is large, with an estimated global annual cost of US$1 trillion. It is ranked as the seventh leading cause of death worldwide (Lott & Head, 2005; Duyckaerts, Charles, & Dennis, 2011; Viña & Sanz-Ros, 2018; Knopman et al., 2021).

Orientation and Directional Terms

Term	Definition	Illustration
Alzheimer's Disease (AD)	Alzheimer's disease (AD) is the most common cause of a decline in cognitive ability. It is a neurodegenerative disorder that usually affects people over the age of 65 with the involvement of language, memory, comprehension, attention, judgment and reasoning.	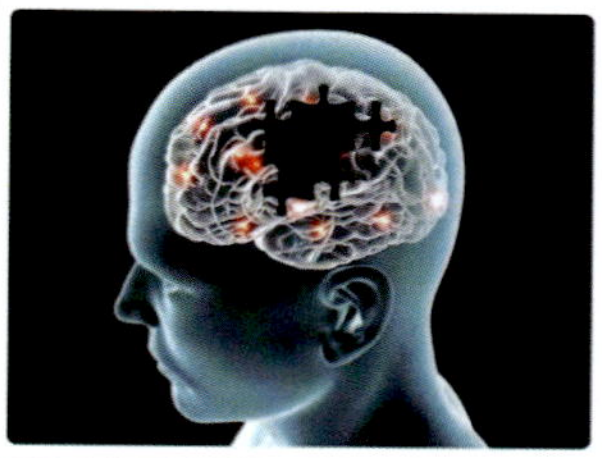
Cerebrospinal Fluid (CSF)	Cerebrospinal fluid is a clear, colorless body fluid found within the tissue that surrounds the brain and spinal cord of all vertebrates. CSF is produced by specialized ependymal cells in the choroid plexus of the ventricles of the brain, and absorbed in the arachnoid granulations.	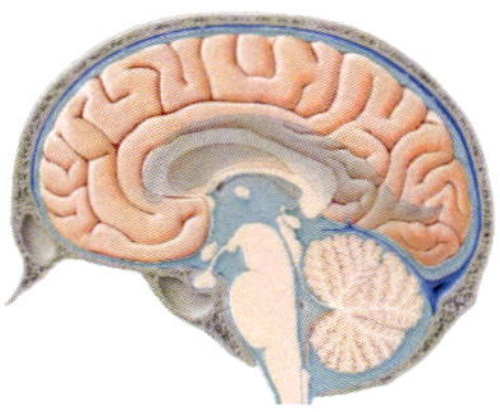
Sleep Apnea	Sleep apnea is a serious sleep disorder that happens when your breathing stops and starts while you're asleep. If it goes untreated, it can cause loud snoring, daytime tiredness, or more serious problems like heart trouble or high blood pressure.	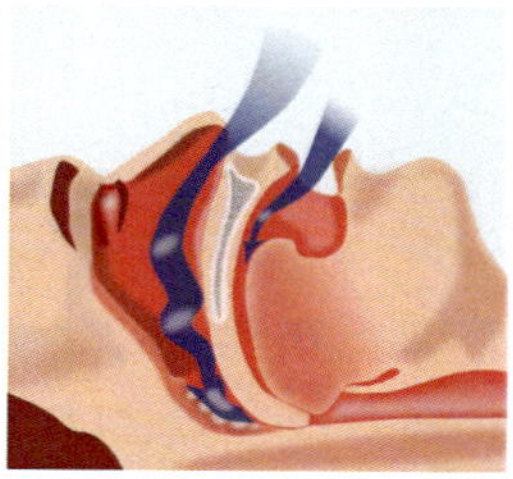
Parkinson's Disease	Parkinson's disease (PD) is a long-term neurodegenerative disease of mainly the central nervous system that affects both the motor system and non-motor systems. The symptoms usually emerge slowly, and as the disease progresses, non-motor symptoms become more common.	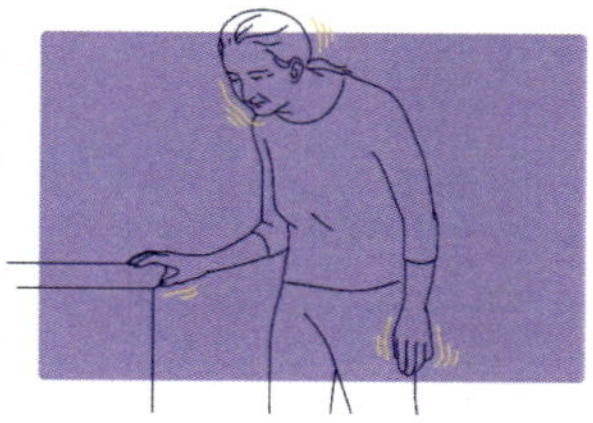
Amyloid-beta Precursor Protein (APP)	Amyloid-beta precursor protein (APP) is an integral membrane protein expressed in many tissues and concentrated in the synapses of neurons. It functions as a cell surface receptor and has been implicated as a regulator of synapse formation, neural plasticity, antimicrobial activity, and iron export.	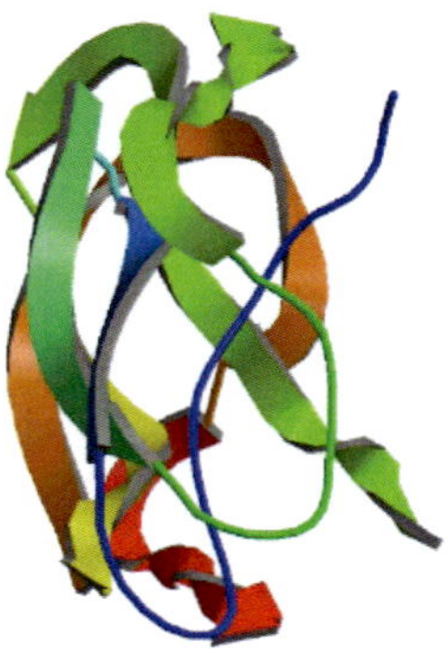

1.1. OVERVIEW OF ALZHEIMER'S DISEASE

Alzheimer's is a disease that causes memory loss in patients. People initially have difficulty recalling recent events, but they may be able to recall events from years past with ease.

As time goes on, other symptoms can appear, including:

- Trouble focusing
- A hard time doing ordinary activities
- Feeling confused or frustrated, especially at night
- Dramatic mood swings – outbursts of anger, anxiety, and depression
- Feeling disoriented and getting lost easily
- Physical problems, such as an odd walk or poor coordination
- Trouble communicating

People with Alzheimer's might forget their loved ones. They might forget how to dress themselves, feed themselves, and use the toilet.

Alzheimer's disease causes progressive deterioration of brain tissue, typically affecting individuals over the age of 65. The duration of the disease can vary, with some living with it for only a few years while others may suffer for decades. On average, individuals with Alzheimer's live with the disease for around 9 years. Approximately 1 in 8 people aged 65 and older are affected by Alzheimer's disease, with women being more likely than men to develop the condition.

1.1.1. How Does Alzheimer's Disease Affect the Brain?

The intricate alterations in the brain that cause Alzheimer's are still being studied by scientists. A decade or more before symptoms manifest, the brain may start to change. Toxic alterations, such as aberrant protein accumulations that result in tau tangles and amyloid plaques, are occurring in the brain during this extremely early stage of Alzheimer's. Formerly healthy neurons die, cease to function, and lose their connections to other neurons. Alzheimer's disease is believed to be influenced by numerous additional intricate brain alterations. The entorhinal cortex and the hippocampus, two regions of the brain crucial for memory formation, appear to be the first areas affected. The brain shrinks as more areas become affected and more neurons die. There has been extensive damage and significant shrinkage of brain tissue by the time Alzheimer's reaches its final stage.

1.1.2. Stages of Alzheimer's Disease

- **Mild Alzheimer's Disease:** People with Alzheimer's disease have more memory loss and other cognitive problems as the disease progresses. Issues may include straying and getting lost, having problems managing finances and paying bills, asking the same questions repeatedly, taking longer than usual to finish everyday tasks, and experiencing behavioral and personality changes. People in this stage are frequently diagnosed.
- **Moderate Alzheimer's Disease:** This stage is characterized by damage to brain regions responsible for language, reasoning, conscious thought, and sensory processing, including accurate sound and smell detection. As confusion and memory loss worsen, people start to have trouble identifying friends and family. They might not be able to pick up new skills, complete

complicated tasks like putting on clothes, or deal with unfamiliar circumstances. People in this stage may also act impulsively and experience hallucinations, delusions, and paranoia.

- **Severe Alzheimer's Disease:** In the end, the brain becomes completely covered in plaques and tangles, and the brain tissue gets much smaller. Individuals suffering from advanced Alzheimer's disease are utterly reliant on others for care and are unable to communicate. When the body shuts down toward the end of life, the person may spend most or all of their time in bed.

1.1.3. How Long Can a Person Live with Alzheimer's Disease?

Alzheimer's is a slowly progressing disease that manifests itself in three stages: mild cognitive impairment in the middle, an early preclinical stage without symptoms, and Alzheimer's dementia in the final stage. A person diagnosed with the disease at any age can pass away in as little as three or four years, whereas a person diagnosed at a younger age may need to live for ten or more years. Though recent estimates suggest that Alzheimer's may rank third among older people's causes of death, right behind cancer and heart disease, the disorder is currently listed as the sixth most common cause of death in the United States.

1.1.4. Brain Changes of Alzheimer's Disease

There are billions of neurons in an adult, healthy brain, and each one has long, branching extensions. Individual neurons can connect with other neurons thanks to these extensions. Information is transferred at these connections, known as synapses, by brief chemical bursts that are released by one neuron and absorbed by another. There are trillions of synapses in the brain. They facilitate fast signal transmission throughout the brain. Memories, thoughts, sensations, emotions, movements, and skills are all based on these signals. Numerous alterations in the brain that may disrupt chemical signaling and cause issues with cognition, learning, and daily functioning have been discovered by researchers over the years as a consequence of Alzheimer's disease. Alzheimer's disease is associated with several brain changes, including the accumulation of the protein fragment beta-amyloid into clumps (called beta-amyloid plaques) outside neurons and the accumulation of an aberrant form of the protein tau (called tau tangles) inside neurons.

Beta-amyloid and tau have different roles in Alzheimer's. Plaques and smaller accumulations of beta-amyloid may damage neurons by interfering with neuron-to-neuron communication at synapses. Inside neurons, tau tangles block the transportation of nutrients and other molecules essential for the normal function and survival of neurons while harming connections between neurons.

Neurodegeneration, or the damage and death of neurons and other brain cells, is the result of beta-amyloid and tau accumulation. Alzheimer's disease is characterized by neurodegeneration, beta-amyloid buildup, and tau accumulation. It is thought that the presence of toxic beta-amyloid and tau proteins activates microglia, which are immune system cells found in the brain. Microglia attempt to remove waste products and hazardous proteins from dead and dying cells. When the microglia are unable to process and eliminate everything, chronic inflammation may result.

Atrophied brain tissue, which results from neurodegeneration and other causes, is another alteration linked to Alzheimer's disease. While some degree of brain atrophy is normal as people age, even in cognitively healthy individuals, Alzheimer's patients experience an accelerated rate of brain atrophy. Reduced brain's capacity to metabolize glucose, its primary fuel, further jeopardizes normal brain function.

1.1.5. Timing of Brain Changes

The timing of these alterations in the brain as become clearer to researchers. Researchers have discovered that levels of beta-amyloid significantly increased beginning 22 years before symptoms were expected to appear in people with rare genetic mutations that cause Alzheimer's disease for whom long-term data have been collected (individuals with these genetic mutations typically develop symptoms at the same or nearly the same age as their parent with Alzheimer's). In a separate investigation, it was discovered that aberrant levels of the neurofilament light chain protein, a biomarker of neurodegeneration, began 22 years before symptoms were predicted to appear. Researchers from a third group discovered that when beta-amyloid clumps together to form amyloid plaques, levels of various tau protein types increase. These tau levels can rise as early as two decades before the typical mature tau tangles associated with Alzheimer's disease manifest. Additionally, researchers discovered that brain atrophy starts 13 years before expected symptom onset and that glucose metabolism starts to decline 18 years before expected symptom onset.

1.1.6. Brain Changes as Biomarkers

Alzheimer's disease biomarkers are these alterations in the brain. Biological alterations known as biomarkers are quantifiable indicators of the existence, absence, or likelihood of a disease. For instance, blood glucose levels are biomarkers of diabetes, and cholesterol levels are biomarkers of the risk of cardiovascular disease. Measuring the biomarkers for Alzheimer's disease has advanced significantly. For instance, we can now detect aberrant levels of tau and beta-amyloid in cerebrospinal fluid (CSF), the fluid that surrounds the brain, and positron emission tomography (PET) imaging can produce images that indicate the locations in the brain where tau and beta-amyloid have accumulated. Blood tests for Alzheimer's disease are also being developed by numerous research teams. The diagnosis of Alzheimer's disease may be made much simpler and faster if these blood tests prove to be successful (Lott & Head, 2005; Duyckaerts, Charles, & Dennis, 2011; Viña & Sanz-Ros, 2018; Knopman et al., 2021).

1.2. CAUSES OF ALZHEIMER'S DISEASE

The pathophysiology of Alzheimer's disease is thought to be caused by aberrant levels of amyloid beta (Aβ), which build up in the brain and affect neuronal connectivity and function, eventually causing a progressive loss of brain function. Aβ can accumulate extracellularly in the form of tau proteins and amyloid plaques or intracellularly as neurofibrillary tangles. This reduced capacity for protein clearance is linked to various neurodegenerative diseases, controlled by brain cholesterol, and ages. Except for 1–2 percent of cases where deterministic genetic differences have been found, the cause of the majority of Alzheimer's cases is still largely unknown. A number of rival theories endeavor to elucidate the fundamental reason; the most widely accepted theory is the amyloid beta (Aβ) hypothesis.

The cholinergic hypothesis, which contends that decreased synthesis of the neurotransmitter acetylcholine is the cause of Alzheimer's disease, is the oldest and the foundation for the majority of pharmacological treatments. One of the main characteristics of Alzheimer's disease progression is the loss of cholinergic neurons, which is observed in the cerebral cortex and limbic system. According to the 1991 amyloid hypothesis, the disease is primarily caused by extracellular deposits of amyloid beta (Aβ). The APP gene's location on chromosome 21 and the nearly universal manifestation of the early signs of Alzheimer's disease by the age of 40 in individuals with trisomy 21 (Down syndrome), who carry an extra copy of the gene, provide evidence in favor of this theory. The apolipoprotein APOE4 isoform is a significant genetic risk factor for Alzheimer's disease. While apolipoproteins aid in the breakdown of beta-amyloid, some isoforms—like APOE4—are less efficient in this regard, which causes an excess of amyloid to accumulate in the brain.

1.2.1. Aging and Alzheimer's Risk

Age is the most significant known risk factor for Alzheimer's disease, but it does not cause the disease. About every five years after the age of 65, the number of people with Alzheimer's disease doubles. Alzheimer's disease may afflict roughly one-third of all adults over 85. Researchers are discovering new ways in which age-related alterations in the brain can damage neurons and other kinds of brain cells, aggravating the damage caused by Alzheimer's. Atherosclerosis, vascular damage, the generation of unstable molecules known as free radicals, the disintegration of energy production within cells, and inflammation are some of these age-related alterations. Age alone, though, does not exclusively increase the risk of Alzheimer's. Dementia never strikes many people who live to be 90 years old or older.

1.2.2. Genetics of Alzheimer's Disease

A lot of people fear getting Alzheimer's, particularly if a family member has already experienced the illness. It's not a guarantee that you will get the illness just because someone in your family has had it before. Still, it might indicate a higher chance of developing it. Alzheimer's disease risk can be influenced by an individual's genes, which are inherited from their biological parents. Gene alterations or variations that can affect an individual's risk of developing a disease are known as genetic risk factors. Some diseases run in families because of these risk factors. Alzheimer's disease comes in two flavors: early-onset and late-onset. There is a genetic component to both kinds.

1.2.2.1. Late-Onset Alzheimer's Disease

About 70% of cases of late-onset Alzheimer's are inherited. In 2020, 90% of accurate predictions of Alzheimer's disease were made by genetic models. Sporadic Alzheimer's disease refers to the majority of Alzheimer's cases, which are not related. The majority of sporadic Alzheimer's cases start later in life, usually after the age of 65. APOEε4 is the most powerful genetic risk factor for sporadic Alzheimer's disease. One of the four alleles of apolipoprotein E (APOE) is APOEε4. The ε4 allele impairs APOE's ability to bind lipids in lipoprotein particles, which is a significant function. Of those who have Alzheimer's disease, 40 to 80% have at least one APOEε4 allele. The homozygote's risk of the disease is increased by 15 times, while heterozygotes' risk is increased by three times due to the APOEε4 allele. Completion penetrance is caused by genetic modifiers and environmental factors, as is the case with many human diseases. For example, Nigerian Yoruba people do not show the relationship between the dose of APOEε4 and incidence or age-of-onset for Alzheimer's disease seen in other human populations.

1.2.2.2. Early Onset Alzheimer's Disease

Because Alzheimer's is highly polygenic, only 1–2 percent of cases are inherited due to autosomal dominant effects. The condition, which is rarer and progresses more quickly, is referred to as early-onset familial Alzheimer's disease when it is brought on by autosomal dominant variants. The early onset of Alzheimer's disease accounts for less than 5% of cases of sporadic Alzheimer's disease, and it is approximately 90% heritable. FAD typically denotes a number of individuals impacted over one or more generations. Three genes—the ones encoding the presenilins PSEN1 and PSEN2, the amyloid-beta precursor protein (APP), and the early onset familial Alzheimer's disease—can be mutated. The majority of APP and presenilin gene mutations increase the production of amyloid beta (Aβ)42, a small protein that forms the core of amyloid plaques. Certain mutations only modify the proportion of Aβ42 to the other major forms, specifically Aβ40, without elevating the levels of Aβ42 in the brain. ABCA7 and SORL1 are two additional genes linked to autosomal dominant Alzheimer's disease. A three to five times increased risk of Alzheimer's disease has been linked to alleles in the TREM2 gene.

- **Familial and Nonfamilial Alzheimer's Disease:** The most common cause of dementia is Alzheimer's disease (AD), a neurodegenerative condition that typically strikes elderly people. Alzheimer's disease that is inherited and rare is known as familial Alzheimer's disease (FAD or EOFAD for early onset). Typically, familial AD manifests itself earlier in life, that is, before the age of 65. FAD typically indicates that several people in one or more generations are impacted. Sporadic AD refers to non-familial cases of AD in which the genetic risk factors are insignificant or not clear. 10 to 15% of cases of EOAD are related to families. The remaining ones are random and not caused by genetic changes.
- **Signs and Symptoms:** Alzheimer's disease with an early onset occurs when a person is younger than 65 years old, usually between the ages of 30 and 60. Unusual memory loss, especially when it comes to recalling names and recent events, is one of the early indicators of AD (logopenic primary progressive aphasia). The patient experiences more severe issues as the illness worsens, including mood swings and an inability to carry out difficult tasks like driving. Confusion, poor judgment, agitation, withdrawal, hallucinations, seizures, Parkinsonian deficits, decreased muscle tone, myoclonus, fecal incontinence, urine incontinence, and mutism are other common findings. When EOAD progresses, a person may lose the ability to do basic activities like brushing their hair and may need 24-hour care.
- **Causes:** Genetics and additional features, such as the age of onset, are used to identify familial AD, which is inherited in an autosomal dominant manner.
  - **Genetics:** Familial Alzheimer's disease is caused by a mutation in one of at least three genes, which code for presenilin 1, presenilin 2, and APP.
  - **PSEN1 – Presenilin 1:** Numerous mutations have

been found in the presenilin 1 gene (PSEN1, which is found on chromosome 14) that was discovered by Sherrington in 1995. Type 3 familial Alzheimer's is definitely caused by mutations in this gene, and the onset occurs in people under 50. Approximately 30–70% of EOFAD are of this type. As a component of the enzymatic complex that cleaves the amyloid-beta peptide from APP, this protein has been identified. A 60 kb estimate for the coding region of the gene indicates that it has 14 exons. An essential membrane protein is what the gene (PS1) codes for. Koizumi (2001) theorized that it may play a role in somitogenesis in the embryo since, as mentioned by Ikeuchi (2002), it cleaves the protein Notch1. It likely contributes to the pathophysiology of familial AD because it also acts on an amyloid precursor protein. Invertebrates, plants, and other vertebrates have all been found to have homologs for PS1.

- Some of the mutations in the gene, of which over 90 are known, include: His163Arg, Ala246Glu, Leu286Val and Cys410Tyr. Most display complete penetrance, but a common mutation is Glu318Gly and this predisposes individuals to familial AD, with a study by Taddei (2002) finding an incidence of 8.7% in patients with familial AD.
- **PSEN2 – Presenilin 2:** The structure and function of the presenilin 2 gene (PSEN2) are strikingly similar to those of PSEN1. This gene, which is found on chromosome 1 (1q31–q42), is mutated to cause type 4 FAD. Less than 5% of all cases of EOFAD are of this type. In mammalian neuronal cells, PS1 and PS2 proteins are expressed in comparable quantities and in the same organelles. Twelve exons made up PSEN2, 10 of which were coding exons. The primary transcript of PSEN2 encodes a 448-amino-acid polypeptide that is 67% similar to PS1. This protein is recognized as a constituent of the enzymatic complex responsible for the cleavage of amyloid beta peptide from APP.
- **APP – Amyloid Beta (A4) Precursor Protein:** Familial Alzheimer's disease is caused by mutations in the amyloid beta A4 precursor protein (APP), which is found on the long arm of chromosome 21 (21q21.3). Additional investigation into molecules such as miR-212–3p may provide fresh insights into possible therapeutic strategies for Alzheimer's disease, potentially in conjunction with APP-targeted interventions. This kind makes up no more than 10% to 15% of EOFAD. There are currently just over 20 known pathogenic APP

mutations. A research team led by John Hardy discovered the most common of these mutations, APP V717I, also referred to as the London Mutation, in Carol Jennings' family in 1991. The Swedish and Arctic mutations are two other noteworthy APP mutations. The pathophysiology of the disease has become considerably clearer thanks to functional analyzes of these mutations. The London mutation, along with other mutations in the APP at codon 717, shifts the ratio of toxic Aβ species to the more aggregate-prone 42 amino-acid length peptide, while the Arctic mutation causes the Aβ peptide to undergo a conformational change and increases the formation of toxic Aβ protofibrils. The Swedish mutation, on the other hand, increases the overall production of Aβ peptides by increasing the β-secretory cleavage.

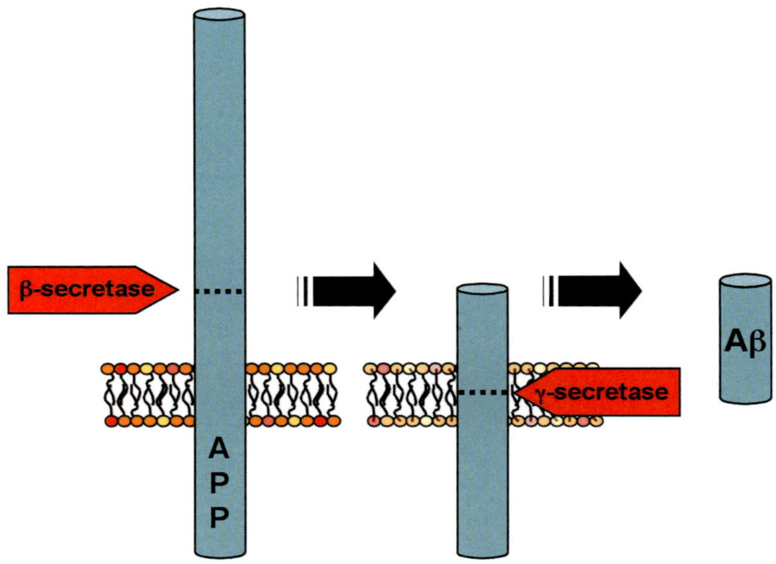

Figure 1.1. *Processing of the amyloid precursor protein.*

Source: https://en.wikipedia.org/wiki/Early-onset_Alzheimer%27s_disease.

- **Non-genetic Risk Factors:** The non-genetic risk factors for early onset dementia, including sporadic Alzheimer's disease and other early-onset dementias are understudied. Nonetheless, new studies indicate that there are several risk factors, both modifiable and nonmodifiable, for dementia with a young onset.
- **Mechanism:** Familial AD is virtually identical to other forms of the disease in terms of histology. Sections of brain tissue have deposits of amyloid. This amyloid protein accumulates in the brain to create neurofibrillary tangles and plaques. Rarely, a

mutation in one of the genes that results in a functional but malformed protein rather than the ineffective gene products that usually result from mutations can cause the plaque to be unique or uncharacteristic of AD. It is only recently that the underlying neurobiology of this disease has begun to be understood.

Scientists are currently studying the pathways of inflammation linked to the development, progression, and degeneration of Alzheimer's disease (AD). Key molecules involved in these pathways include glial cells, such as astrocytes and microglia, beta-amyloid, and proinflammatory compounds. As neurons in the brain become damaged and die, connections between neural networks may deteriorate, leading to the shrinking of various brain regions. Eventually, this process, known as brain atrophy, becomes widespread, resulting in a significant loss of brain volume. This loss of brain volume impacts a person's ability to function and live normally, ultimately leading to fatality. Beta-amyloid is a fragment of a larger protein called amyloid precursor protein (APP). When APP is activated, it is broken down into smaller protein fragments, with β-amyloid being one of them. β-amyloid is particularly sticky compared to other protein fragments, causing it to accumulate in the brain. This accumulation is believed to be caused by a combination of genetic and biochemical issues. Over time, these fragments form oligomers, then fibrils, beta-sheets, and ultimately plaques. The presence of β-amyloid plaques in the brain triggers the recruitment and activation of microglial cells and astrocytes. Through a series of cleavages by various enzymes, APP is ultimately converted into Aβ. Mutations in the APP gene have been linked to early-onset familial Alzheimer's disease, with 21 different mutations identified in the region responsible for encoding the Aβ domain.

- **Genetic testing:** For those with symptoms and their asymptomatic relatives, genetic testing is offered. Between 40 and 80% of EOFAD families will have an APP, PSEN1, or PSEN2 gene mutation that can be detected. As a result, testing may not reveal a mutation in some EOFAD family members.

- **Prognosis:** Early-onset Alzheimer's has unique effects on experience due to its unusual timing. For instance, the illness may have a disastrous impact on a patient's family, caregivers, and career. People who are employed are compelled to retire early because they are unable to carry out their jobs competently. When this is foreseeable, workers need to talk to their employers about their future and the anticipated loss of skills. People who are compelled to retire early might not be eligible for all of the benefits offered to people who retire at the government-set minimum age. In certain professions, a single error can have catastrophic effects on a large number of people, and reports exist of instances where an individual with early-onset Alzheimer's who is not aware of their illness has caused distress. Alzheimer's disease may also cause younger people to lose their capacity for self-care, including handling money. Conceptualizations of aging and Alzheimer's disease have been proposed to challenge the idea that these two conditions are different. The difficulties faced by elderly people may be minimized in a binary model that emphasizes the needs of the younger generation.

1.2.3. Hypotheses

- **Amyloid-Beta and Tau Protein:** The tau hypothesis suggests that the disease cascade is started by abnormalities in tau protein. In this model, tau that has undergone hyperphosphorylation starts to form paired helical filaments with other tau threads. They eventually create neurofibrillary tangles within the cell bodies of nerves. The neuron's transport system collapses as a result of the microtubules breaking down and destroying the cytoskeleton of the cell. Numerous studies link the misfolded tau and amyloid beta proteins to the pathology of Alzheimer's disease by demonstrating how they cause oxidative stress, which in turn triggers neuroinflammation. Other neurodegenerative illnesses like ALS and Parkinson's disease also exhibit this persistent inflammation. Dementia and spirochete infections have also been connected. In AD brains, DNA damage builds up, and reactive oxygen species may be the main cause of this damage.
- **Sleep:** An additional risk factor for inflammation in Alzheimer's disease is thought to be sleep disturbances. Alzheimer's disease was previously thought to be the only cause of sleep disruption, but as of 2020, mounting data indicates that there may be a reciprocal relationship.
- **Metal Toxicity, Smoking, Neuroinflammation and Air Pollution:** Alzheimer's disease disrupts the cellular homeostasis of biometals, including ionic copper, iron, and zinc, though it's not clear if the alterations in proteins produce or contribute to this. One of the main risk factors for Alzheimer's disease is smoking. Late-onset Alzheimer's disease is associated with a higher risk of developing systemic markers of the innate immune system. One possible risk factor for Alzheimer's disease development is exposure to air pollution.
- **Other Hypotheses:** According to the medical theory known as "retrogenesis," individuals with Alzheimer's disease experience a reverse neurodegeneration process in their brains, beginning with demyelination and the death of axons (white matter) and concluding with the death of gray matter. This process is analogous to the neurodevelopment process that a fetus goes through beginning with neurulation and ending with myelination. According to the theory, persons with Alzheimer's disease experience progressive cognitive impairment like that of infants going through stages of cognitive development. One theory holds that as we age, dysfunction of oligodendrocytes and the myelin they produce contributes to axon damage, which in turn causes the production of amyloid and tau hyperphosphorylation. Research has indicated a possible connection between late-life Alzheimer's disease development and viral infection. Notably, a large-scale study involving 6,245,282 patients revealed that cognitively normal adults over 65

who contracted COVID-19 had a higher chance of developing Alzheimer's disease later in life.

1.2.4. Health, Environmental, and Lifestyle Factors that May Contribute to Alzheimer's

Numerous variables other than heredity may contribute to the onset and progression of Alzheimer's disease, according to research. For instance, the connection between metabolic disorders like diabetes and obesity and vascular diseases like high blood pressure, heart disease, and stroke, as well as cognitive decline, is of great interest. We will learn more about whether and how lowering risk factors for these illnesses may also lower the risk of Alzheimer's disease through ongoing research. A balanced diet, regular exercise, social interaction, rest, and mentally challenging activities have all been linked to maintaining good health as one ages. Additionally, these factors may lessen the chance of Alzheimer's disease and cognitive decline. Some of these theories are being tested in clinical trials. Early-life circumstances might also be important. For instance, research has connected a lower risk of dementia with greater educational attainment. Research is being done on these variations in dementia risk among sexes and racial groups to better understand the causes of Alzheimer's disease and create preventative and treatment strategies that work for everyone (Lott & Head, 2005; Duyckaerts, Charles, & Dennis, 2011; Viña & Sanz-Ros, 2018; Knopman et al., 2021).

1.3. SIGNS AND SYMPTOMS OF ALZHEIMER'S DISEASE

0One of the first indications of cognitive impairment associated with Alzheimer's disease is usually memory problems. Mild cognitive impairment (MCI) is a condition that affects some persons who have memory issues. Although patients with MCI experience more memory issues than is typical for their age, their symptoms do not significantly affect their day-to-day activities. MCI has also been associated with issues related to movement and smell. Alzheimer's disease is more likely to strike older adults with MCI, though not all of them do. Some might even return to thinking normally. The initial signs of Alzheimer's disease differ from person to person. Many people believe that the very early stages of Alzheimer's disease may be indicated by a decline in non-memory aspects of cognition, such as word finding, vision/spatial problems, and impaired reasoning or judgment. To determine whether biomarkers can identify early changes in the brains of individuals with MCI and cognitively normal individuals who may be more susceptible to Alzheimer's disease, researchers are examining biomarkers, which are biological indicators of disease found in brain images, cerebrospinal fluid, and blood. Although some research suggests that this kind of early detection might be feasible, more studies are required before these methods can be depended upon to diagnose Alzheimer's disease in routine medical practice.

- **Signs of Mild Alzheimer's Disease:** In mild Alzheimer's disease, a person may seem to be healthy but has more and more trouble making sense of the world around him or her. The realization that something is wrong often comes gradually to the person and his or her family. Problems can include:
  - Memory loss
  - Poor judgment leading to bad decisions
  - Loss of spontaneity and sense of initiative

- Taking longer to complete normal daily tasks
- Repeating questions
- Trouble handling money and paying bills
- Wandering and getting lost
- Losing things or misplacing them in odd places
- Mood and personality changes
- Increased anxiety and/or aggression

Alzheimer's disease is often diagnosed at this stage.

- **Signs of Moderate Alzheimer's Disease:** In this stage, more intensive supervision and care become necessary, which can be difficult for many spouses and families. Symptoms may include:
  - Increased memory loss and confusion
  - Inability to learn new things
  - Difficulty with language and problems with reading, writing, working with numbers
  - Difficulty organizing thoughts and thinking logically
  - Shortened attention span
  - Problems coping with new situations
  - Difficulty carrying out multistep tasks, such as getting dressed
  - Problems recognizing family and friends
  - Hallucinations, delusions, and paranoia
  - Impulsive behavior such as undressing at inappropriate times or places or using vulgar language
  - Inappropriate outbursts of anger
  - Restlessness, agitation, anxiety, tearfulness, wandering—especially in the late afternoon or evening
  - Repetitive statements or movement, occasional muscle twitches
- **Signs of Severe Alzheimer's Disease:** People with severe Alzheimer's cannot communicate and are completely dependent on others for their care. Near the end, the person may be in bed most or all of the time as the body shuts down. Their symptoms often include:
- Inability to communicate
- Weight loss
- Seizures
- Skin infections
- Difficulty swallowing

- Groaning, moaning, or grunting
- Increased sleeping
- Loss of bowel and bladder control

A common cause of death for people with Alzheimer's disease is aspiration pneumonia. This type of pneumonia develops when a person cannot swallow properly and takes food or liquids into the lungs instead of air.

There is currently no cure for Alzheimer's, though there are medicines that can treat the symptoms of the disease.

- **Symptoms of Mild Cognitive Impairment:** Some people have a condition called mild cognitive impairment, or MCI. It can be an early sign of Alzheimer's. But, not everyone with MCI will develop Alzheimer's disease. People with MCI can still take care of themselves and do their normal activities. MCI memory problems may include:
  - Losing things often
  - Forgetting to go to events or appointments
  - Having more trouble coming up with words than other people the same age (Lott & Head, 2005; Duyckaerts, Charles, & Dennis, 2011; Viña & Sanz-Ros, 2018; Knopman et al., 2021).

1.4. DIAGNOSIS OF ALZHEIMER'S DISEASE

Alzheimer's disease can be identified in several ways. Alzheimer's is frequently identified through testing performed by a member of your medical team. After assessing your symptoms, the medical practitioner might recommend several tests. To learn more about your symptoms and behavior, the medical professional might speak with your friends and family. The most prevalent kind of dementia, Alzheimer's, requires a precise diagnosis. Obtaining the proper diagnosis is a crucial first step in receiving the right care, treatment, family education, and future planning.

1.4.1. Early Symptoms of Alzheimer's Dementia

Early symptoms of Alzheimer's dementia include:

- Memory impairment, such as trouble remembering events.
- Having a hard time concentrating, planning or problem-solving.
- Trouble finishing daily tasks at home or at work, such as writing or using eating utensils.
- Confusion with location or passage of time.
- Having visual or spatial issues, such as not understanding distance in driving, getting lost or misplacing items.
- Trouble with language, such as not being able to find the right word or having a reduced vocabulary in speech or writing.
- Using poor judgment in decisions.

- Withdrawal from work events or social engagements.
- Changes in mood, such as depression or other behavior and personality changes.

Alzheimer's dementia can affect several aspects of your daily life.

When warning signs of Alzheimer's dementia appear, it's important that you get a prompt and accurate diagnosis.

1.4.2. Diagnosing Alzheimer's Dementia

You may see a healthcare provider to get an Alzheimer's diagnosis. Alternatively, you may see a geriatrician, a medical professional trained in treating elderly patients, or a neurologist, a medical professional trained in treating brain disorders. The physician or other healthcare provider examines your medical history, medication history, and symptoms. A close friend or family member is one person your health professional might speak with. There will also be multiple tests and a physical examination.

During your appointment, your healthcare professional looks at the following:

- Whether you have impaired memory or thinking skills, also known as cognitive skills.
- Whether you exhibit changes in personality or behaviors.
- The degree of your memory or thinking impairment or changes.
- How thinking impairment affects your ability to function in daily life.
- The cause of your symptoms.
- You may need lab tests, brain-imaging tests or detailed memory testing. These tests can provide useful information for a diagnosis. They also can rule out other conditions that cause similar symptoms.

1.4.3. Ruling out Other Conditions

In addition to performing a physical examination, doctors and other medical professionals make sure you don't have any other medical conditions that could be the source or aggravate your symptoms. They might search for indications of previous strokes, depression, sleep apnea, Parkinson's disease, or other illnesses.

1.4.4. Testing Memory Loss and Other Symptoms

You might be asked to complete tasks or questions by your healthcare provider that assess your cognitive abilities. Your memory, abstract thought, problem-solving, language use, and related skills are all assessed by these tasks. Mental status testing. This test focuses on your memory and cognitive abilities, or how you think. The level of cognitive impairment can be inferred from the test results. neuropsychological evaluations. You might consult a neuropsychologist, or a specialist with training in mental health and brain disorders. This expert can perform comprehensive evaluations of your cognitive and memory abilities. The tests assist medical professionals, including your doctor, in determining whether you have dementia. They assist your medical team in determining whether you are capable of carrying out regular activities, like taking your medication on time and handling your money, in a safe manner. These tests also tell you what you might have lost and what you can still do. Additionally, they can let your doctor know if depression might be the reason behind your symptoms.

Conversations with loved ones and friends. Your family members or friends may be questioned by doctors and other medical professionals about you and your conduct. Experts in healthcare look for information that doesn't align with your previous level of functioning. It's common for friends or family to be able to explain how your behaviors, functional skills, and cognitive abilities have evolved over time. Alzheimer's dementia can often be diagnosed with these tests, a physical examination, and details regarding the patient's age and the length of time that symptoms have gotten worse. But in cases where the diagnosis is unclear, medical practitioners might have to request more testing.

1.4.5. Laboratory Tests

To rule out other conditions that cause symptoms similar to Alzheimer's dementia, you might need to undergo lab tests. For instance, you might undergo testing to determine whether your body needs more vitamin B-12 or if you have a thyroid issue. To diagnose Alzheimer's, a cerebrospinal fluid test might be suggested. The fluid can be used to measure the proteins tau and amyloid. You can tell if you have Alzheimer's dementia by looking at the ratio of these proteins. Cerebrospinal fluid testing is typically not required for a diagnosis. However, if symptoms are worsening quickly or in some other situation, the test might be helpful.

1.4.6. Brain Imaging Tests

The progressive death of brain cells leads to Alzheimer's dementia. Degeneration is the term for this. Brain scans may show degeneration in many different ways. Still, a diagnosis cannot be reached with these scans alone. Because there is an overlap between what is thought to be normal age-related brain changes and changes associated with Alzheimer's, brain scans are not used to diagnose dementia.

However, brain imaging can help:

- Rule out other causes, such as heavy bleeding, brain tumors or strokes.
- Distinguish between different types of degenerative brain disease.
- Establish a baseline about the degree of degeneration.

The brain-imaging technologies most often used are:

- **Magnetic Resonance Imaging (MRI):** An MRI uses powerful radio waves and magnets to create a detailed view of your brain.
- **Computerized Tomography (CT):** A CT scan uses X-rays to obtain cross-sectional images of your brain.
- **Positron Emission Tomography (PET):** A PET scan uses a radioactive substance known as a tracer to detect substances in the body. There are different types of PET scans. The most commonly used PET scan is a fluorodeoxyglucose (FDG) PET scan. This scan can identify brain regions with decreased glucose metabolism. The pattern of metabolism change can distinguish between different types of degenerative brain disease.

Recently, PET scans have been developed to identify tau, also known as neurofibrillary tangles, or clusters of amyloid proteins, also known as plaques. Both have a connection to dementia caused by Alzheimer's. Usually, research settings are where these kinds of PET scans are employed.

1.4.7. Future of Diagnosis

Researchers are attempting to develop new methods for early Alzheimer's dementia diagnosis. It may be possible to diagnose the illness with new tests even in the absence of symptoms or at very mild stages. Scientists are currently working on assays to quantify tau or amyloid in the blood. These tests show promise in identifying individuals at risk for Alzheimer's disease and determining whether Alzheimer's disease is the cause of dementia. Numerous disease markers and diagnostic procedures are being studied by scientists. These biomarkers include tau and other Alzheimer's-related genes and proteins. Additionally, new imaging tests are being created. These could provide insight into the severity of your Alzheimer's disease and whether you have it or not. Still, more investigation into these tests is required.

1.4.8. Benefit of an Early Diagnosis

When they or a family member has memory problems, some people are anxious to visit a medical professional. Some people pretend their symptoms are real, or family members take their place. The losses that come with Alzheimer's dementia, like losing one's independence and driving ability, can be difficult to cope with. Alzheimer's disease cannot be cured, but early detection can still have benefits.

It's crucial to understand your strengths and limitations alike. Your healthcare team can begin treating memory loss if it is being caused by another treatable condition. Early medication administration can help prevent memory loss and other cognitive deficits in people with Alzheimer's dementia. Additional medications and therapies may aid in symptom management. Clinical trials are another option that might be available to you.

Alzheimer's dementia can lessen its impact on daily life and you and your carers can learn strategies to manage your changing skills. Learning how to create routines, schedule activities, and make your home safer are examples of strategies.

An early diagnosis also helps you, your family and caregivers plan for the future. You'll have the chance to make informed decisions on many issues, such as:

- Appropriate community services and resources.
- Options for residential and at-home care.
- Plans for handling financial issues.
- Expectations for future care and medical decisions.

When healthcare professionals diagnose you or a family member with Alzheimer's, they can help you understand the disease. They can answer your questions and explain what to expect. Your healthcare team can help you figure out ways to maintain independence, health and safety (Lott & Head, 2005; Duyckaerts, Charles, & Dennis, 2011; Viña & Sanz-Ros, 2018; Knopman et al., 2021).

1.5. TREATMENT OF ALZHEIMER'S DISEASE

Because Alzheimer's disease is so complicated, it is unlikely that it can be effectively treated with a single medication or other strategy. The current strategies concentrate on assisting patients in preserving mental capacity, controlling behavioral symptoms, and delaying the progression of medical conditions. The U.S. currently approves several prescription medications. The FDA is responsible for treating individuals who have been diagnosed with Alzheimer's disease. Alzheimer's patients who receive treatment can live longer, more comfortable lives with dignity and independence. They can also benefit and support their carers. For most people with Alzheimer's, the early or middle stages are the best times to take medication. For instance, they may momentarily lessen the severity of some symptoms, like memory loss. It is crucial to realize that none of these drugs treat the illness directly.

1.5.1. Treatment for Mild to Moderate Alzheimer's

A combination of pharmacological and non-pharmacological treatments is usually used to treat mild to moderate Alzheimer's disease to control symptoms and delaying the disease's progression. Medications known as cholinesterase inhibitors, which include galantamine, rivastigmine, and donepezil, are frequently prescribed drugs that function by raising acetylcholine levels, a neurotransmitter important in memory and learning. Another drug approved for moderate to severe Alzheimer's is memantine, a N-methyl-D-aspartate (NMDA) receptor antagonist that helps control glutamate activity in the brain. Non-pharmacological methods like cognitive stimulation, physical activity, and social interaction are crucial parts of treatment in addition to medication because they support cognitive function, elevate mood, and improve quality of life for both Alzheimer's patients and their carers. Additionally, to address specific functional impairments and communication difficulties related to the disease, supportive therapies like occupational therapy and speech therapy may be suggested. Although there is no known cure for Alzheimer's, these treatments can improve the quality of life and offer significant support to those who are affected. The secret to improving treatment outcomes and enhancing the quality of life for individuals with Alzheimer's disease is early diagnosis and proactive management.

1.5.2. Treatment for Moderate to Severe Alzheimer's

Since there is presently no known cure for moderate-to-severe Alzheimer's disease, treatment for the illness focuses on symptom management and quality of life enhancement. Cholinesterase inhibitors like donepezil, rivastigmine, and galantamine are frequently prescribed with medications like memantine, which controls glutamate activity in the brain. These drugs may help control behavioral symptoms like agitation and aggression as well as slow cognitive aging. Even in the advanced stages of the disease, non-pharmacological interventions like social interaction, physical activity, and cognitive stimulation are crucial parts of treatment. Supportive therapies can also help with functional impairments and communication issues. Examples of these therapies are occupational therapy and speech therapy. To handle the growing demands of caregiving, caregivers may need more resources and support as the disease worsens. Palliative care and hospice services, which concentrate on symptom management and enhancing quality of life during the later stages of the disease, can offer consolation and support to people with Alzheimer's and their families. Healthcare professionals must collaborate closely with patients and their carers to create a thorough care plan that is customized to each patient's unique requirements and preferences.

Drug Name	Drug Type & Use	How It Works	Common Side Effects
Aricept (donepezil)	Cholinesterase inhibitor prescribed to treat symptoms of mild, moderate, and severe Alzheimer's	Prevents the breakdown of acetylcholine in the brain	Nausea, vomiting, diarrhea, muscle cramps, fatigue, weight loss
Exelon (rivastigmine)	Cholinesterase inhibitor prescribed to treat symptoms of mild to moderate Alzheimer's (patch is also for severe Alzheimer's)	Prevents the breakdown of acetylcholine and butyrylcholine (a brain chemical similar to acetylcholine) in the brain	Nausea, vomiting, diarrhea, weight loss, indigestion, muscle weakness

Namenda (memantine)	N-methyl D-aspartate (NMDA) antagonist prescribed to treat symptoms of moderate to severe Alzheimer's	Blocks the toxic effects associated with excess glutamate and regulates glutamate activation	Dizziness, headache, diarrhea, constipation, confusion
Namzaric (memantine and donepezil)	NMDA antagonist and cholinesterase inhibitor prescribed to treat symptoms of moderate to severe Alzheimer's	Blocks the toxic effects associated with excess glutamate and prevents the breakdown of acetylcholine in the brain	Headache, nausea, vomiting, diarrhea, dizziness, anorexia
Razadyne (galantamine)	Cholinesterase inhibitor prescribed to treat symptoms of mild to moderate Alzheimer's	Prevents the breakdown of acetylcholine and stimulates nicotinic receptors to release more acetylcholine in the brain	Nausea, vomiting, diarrhea, decreased appetite, dizziness, headache

1.5.3. Dosage and Side Effects of Alzheimer's Medications

Depending on how well a patient tolerates the medication, doctors typically start their patients on low dosages and progressively increase it. There is some evidence to suggest that higher doses of cholinesterase inhibitors may be beneficial for some individuals. However, side effects are more likely to occur at higher doses. When starting a medication, patients need to be closely watched. Potential adverse effects of all these medications include nausea, vomiting, diarrhea, and appetite loss. Notify the prescribing physician of any strange symptoms straight away. It is important to follow the doctor's instructions when taking any medication, including vitamins and herbal supplements. Also, let the doctor know before adding or changing any medications.

1.5.4. Managing Behavioral Symptoms of Alzheimer's Disease

Alzheimer's disease frequently causes restlessness, depression, agitation, anxiety, aggression, insomnia, and wandering. Researchers are figuring out why these symptoms happen and looking into new medication and non-drug approaches to treat them. Treatment for behavioral symptoms of Alzheimer's disease has been found to improve the quality of life for patients with the disease as well as ease the burden on carers. Experts concur that using medication to address these behavioral issues should come only after non-pharmacological treatment options have been exhausted. Find out more about coping mechanisms and behavioral changes in individuals with Alzheimer's disease.

1.5.5. Medicines to Be Used with Caution in People with Alzheimer's Disease

There are some medicines, such as sleep aids, anti-anxiety drugs, anticonvulsants, and antipsychotics, that a person with Alzheimer's disease should take only:

- After the doctor has explained all the risks and side effects of the medicine
- Other, safer non-medication options have not helped treat the problem

- You will need to watch closely for side effects from these medications.

Sleep aids are used to help people get to sleep and stay asleep. People with Alzheimer's disease should NOT use these drugs regularly because they make the person more confused and more likely to fall. There are lifestyle changes people can make to improve their sleep.

Anti-anxiety drugs are used to treat agitation. These drugs can cause sleepiness, dizziness, falls, and confusion. For this reason, doctors recommend they should only be used for short periods of time.

Anticonvulsants are drugs sometimes used to treat severe aggression. Side effects may cause sleepiness, dizziness, mood swings, and confusion.

Antipsychotics are drugs used to treat paranoia, hallucinations, agitation, and aggression. Side effects of using these drugs can be serious, including an increased risk of death in some older people with dementia. They should only be given to people with Alzheimer's disease when the doctor agrees that the symptoms are severe.

1.5.6. The Future of Alzheimer's Disease Treatments

The state of research on Alzheimer's disease has advanced to the point where experts can consider addressing underlying disease processes rather than just treating symptoms. Scientists are creating and testing many potential interventions in ongoing clinical trials, such as medication therapies, physical activity, cognitive training, immunization therapy, and treatments for diabetes and cardiovascular disease (Lott & Head, 2005; Duyckaerts, Charles, Dennis, 2011; Viña & Sanz-Ros, 2018; Knopman et al., 2021).

1.6. PREVENTION OF ALZHEIMER'S DISEASE

As a result of the lack of disease-modifying therapies for Alzheimer's disease, research on the condition has concentrated on interventions meant to stop its onset and progression. No specific intervention has been shown to be effective in preventing Alzheimer's, and research on interventions to delay the disease's onset or progression has yielded mixed results. A person's risk of developing AD may be influenced by modifiable factors like diet, lifestyle, and medication, according to epidemiological studies. Deciding whether Alzheimer's disease interventions serve as a secondary prevention strategy, identifying the disease in its early stages, or a primary prevention strategy, preventing the disease itself, presents certain challenges. The length of the intervention, the various disease stages at which it starts, and the lack of standardization in the inclusion criteria for biomarkers unique to Alzheimer's disease are some of these challenges. To identify the risk factors for Alzheimer's disease, more research is required.

1.6.1. Medication

Cardiovascular risk factors include smoking, diabetes, high blood pressure, high cholesterol, and high blood pressure are linked to an increased chance of developing AD and a worsened course of the disease. In Alzheimer's disease, statin use for cholesterol reduction may be beneficial. By influencing cerebrovascular pathology, antihypertensive and antidiabetic medications may reduce the risk of dementia in people without overt cognitive impairment. More investigation is required to specifically look at the connection with Alzheimer's disease; it's also necessary to clarify the exact role that medications play in comparison to other concurrent lifestyle changes (such as diet, exercise, and smoking). Since depression is linked to a higher risk of Alzheimer's, antidepressant treatment may offer a preventative measure.

Because they reduce inflammation, non-steroidal anti-inflammatory drugs (NSAIDs) have historically been linked to a lower risk of Alzheimer's disease; however, they don't seem to be very effective as a treatment. In addition, it was previously believed that a lack of estrogen during menopause was a risk factor for Alzheimer's disease because women are more likely than men to develop the disease. Hormone replacement therapy (HRT) during menopause does not, however, appear to reduce the risk of cognitive decline.

1.6.2. Lifestyle

Alzheimer's risk may be impacted by several lifestyle factors, including stress, sleep, cigarette smoking, higher education and professional achievement, physical and cognitive exercise, and managing other comorbidities like diabetes and hypertension. Exercise is beneficial in lessening the severity of symptoms in AD patients and is linked to a lower incidence of dementia. Aerobic activities such as brisk walking for 40 minutes three times a week can help with memory and cognitive functions. It might also cause the brain to become more neuroplastic. Engaging in cognitive activities like crossword puzzles, chess, and reading has demonstrated potential as a preventive measure. AD risk is lowered when physical activity levels meet WHO recommendations.

Engaging in recreational activities, along with achieving higher levels of education and occupation, can either delay or prevent the onset of Alzheimer's symptoms. This is consistent with the theory of cognitive reserve, which postulates that certain experiences in life lead to more effective brain activity, thereby granting an individual a cognitive reserve that postpones the onset of dementia symptoms. Without affecting how long the disease takes to manifest, education can postpone the onset of Alzheimer's disease. Giving up smoking may lower the risk of Alzheimer's, especially for people with the APOE 4 allele. Smoking increases oxidative stress, which in turn causes neurodegenerative or inflammatory processes that may raise the risk of AD. It is advised to abstain from smoking, to use medication and counseling to help quit, and to keep oneself away from tobacco smoke in the surrounding air.

Although the exact correlation between sleep disorders and Alzheimer's disease is unknown, it is known to exist. It used to be believed that the risk of both AD and sleep disorders increased separately with age, but current research is looking at the possibility that AD may become more common as a result of sleep disorders. One theory suggests that mechanisms involved in increasing the clearance of toxic substances, such as Aβ, are active when you're sleeping. A person who gets less sleep produces more Aβ and has less Aβ clearance, which leads to an accumulation of Aβ. Getting enough sleep each night—roughly 7 to 8 hours—has emerged as a promising lifestyle intervention to stop the onset of AD. Alzheimer's disease development is influenced by stress. It is unclear how stress predisposes a person to Alzheimer's disease, but it has been hypothesized that stressors experienced throughout life may alter an individual's epigenome, causing certain genes to express themselves either excessively or insufficiently. Although the exact link between stress and Alzheimer's disease is unknown, there may be ways to slow the disease's progression by practicing stress management and mental relaxation techniques. For example, although more research is required to assess long-term effects, meditation is a helpful lifestyle change to support cognition and well-being (Lott &

Head, 2005; Duyckaerts, Charles, Dennis, 2011; Viña & Sanz-Ros, 2018; Knopman et al., 2021).

1.7. MANAGEMENT OF ALZHEIMER'S DISEASE

Alzheimer's disease has no known cure; the only treatments that are currently available are palliative in nature and only slightly improve symptoms. There are three categories of treatments: pharmacological, psychosocial, and caregiving.

1.7.1. Pharmaceutical

Memantine, an NMDA receptor antagonist, and four acetylcholinesterase inhibitors—tacrine, rivastigmine, galantamine, and donepezil—are among the medications used to treat the cognitive symptoms of Alzheimer's disease rather than the underlying cause. Memantine is meant for people with moderate to severe Alzheimer's disease, while acetylcholinesterase inhibitors are meant for those with mild to severe Alzheimer's. The advantage of using them is negligible. One well-known characteristic of Alzheimer's disease is a decrease in cholinergic neuron activity. To counteract the loss of acetylcholine (ACh) brought on by the death of cholinergic neurons and raise the concentration of ACh in the brain, acetylcholinesterase inhibitors are used to slow down the rate at which ACh is broken down. These drugs have been shown to be effective in treating mild to moderate Alzheimer's disease, and there is also some evidence supporting their use in more advanced stages of the illness. There has been no evidence that using these medications to treat mild cognitive impairment can postpone the onset of Alzheimer's disease. The most frequent adverse effects are vomiting and nausea, which are both related to excess cholinergic function. About 10–20% of users experience these side effects, which range in severity from mild to moderate and are manageable with gradual dosage adjustments. Muscle spasms, bradycardia (low heart rate), decreased appetite and weight, and increased gastric acid production are less frequent secondary effects.

Although glutamate is an excitatory neurotransmitter in the nervous system, excessive levels in the brain can cause excitotoxicity, or the overstimulation of glutamate receptors, which can result in cell death. In addition to Alzheimer's disease, other neurological conditions like multiple sclerosis and Parkinson's disease also exhibit excitotoxicity. Memantine is a noncompetitive antagonist of the NMDA receptor that was initially prescribed to treat influenza. By blocking NMDA receptors and preventing glutamate from overstimulating them, it affects the glutamatergic system. It has been demonstrated that memantine offers a slight advantage when treating moderate-to-severe Alzheimer's disease. Memantine side effects that have been reported are rare and mild, and they include headaches, fatigue, dizziness, and hallucinations. It has been demonstrated that donepezil and memantine together have statistically significant but clinically marginal efficacy.

Alzheimer's disease and other neuropsychiatric conditions have been treated with EGb 761, an extract of ginkgo biloba. Europe as a whole has approved its use. EGb 761 is listed in the World Federation of Biological Psychiatry guidelines with the same weight of evidence (level B) as memantine and acetylcholinesterase inhibitors. The only one to show improvement in vascular dementia and Alzheimer's disease symptoms was EGb 761. If other treatments don't work, EGb 761 might be useful either by itself or as an adjunct. A 2016 review concluded that there was not enough evidence from Ginkgo biloba clinical trials to support its use in treating Alzheimer's disease. The benefits of atypical antipsychotics in lowering psychosis and aggression in Alzheimer's patients are somewhat outweighed by their major side effects, which include stroke, impaired mobility, and cognitive decline. Long-term use has been demonstrated to be associated with higher mortality rates. In this group of individuals, stopping antipsychotic use seems safe.

1.7.2. Psychosocial

Psychosocial interventions fall into one of four categories: behavior-, emotion-, cognition-, or stimulation-oriented approaches. They are used in addition to pharmaceutical treatment. Behavioral interventions aim to pinpoint and mitigate the causes and effects of problematic behaviors. While it hasn't been successful in enhancing general functioning, this method can lessen some particular problematic behaviors, like incontinence. High-quality research on the efficacy of these methods in treating other behavioral issues like wandering is lacking. The reduction of behavioral and psychological symptoms is a successful outcome of music therapy. Reminiscence therapy, validation therapy, supportive psychotherapy, sensory integration—also known as snoezelen—and simulated presence therapy are examples of emotion-oriented interventions. According to a Cochrane review, there is no proof that this works. In reminiscence therapy (RT), people talk about their past experiences either alone or in groups, frequently using old-fashioned pictures, household objects, audio recordings, and other familiar objects. According to a 2018 evaluation of its efficacy, its effects were situation-specific, uneven, small-scale, and doubtfully clinically significant. Based on attachment theories, simulated presence therapy (SPT) plays a recording featuring the voices of the patient's closest family members. A small body of research suggests that SPT might lessen problematic behaviors.

Reducing cognitive deficits is the goal of cognition-oriented therapies, such as reality orientation and cognitive retraining. Presenting facts about a person, place, or time to help someone understand their surroundings and their role in them is known as reality orientation. Conversely, cognitive retraining uses mental exercises to help improve impaired capacities. Both have demonstrated some effectiveness in enhancing cognitive abilities. Exercise, any form of recreational activity, music, art, and pet therapy are examples of stimulation-oriented treatments. There is some evidence that stimulation can enhance behavior, mood, and, to a lesser degree, function. Even so, the shift in the patient's routine serves as the primary argument in favor of the use of stimulation therapies.

1.7.3. Caregiving

Caregiving is essentially the treatment for Alzheimer's disease and needs to be closely monitored throughout the disease because there is no cure and the condition gradually makes people unable to tend to their own needs. Changes to lifestyle and living conditions can lessen caregiver stress and improve safety in the early and moderate stages.

Some examples of these adjustments include using modified everyday objects, labeling household items to alert the person with the illness, installing safety locks, and adhering to simplified routines. Food may need to be prepared in smaller portions or even puréed if eating becomes difficult. It could be necessary to use feeding tubes when swallowing issues occur. In these situations, the family members and caregivers must weigh the medical necessity and morality of continuing feeding. Physical restraints are rarely recommended at any stage of the disease, though there are instances in which they are required to protect the Alzheimer's patient or their carers. The goal of treatment in the latter stages of the illness is to minimize suffering until death, frequently with hospice assistance.

1.7.4. Diet

Alzheimer's disease risk factors that can be changed include diet. Reduced cognitive decline is linked to both the DASH and Mediterranean diets. A different strategy has been to combine components of these two diets into the MIND diet. Research on specific dietary elements, minerals, and supplements has produced conflicting results regarding their ability to fend off AD or cognitive decline (Lott & Head, 2005; Duyckaerts, Charles, Dennis, 2011; Viña & Sanz-Ros, 2018; Knopman et al., 2021).

1.8. BIOCHEMISTRY OF ALZHEIMER'S DISEASE

The most common cause of dementia, Alzheimer's disease, has poorly understood biochemistry. The accumulation of aberrantly folded amyloid beta (Aβ) protein in the brain has led to the identification of Alzheimer's disease (AD) as a proteinopathy, or protein misfolding disease. A short peptide known as amyloid beta is an aberrant byproduct of amyloid-beta precursor protein (APP), a transmembrane protein whose exact role in neuronal development is unknown. Presenilins are parts of a proteolytic complex that breaks down and processes APP. Though mostly alpha helical in membranes, amyloid beta monomers are soluble and contain brief regions of beta-sheet and polyproline II helix secondary structures in solution. However, at high enough concentrations, they dramatically alter their conformation to form a tertiary structure that is rich in beta sheets and aggregates to form amyloid fibrils. The deposits of these fibrils and oligomeric forms of Aβ outside of neurons are referred to as senile plaques. Different types of plaques exist, such as diffuse, compact, cored, or neuritic plaque types. Cerebral amyloid angiopathy is the term for Aβ deposits in the walls of small blood vessels in the brain.

Due to aberrant tau protein aggregation—a microtubule-associated protein expressed in neurons that typically functions to stabilize microtubules in the cell cytoskeleton—AD is also regarded as a tauopathy. Like most microtubule-associated proteins, tau is normally controlled by phosphorylation. However, hyperphosphorylated tau builds up as paired helical filaments in Alzheimer's disease, which subsequently combine to form masses called neurofibrillary tangles inside nerve cell bodies and dystrophic neurites linked to amyloid plaques. The depletion of a prolyl isomerase protein belonging to the parvulin family has been observed to hasten the accumulation of abnormal tau, although little is known about the process of filament assembly. Another factor in the intricate chain of events that results in AD pathology and symptoms is neuroinflammation. Significant pathological and clinical data demonstrates immunological alterations linked to AD, such as elevated levels of pro-inflammatory cytokines in the blood and CSF. The pathophysiology and progression of AD have been linked to inflammation within the brain, including increased reactivity of the resident microglia towards amyloid deposits. Whether these changes are a cause or consequence of AD is still unclear. Research employing experimental models of Alzheimer's disease has helped to unravel much of the disease's known biochemistry.

1.8.1. Neuropathology

The loss of neurons and synapses in the cerebral cortex and some subcortical regions is the macroscopic hallmark of AD. This causes the afflicted areas to atrophy severely, including the temporal and parietal lobes as well as portions of the frontal cortex and cingulate gyrus. Under a microscope, AD brains exhibit both neurofibrillary tangles and amyloid plaques. Plaques are thick, mostly insoluble accumulations of cellular debris and protein that surround and surround neurons. Inside the nerve cell, tangles are made up of insoluble twisted fibers. While plaques and tangles are common in the brains of the elderly, AD patients' brains exhibit a significantly higher concentration of these lesions in various brain regions.

1.8.2. Biochemical Characteristics

The biochemical processes that result in the buildup of tau-protein tangles and amyloid-beta plaques are essential to our comprehension of Alzheimer's disease. The buildup of amyloid-beta is controlled by a fine balance of secretases, which are enzymes. Alpha-secretase activity and cholinergic neuronal activity have recently been linked, and this may prevent the buildup of amyloid-beta proteins in the brains of Alzheimer's disease patients. Because of the build-up of aberrantly folded amyloid-beta proteins in AD patients' brains, the disease has been classified as a proteopathy, or protein misfolding disease. Cerebrospinal fluid analysis and positron emission tomography (PET) are two methods that can be used to identify abnormal amyloid-beta accumulation.

While AD and prion diseases have similar pathophysiological mechanisms, AD cannot spread in the wild like prion diseases do. Any transmissibility it might have is restricted to incredibly rare iatrogenic events resulting from discontinued donor-derived therapies. Although its exact role is unknown, amyloid-beta, also written Aβ, is a brief peptide that is produced as a proteolytic byproduct of the transmembrane protein amyloid precursor protein (APP). It is believed to play a role in the development of neurons. Presenilins are parts of a proteolytic complex that breaks down and processes APP. Though innocuous, amyloid beta monomers experience a profound conformational shift at high enough concentrations to generate a beta sheet-rich tertiary structure. This structure then aggregates to form amyloid fibrils, which deposit outside neurons in dense formations called neuritic or senile plaques, in less dense aggregates called diffuse plaques, and occasionally in the walls of small blood vessels in the brain in a condition known as amyloid angiopathy or congophilic angiopathy.

Because of the aberrant aggregation of tau protein—a microtubule-associated protein that is expressed in neurons and is normally responsible for stabilizing microtubules in the cell cytoskeleton—AD is also regarded as a tauopathy. Tau is normally controlled by phosphorylation, like most other microtubule-associated proteins. However, in Alzheimer's disease (AD) patients, hyperphosphorylated tau builds up as paired helical filaments, which then combine to form masses inside nerve cell bodies called neurofibrillary tangles and dystrophic neurites linked to amyloid plaques. Acetylcholine (ACh) levels, a neurotransmitter, are lowered. Serotonin, norepinephrine, and somatostatin levels—three other neurotransmitters—are frequently decreased as well. The FDA has approved the use of anti-cholinesterases to replenish the ACh. As a next-generation cholinomimetic for Alzheimer's disease, an alternate strategy for activating ACh receptors of the M1–M3 types has been proposed. These synthetic agonists have a slower rate of dissociation from the receptor.

1.8.3. Disease Mechanisms

Although the gross histological characteristics of AD in the brain have been thoroughly described, various theories have been put forth concerning the underlying cause. The cholinergic hypothesis, one of the oldest theories, postulates that a lack of cholinergic signaling causes the disease to progress. According to current theories, the cascade that leads to AD pathology is triggered by both amyloid beta aggregation outside the cell and tau protein misfolding inside the cell. According to more recent potential theories, AD may be influenced by metabolic variables, vascular disruption, and persistently high levels of inflammation in the brain. To date, the amyloid beta hypothesis of molecular initiation has gained traction among a large number of researchers. The two most widely accepted theories are the tau and amyloid ones.

1.8.3.1. Amyloid Hypothesis

The amyloid hypothesis was found because chromosome 21 contains the gene for the amyloid beta precursor or APP, and individuals with trisomy 21, or Down syndrome, who have an extra copy of the gene show symptoms of AD by the time they are 40 years old. According to the amyloid hypothesis, the toxic form of the protein that upsets the calcium ion balance of the cell and causes apoptosis is mature aggregated amyloid fibrils. These fibrils are thought to be cytotoxic. The finding that increased levels of a beta-amyloid protein variant known to form fibrils more quickly in vitro correlate with an earlier onset and more severe cognitive impairment in mouse models as well as with the diagnosis of AD in humans supports this theory. However, it is unclear how mature fibrils cause the induced calcium influx or what other cytotoxic mechanisms they might suggest. According to a more recent version of the amyloid hypothesis, the cytotoxic species is an intermediate misfolded form of amyloid beta. It is an oligomeric species, possibly toroidal or star-shaped, with a central channel that may physically pierce the cell membrane and cause apoptosis. Instead of being a soluble monomer or mature aggregated polymer. According to the ion channel hypothesis, soluble, non-fibrillar Aβ oligomers form membrane ion channels that permit uncontrollably high levels of calcium influx into neurons. A related alternative proposes that the cytotoxic species is a globular oligomer localized to neuronal axons and dendritic processes. It was demonstrated that the prefibrillar aggregates could damage the membrane.

The cytotoxic-fibril hypothesis provides a well-defined target for drug discovery: impede the process of fibrillization. The toxic-oligomer theory would suggest that preventing oligomeric assembly is the more important process or that a better target lies upstream, for example in the inhibition of APP processing to amyloid beta. Much of the early development work on lead compounds has focused on this inhibition; most are also reported to reduce neurotoxicity.

- **Soluble Intracellular (o)Aβ42:** Two studies have demonstrated that by activating casein kinase 2, oligomeric (o)Aβ42, a species of Aβ, in soluble intracellular form, acutely inhibits synaptic transmission—a pathophysiology that characterizes AD (in its early stages).

1.8.3.2. Inflammatory Hypothesis

A growing body of research indicates that AD pathology is primarily modified by a persistent inflammatory response in the brain, which may also play a significant role in the pathophysiology of the disease. Patients with AD have brains that show multiple indicators of elevated inflammatory signaling. According to the inflammatory hypothesis, persistently high levels of inflammation in the brain boost the severity of the disease in the later stages of AD and are essential to the amyloid cascade in the early stages of the disease. It is unknown how Aβ production begins to exceed the brain's clearance capacity and causes AD progression, but it is present in healthy brains and plays a critical physiological role in the blood-brain barrier repair, neuronal injury recovery, and infection prevention. One theory is that Aβ activates the brain's resident immune cells, called microglia, causing them to release pro-inflammatory signaling molecules called cytokines that draw in more nearby microglia. Acute activation of microglia in response to injury is advantageous as it enables the microglia to phagocytose Aβ and other cellular debris; however, chronically activated microglia are less effective in clearing Aβ. Reactive oxygen species and pro-inflammatory cytokines such as interleukins 1β and 6 (IL-6, IL-1β) and tumor necrosis factor-alpha (TNF-a) are secreted by activated microglia despite their decreased ability to clear AB. These cytokines impair normal synaptic functioning and ultimately result in neuronal death. The cognitive deficits and volume loss in important brain regions linked to AD are caused by a loss of synaptic functioning and ultimately by neuronal death. Further Aβ oligomer production and tau hyperphosphorylation are brought on by IL-1B, IL-6, and TNF-a. This results in microglia activation and a feed-forward mechanism that eventually causes Aβ production to increase and Aβ clearance to decrease, forming Aβ plaques.

1.8.3.3. Historical Cholinergic Hypothesis

The cholinergic hypothesis of AD development was first proposed in 1976 by Peter Davies and A.J.F Maloney. It claimed that Alzheimer's begins as a deficiency in the production of acetylcholine, a vital neurotransmitter. Much early therapeutic research was based on this hypothesis, including restoration of the "cholinergic nuclei." The possibility of cell-replacement therapy was investigated based on this hypothesis. All of the first-generation anti-Alzheimer medications are based on this hypothesis and work to preserve acetylcholine by inhibiting acetylcholinesterases (enzymes that break down acetylcholine). These medications, though sometimes beneficial, have not led to a cure. In all cases, they have served to only treat symptoms of the disease and have neither halted nor reversed it. These results and other research have led to the conclusion that acetylcholine deficiencies may not be directly causal, but are a result of widespread brain tissue damage, damage so widespread that cell-replacement therapies are likely to be impractical. More recent findings center on the effects of the misfolded and aggregated proteins, amyloid beta and tau: tau protein abnormalities may initiate the disease cascade, then beta amyloid deposits progress the disease.

1.8.3.4. Glucose Consumption

One of the body's most metabolically active organs, the human brain uses a lot of glucose to create adenosine triphosphate (ATP), which is used by cells as energy. The brain is largely dependent on circulating glucose for energy, even with its high energy demands. It is relatively rigid in its ability to use substrates for energy production. Due to its reliance on glucose, the brain is vulnerable to damage from a disruption in glucose supply or a malfunction in its metabolism. Cognitive function is eventually compromised if the brain is unable to produce ATP, which maintains synapses and cells.

The brains of Alzheimer's patients use glucose less when the disease is still in its early stages, even before symptoms of cognitive impairment appear. This is demonstrated by imaging studies. As clinical symptoms appear and the disease worsens, this decline in glucose metabolism gets worse. Comparing Alzheimer's patients to age-matched controls, research has revealed a decline in cerebral glucose metabolism of 17–24%. This finding has subsequently been validated by numerous imaging studies. In particular, the posterior cingulate, parietal, temporal, and prefrontal cortices exhibit abnormally low rates of cerebral glucose metabolism in a pattern characteristic of Alzheimer's disease brain disease. Many facets of memory and cognition are thought to be regulated by these brain areas. It has even been suggested that this metabolic pattern can be used to diagnose Alzheimer's disease because it is repeatable. In addition, in patients with more advanced disease, diminished cerebral glucose metabolism (DCGM) correlates with plaque density and cognitive deficits.

Since diminished cerebral glucose metabolism (DCGM) can occur in both inherited forms of Alzheimer's disease and asymptomatic patients at risk for the disease, such as those homozygous for the epsilon 4 variant of the apolipoprotein E gene (APOE4, a genetic risk factor for the disease), it may not be exclusively an artifact of brain cell loss. Since DCGM happens before other pathological and clinical changes, the large-scale cell loss linked to Alzheimer's disease is unlikely to be the cause. The same brain regions as older Alzheimer's disease patients showed diminished cerebral glucose metabolism (DCGM) in imaging studies involving young adult APOE4 carriers who showed no signs of cognitive impairment. DCGM is not limited to APOE4 carriers, though. In genotypes APOE3/E4, APOE3/E3, and APOE4/E4, DCGM occurs by the time Alzheimer's disease is diagnosed. DCGM is a metabolic biomarker for the illness state as a result.

1.8.3.5. Insulin Signaling

Over the past 10 years, there has been evidence linking diabetes to Alzheimer's disease, as subjects with Alzheimer's disease have also shown signs of insulin resistance, a characteristic hallmark of the disease. Neurotoxic oligomeric amyloid-β species eliminate neuronal insulin signaling and reduce the expression of insulin receptors on the cell surface of neurons. It has been proposed that the removal of insulin receptors from the neuronal surface caused by amyloid-β is facilitated by neuronal gangliosides, which are involved in the formation of membrane lipid microdomains. TNF-α signaling is triggered by oligomeric amyloid-β species in Alzheimer's disease. TNF-α-induced activation of c-Jun N-terminal kinase then triggers stress-related kinases and leads to serine phosphorylation of IRS-1, which stops insulin signaling downstream. Insulin resistance that develops as a result exacerbates cognitive decline. Thus, boosting insulin sensitivity and signaling in neurons could be a novel therapeutic strategy for Alzheimer's disease.

1.8.3.6. Oxidative Stress

One of the main players in the etiology of AD is now thought to be oxidative stress. The overproduction of reactive oxygen species (ROS) is believed to be a major factor in the build-up and deposit of amyloid beta in AD. Both nuclear and mitochondrial DNA in the brains of AD patients exhibit high levels of oxidative DNA damage; however, the levels of damage to mitochondrial DNA are about 10 times higher than those to nuclear DNA. An important contributing factor to the onset of neurodegeneration in AD may be aged mitochondria. Increased oxidative damage has been found in the nuclear and mitochondrial brain DNA of even those with mild cognitive impairment, which is a stage between normal aging and early dementia (see Aging brain). The majority of naturally occurring double-strand breaks (DSBs) in human cells result from single-strand breaks that are caused by a variety of factors, such as the activity of topoisomerases, reactive oxygen species, and hydrolysis brought on by temperature fluctuations. A type II topoisomerase causes DSBs in neurons as a part of the physiological process of memory formation. DSBs are more prevalent in astrocytes and neurons in the postmortem human hippocampal regions of AD patients compared to those in non-AD patients. Early on in the disease's progression, AD is linked to a buildup of DSBs in the neurons and astrocytes of the hippocampus and frontal cortex. In the hippocampus, DSB accumulation is elevated in the vicinity of amyloid plaques, suggesting a possible involvement of Aβ in DSB accumulation or the opposite. The DNA-dependent protein kinase (DNA-PK) complex is utilized in non-homologous end joining (NHEJ), the main mechanism for repairing DNA double-strand breaks. In comparison to normal brains, AD brains exhibit significantly lower levels of

DNA-PK catalytic subunit protein and end joining activity.

1.8.3.7. Cholesterol Hypothesis

The tau hypothesis, the inflammatory hypothesis, and the amyloid hypothesis are combined to form the cholesterol hypothesis. It has been demonstrated that tau and amyloid production occur upstream of cholesterol. The astrocytes produce the cholesterol, which is then transported to the neurons via a process known as substrate presentation, where it triggers the production of amyloid. The procedure called for apoE. Although the exact mechanism by which cholesterol regulates the production of Tau is unknown, Tau phosphorylation was reduced when the cholesterol synthesis enzyme SREBP2 was deleted. Cells absorb the cholesterol after innate immunity starts the synthesis of cholesterol. It is thought that as people age, a brain cell dies and initiates innate immunity. To directly link the inflammatory theory to the synthesis of cholesterol in the brain, more research is required.

1.8.3.8. Reelin Hypothesis

According to a 1994 study, Alzheimer's disease cannot be considered a consequence of premature aging because the isoprenoid changes it causes are different from those that occur during normal aging. The human brain exhibits a gradual rise in dolichol levels, a fall in ubiquinone levels, and essentially stable concentrations of cholesterol and dolichyl phosphate as it ages. The situation is reversed in Alzheimer's disease, with elevated ubiquinone levels and decreased dolichol levels. While cholesterol stays the same, dolichyl phosphate concentrations rise as well. An increased rate of glycosylation in the diseased brain and an attempt to shield the brain from oxidative stress, such as that caused by lipid peroxidation, may be the causes of the rise in the sugar carrier dolichyl phosphate and endogenous antioxidant ubiquinone. In a rat model of Alzheimer's disease, the previously discovered compound rovetin exhibits neuroprotective properties.

A relatively recent theory, primarily based on rodent studies, connects the hypofunction of the large extracellular protein reelin to the development of Alzheimer's disease. Reelin levels in the human entorhinal cortex, where the disease usually starts, are clearly declining, but there is also evidence of compensatory increases in reelin levels in the patients' other brain structures. The ability of reelin overexpression to restore cognitive function in mice modeling Alzheimer's disease and τ-protein overexpressing mice is crucial. The reelin hypothesis was theoretically supported by a recent circuit level model that suggested a mechanism for how reelin depletion causes early deterioration of episodic memory.

1.8.3.9. Large Gene Instability Hypothesis

0In 2017, a bioinformatics analysis found that the brain exhibits a significant over-expression of extremely large human genes, which are involved in postsynaptic architecture. Moreover, these genes frequently map to chromosomal fragile sites and have a high enrichment in cell adhesion Gene Ontology (GO) terms. Cell adhesion mechanisms are shared by the majority of known Alzheimer's disease risk gene products, such as gamma-secretase and amyloid precursor protein (APP), as well as the APOE receptors and GWAS risk loci. It was determined that mutational instability of large synaptic adhesion genes may be the etiological trigger of neurotransmission disruption and synaptic loss in brain aging and that dysfunction of cell and synaptic adhesion is central to the pathogenesis of Alzheimer's disease. This theory, as a typical example, explains the APOE risk locus of AD in terms of signaling of its giant lipoprotein receptor, LRP1b, a large tumor-suppressor gene that maps to an unstable chromosomal fragile site and is expressed specifically in the brain. The DNA damage mechanism is central to the pathophysiology of Alzheimer's disease, according to the large gene instability hypothesis (Lott & Head, 2005; Duyckaerts, Charles, Dennis, 2011; Viña & Sanz-Ros, 2018; Knopman et al., 2021).

A Closer Look

Alzheimer's and Dementia

As of 2020, dementia and Alzheimer's combined will affect about 55 million people globally, but most people are only aware of how these conditions affect memory loss. Though their symptoms are similar, dementia and Alzheimer's disease are not the same. A lot of brain diseases that cause memory loss can be grouped together under the general term "dementia," which describes a set of symptoms that negatively impact memory. A particular type of neurodegenerative illness called Alzheimer's also results in a decline in cognitive function in addition to memory loss. Depending on which part of the brain is affected, both of these conditions can have different effects on a person.

The two primary indicators of Alzheimer's disease, or AD, are beta-amyloid plaques and neurofibrillary tangles. Simply expressed, Alzheimer's disease is a brain ailment that obstructs the channels via which neurons, or nerve cells, in the brain, can communicate with one another, thereby impairing the brain's ability to transmit messages. Alzheimer's disease causes the progressive death of brain cells, which makes it difficult to do everyday tasks like eating or speaking. Dementia is not a specific disease but rather a much broader umbrella term than Alzheimer's. But there are several varieties of dementia, such as frontotemporal, Lewy body, and vascular dementia.

Considering the variety of dementias that people can develop, illuminating some of the more well-known varieties will offer a deeper understanding of some of the complexities associated with the illness. These three forms of dementia affect not only memory loss but also physical, cognitive, and social functioning. When problems with the blood supply that is meant to reach the brain cause damage to the brain, it is known as vascular dementia. It usually results in decreased analytical and communication abilities, difficulty focusing, and organizational difficulties. One of the most prevalent types of dementia is Lewy body dementia (LBD), which is caused by abnormal masses of the alpha-synuclein protein (called Lewy bodies after FH Lewy, who discovered them) and chemical alterations in the brain that impair thinking, movement, and behavior. Lewy body dementia develops symptoms quickly in the early stages and advances more quickly than Alzheimer's disease.

The frontal and temporal lobes are two distinct regions of the brain that are associated with frontotemporal dementia (FTD). A collection of illnesses known as FTD is brought on by the death of neurons in certain areas. This causes lobe shrinkage and behavioral changes, which raises the possibility that the patient will withdraw socially or begin to lose interest in their hobbies and loved ones. The effects of dementia or Alzheimer's disease can also be felt by a person's loved ones. It's possible that the family member played a significant role in the home, making it difficult to pay for the medical expenses. Even scheduling the family's transportation to appointments can cause stress.

While dementia and HIV/AIDS are both illnesses that should be acknowledged, dementia is more commonly associated with old age than HIV/AIDS and other conditions that can affect a wide range of people, not just those in a particular age range. As such, dementia is less relevant to adolescents and young adults. Conditions outside of the brain receive far less attention and education than conditions inside the brain, primarily those affecting other parts of the body. In general, getting enough sleep, exercising to keep the heart healthy and, consequently, the blood supply to the brain healthy, eating a well-balanced diet, and quitting bad habits like smoking can all help prevent or at least delay the onset of Alzheimer's and dementia. Additionally, acquiring new knowledge is a key component of prevention. New connections between neurons and even different connections made on a single subject can be made through the intake of new information. In general, multiple pieces of information related to a subject increase the likelihood that the person will remember it. Official treatments for dementia and Alzheimer's disease vary widely. In addition to medication, family members of the patient may choose to engage in therapy or other more informal forms of care when looking after the patient. One pharmaceutical approach is the use of cholinesterase inhibitors. These inhibitors increase a chemical messenger's levels in the brain, delaying the process by which the messengers become more impeded as Alzheimer's disease symptoms worsen. Glutamate is a different chemical messenger primarily involved in memory and learning that is regulated by memantine. Memantine is occasionally prescribed in addition to the previously mentioned inhibitor.

Another available treatment is occupational therapy, where an occupational therapist teaches the patient's caretakers how to modify their home into a safer space and teaches coping behavior that serves to prevent accidents and manage the patient's behavior as their symptoms progress.

Another exceptional case is that of an elderly woman who remembers and acts out her ballet routine from her youth. The classical music being played brings this woman back to a time filled with joy and activity. Though the implications behind the quick progression of her symptoms are heart-wrenching, it is touching to see her tap back into such an important part of life that was deep within her memory.

Summary

- The tau hypothesis proposes that tau protein abnormalities initiate the disease cascade. In this model, hyperphosphorylated tau begins to pair with other threads of tau as paired helical filaments.
- The cellular homeostasis of biometals such as ionic copper, iron, and zinc is disrupted in Alzheimer's disease, though it remains unclear whether this is produced by or causes the changes in proteins. Smoking is a significant Alzheimer's disease risk factor.
- Alzheimer's disease is complex, and it is unlikely that any one drug or other intervention will successfully treat it. Current approaches focus on helping people maintain mental function, manage behavioral symptoms, and slow down the symptoms of disease.
- Anticonvulsants are drugs sometimes used to treat severe aggression. Side effects may cause sleepiness, dizziness, mood swings, and confusion.
- The biochemistry of Alzheimer's disease, the most common cause of dementia, is not yet very well understood. Alzheimer's disease (AD) has been identified as a proteinopathy: a protein misfolding disease due to the accumulation of abnormally folded amyloid beta (Aβ) protein in the brain.
- At a macroscopic level, AD is characterized by the loss of neurons and synapses in the cerebral cortex and certain subcortical regions. This results in gross atrophy of the affected regions, including degeneration in the temporal lobe and parietal lobe, and parts of the frontal cortex and cingulate gyrus.
- The amyloid hypothesis points to the cytotoxicity of mature aggregated amyloid fibrils, which are believed to be the toxic form of the protein responsible for disrupting the cell's calcium ion homeostasis and thus inducing apoptosis.
- The human brain is one of the most metabolically active organs in the body and metabolizes a large amount of glucose to produce cellular energy in the form of adenosine triphosphate (ATP).
- Oxidative stress is emerging as a key factor in the pathogenesis of AD. Reactive oxygen species (ROS) over-production is thought to play a critical role in the accumulation and deposition of amyloid beta in AD.
- The cholesterol hypothesis is a combination of the amyloid hypothesis, the tau hypothesis, and potentially the inflammatory hypothesis. Cholesterol was shown to be upstream of both amyloid and tau production.

REFERENCES

1. Agostinho, P., Cunha, R. A., & Oliveira, C. (2010). Neuroinflammation, oxidative stress and the pathogenesis of Alzheimer's disease. *Current Pharmaceutical Design, 16*(25), 2766–2778. https://doi.org/10.2174/138161210793176098.
2. Akiyama, H., Barger, S., Barnum, S., Bradt, B., Bauer, J., Cole, G. M., et al. (2000). Inflammation and Alzheimer's disease. *Neurobiology of Aging, 21*(3), 383–421. https://doi.org/10.1016/S0197-4580(00)00124-X.
3. Borchelt, D. R. (1998). Metabolism of presenilin 1: Influence of presenilin 1 on amyloid precursor protein processing. *Neurobiology of Aging, 19*(1 Suppl), S15–S18. https://doi.org/10.1016/S0197-4580(98)00026-1.
4. Cai, D., Netzer, W. J., Zhong, M., Lin, Y., Du, G., Frohman, M., et al. (2006). Presenilin-1 uses phospholipase D1 as a negative regulator of beta-amyloid formation. *Proceedings of the National Academy of Sciences of the United States of America, 103*(6), 1941–1946. https://doi.org/10.1073/pnas.0510658103.
5. Craft, S. (2012). Alzheimer's disease: Insulin resistance and AD–extending the translational path. *Nature Reviews. Neurology, 8*(7), 360–362. https://doi.org/10.1038/nrneurol.2012.97.
6. Danielsson, J., Andersson, A., Jarvet, J., & Gräslund, A. (2006). 15N relaxation study of the amyloid beta-peptide: Structural propensities and persistence length. *Magnetic Resonance in Chemistry, 44* (Spec No), S114–S121.
7. Davies, P., & Maloney, A. J. (1976). Selective loss of central cholinergic neurons in Alzheimer's disease. *Lancet, 2*(8000), 1403. https://doi.org/10.1016/S0140-6736(76)92159-4.
8. De Felice, F. G. (2013). Alzheimer's disease and insulin resistance: Translating basic science into clinical applications. *The Journal of Clinical Investigation, 123*(2), 531–539. https://doi.org/10.1172/JCI64077.
9. Duyckaerts, C., & Dickson, D. W. (2011). *Neurodegeneration: The Molecular Pathology of Dementia and Movement Disorders*. Oxford: Wiley-Blackwell.
10. Hashimoto, M., Rockenstein, E., Crews, L., & Masliah, E. (2003). Role of protein aggregation in mitochondrial dysfunction and neurodegeneration in Alzheimer's and Parkinson's diseases. *Neuromolecular Medicine, 4*(1–2), 21–36. https://doi.org/10.1385/NMM:4:1-2:21.
11. Kerr, M. L., & Small, D. H. (2005). Cytoplasmic domain of the beta-amyloid protein precursor of Alzheimer's disease: Function, regulation of proteolysis, and implications for drug development. *Journal of Neuroscience Research, 80*(2), 151–159. https://doi.org/10.1002/jnr.20450.
12. Knopman, D. S., Amieva, H., Petersen, R. C., Chételat, G., Holtzman, D. M., Hyman, B. T., et al. (2021). Alzheimer's disease. *Nature Reviews Disease Primers, 7*(1), 33. https://doi.org/10.1038/s41572-021-00278-5.
13. Liu, Z., Zhou, T., Ziegler, A. C., Dimitrion, P., & Zuo, L. (2017). Oxidative stress in neurodegenerative diseases: From molecular mechanisms to clinical applications. *Oxidative Medicine and Cellular Longevity, 2017*, Article 2525967. https://doi.org/10.1155/2017/2525967.
14. Lott, I. T., & Head, E. (2005). Alzheimer's disease and Down syndrome: Factors in pathogenesis. *Neurobiology of Aging, 26*(3), 383–389. https://doi.org/10.1016/j.neurobiolaging.2004.09.011.

15. Mendez, M. F. (2012). Early-onset Alzheimer's disease: Nonamnestic subtypes and type 2 AD. *Archives of Medical Research, 43*(8), 677–685. https://doi.org/10.1016/j.arcmed.2012.11.005.

16. Ohnishi, S., & Takano, K. (2004). Amyloid fibrils from the viewpoint of protein folding. *Cellular and Molecular Life Sciences, 61*(5), 511–524. https://doi.org/10.1007/s00018-003-3316-4.

17. Reiman, E. M., Chen, K., Alexander, G. E., Caselli, R. J., Bandy, D., Osborne, D., et al. (2004). Functional brain abnormalities in young adults at genetic risk for late-onset Alzheimer's dementia. *Proceedings of the National Academy of Sciences of the United States of America, 101*(1), 284–289. https://doi.org/10.1073/pnas.2635903100.

18. Small, G. W., Ercoli, L. M., Silverman, D. H., Huang, S. C., Komo, S., Bookheimer, S. Y., et al. (2000). Cerebral metabolic and cognitive decline in persons at genetic risk for Alzheimer's disease. *Proceedings of the National Academy of Sciences of the United States of America, 97*(11), 6037–6042. https://doi.org/10.1073/pnas.090106797.

19. Viña, J., & Sanz-Ros, J. (2018). Alzheimer's disease: Only prevention makes sense. *European Journal of Clinical Investigation, 48*(10), e13005. https://doi.org/10.1111/eci.13005.

Chapter 2

DEMENTIA DUE TO ALZHEIMER'S DISEASE (AD)

Contents

Introduction 38
2.1. Dementia 40
2.2. Stages of Dementia 46
2.3. Alzheimer's Disease Progression 50
2.4. The Diagnosis of Dementia Due to Alzheimer's Disease 53
2.5. Dementia Caregiving 58
Summary 67
References 68

INTRODUCTION

The term "dementia" refers to a syndrome that can result from several illnesses that gradually damage the brain and kill nerve cells, impairing cognitive function (i.e., the capacity to think critically) more than would be predicted from the normal aging process. Changes in mood, emotional regulation, behavior, or motivation are frequently present along with, and occasionally precede, the impairment in cognitive function, even though consciousness is unaffected.

The physical, psychological, social, and economic aspects of dementia affect not only the person with the disease but also their family, carers, and society at large. Dementia is frequently misunderstood, which leads to stigmatization and obstacles to diagnosis and treatment.

Dementia can have a variety of causes, including Alzheimer's disease. The disorders collectively referred to as "dementia" are brought on by aberrant alterations in the brain. These alterations lead to a reduction in cognitive abilities, or thinking skills, that is severe enough to affect independent function and day-to-day living. They also have an impact on relationships, behavior, and emotions.

Dementia-related brain abnormalities can be momentary, but they are typically permanent and get worse over time, increasing disability and shortening life expectancy. The cause of the dementia, the patient's age at diagnosis, and other medical issues can all have a significant impact on survival.

Worldwide, 6 to 70% of dementia cases are caused by Alzheimer's disease. The two most typical signs of Alzheimer's disease are difficulty finding words and short-term memory loss. Problems with reasoning, judgment, insight, and visuospatial functioning (frequently getting lost). Whether or not a person is aware that they have memory issues is referred to as insight.

The hippocampal region is the area of the brain most impacted by Alzheimer's. Other areas exhibiting atrophy (shrinking) are the parietal and temporal lobes. While this pattern of shrinkage in the brain is suggestive of Alzheimer's disease, it is not conclusive, and a brain scan is not enough to make the diagnosis.

The processes that lead up to and genuinely cause Alzheimer's disease are not well understood. This is because research on brain tissue from disease patients is only possible after the patient has passed away. Nonetheless, it is recognized that a malfunction in the amyloid-producing gene is among the initial features of the illness. Two well-known pathological hallmarks of AD are intracellular neurofibrillary tangles (NFTs), which are formed by hyperphosphorylated tau proteins, and extracellular senile plaques (SPs), which are composed of beta-amyloid (Aβ) peptides. Amyloid produces inflammation in the vicinity of the brain's senile plaques, and an excessive accumulation of this inflammation results in uncontrollable alterations in the brain that cause Alzheimer's symptoms (McKhann et al., 1984; Knopman et al., 2001; Albert et al., 2011; Jack et al., 2011).

Orientation and Directional Terms

Term	Definition	Illustration
Neurofibrillary Tangles (NFTs)	Neurofibrillary tangles (NFTs) are intracellular aggregates of hyperphosphorylated tau protein that are most commonly known as a primary biomarker of Alzheimer's disease. Their presence is also found in numerous other diseases known as tauopathies. Little is known about their exact relationship to the different pathologies.	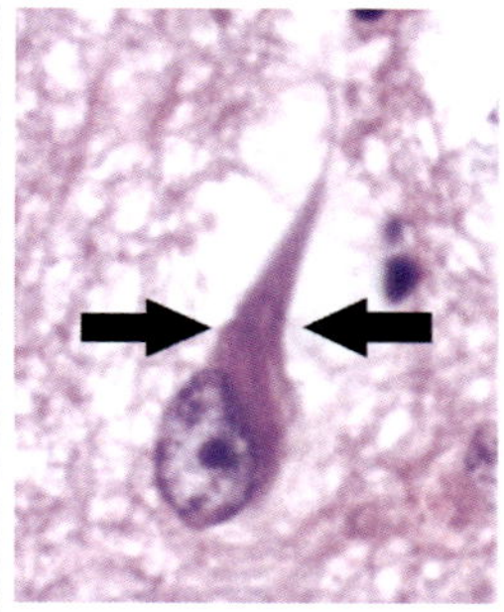
Neurocognitive disorder	Neurocognitive disorder is a general term that describes decreased mental function due to a medical disease other than a psychiatric illness.	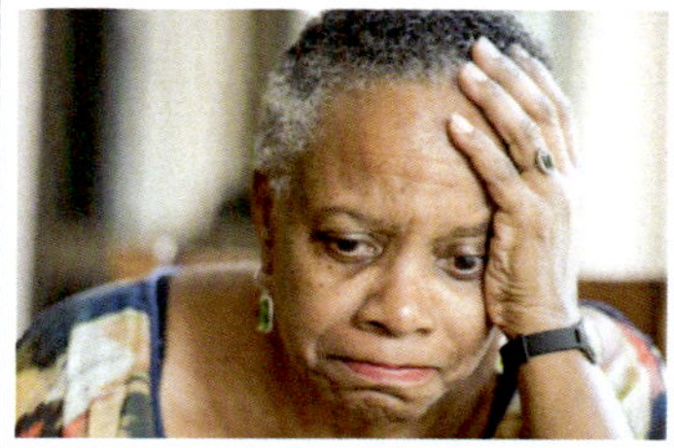
Neurodevelopmental disorder	Neurodevelopmental disorders are a group of conditions that begin to emerge during childhood (or the development of the nervous system).	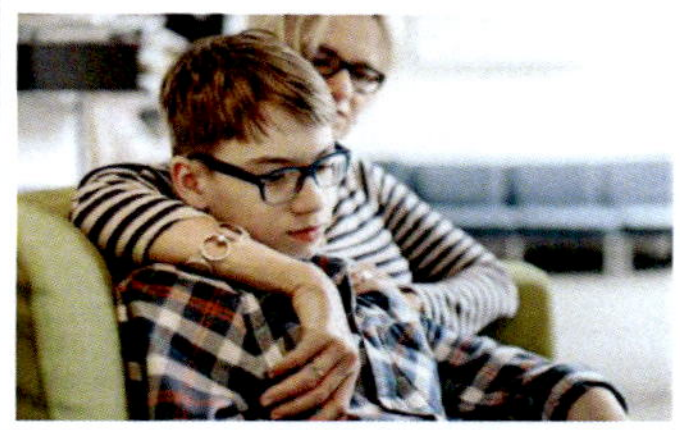
Mild cognitive impairment (MCI)	Mild cognitive impairment (MCI) is the stage between the expected decline in memory and thinking that happens with age and the more serious decline of dementia. MCI may include problems with memory, language or judgment.	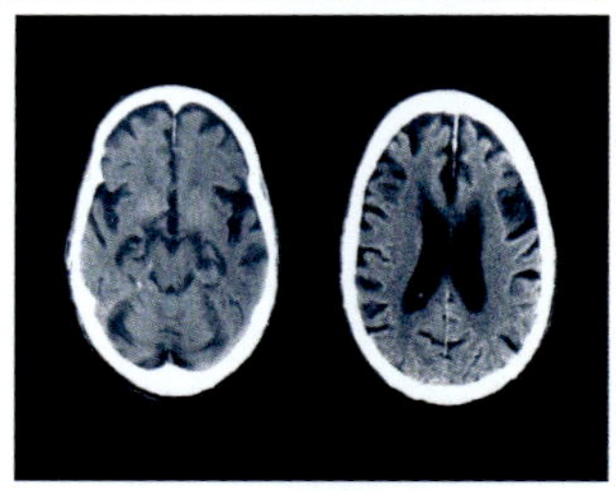
Activities of daily living (ADLs)	Activities of daily living (ADLs) are essential and routine tasks that most young, healthy individuals can perform without assistance. The inability to accomplish essential activities of daily living may lead to unsafe conditions and poor quality of life.	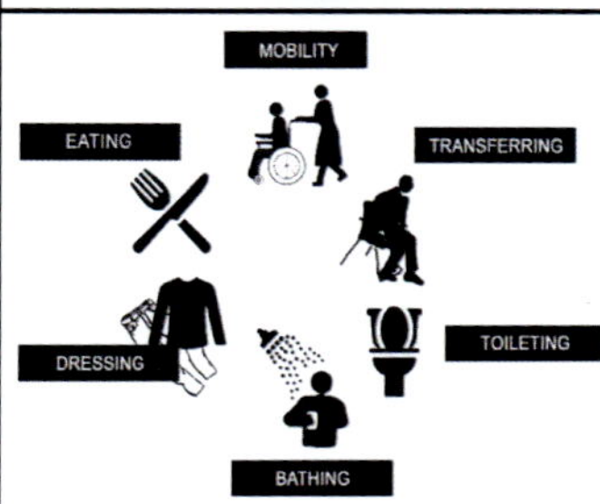

2.1. DEMENTIA

Dementia is a syndrome marked by a general decline in cognitive abilities that affects a person's ability to perform daily activities. It is associated with many neurodegenerative diseases, most commonly Alzheimer's. Usually, memory, thinking, behavior, and motor control issues are involved. In addition to cognitive disruption and memory impairment, emotional issues, language barriers, and low motivation are among the most prevalent symptoms. One way to characterize the symptoms is as a continuum spanning multiple stages. In the end, dementia has a big impact on the person with dementia, their carers, and social interactions in general. To diagnose dementia, a patient must exhibit altered mental functioning and a more marked decline in cognitive function than would be expected with normal aging.

Dementia is classified as a neurocognitive disorder (NCD) with multiple forms or subclasses in the International Classification of Diseases. In contrast to neurodevelopmental disorders, dementia is classified as an acquired brain syndrome and is characterized by a decline in cognitive function. The term "dementia spectrum" can also refer to a group of disorders that cause different subtypes of dementia depending on the underlying cause of the disorder. For example, vascular disease can cause dementia, Parkinson's disease can cause dementia, Huntington's disease can cause dementia, frontotemporal lobar degeneration can cause dementia, Lewy body disease can cause dementia with Lewy bodies, and prion diseases can cause dementia. The pathology of misfolded proteins, such as tauopathies and synucleinopathies, may also underlie subtypes of neurodegenerative dementias. Mixed dementia refers to the coexistence of multiple dementia types.

Brain tumors, subdural hematomas, endocrine disorders like hypothyroidism and hypoglycemia, nutritional deficiencies like thiamine and niacin, infections, immune disorders, liver or kidney failure, metabolic disorders like Kufs disease and some leukodystrophies, and neurological disorders like epilepsy and multiple sclerosis are just a few of the conditions and disorders that can cause neurocognitive disorders. Treatment for the ailment may occasionally result in improvements to some of the neurocognitive deficiencies.

The diagnosis is typically made using imaging-assisted cognitive testing and the patient's medical history. Blood tests may be performed to identify the subtype of dementia and to rule out other potentially treatable causes, such as hypothyroidism (an underactive thyroid). The mini-mental state examination is one frequently used cognitive test. Aging is the biggest risk factor for dementia, but dementia is not a typical aspect of aging. Many adults over 90 don't exhibit any symptoms of dementia. Changes in lifestyle are preventive in the case of smoking and obesity, two risk factors for dementia. It is believed that screening older adults in general for the disorder has no bearing on the result.

10 million new cases of dementia are reported annually, making it the seventh most common cause of death worldwide (one case every 3.4 seconds). Dementia has no known treatment. In mild to moderate disorders, acetylcholinesterase inhibitors, like donepezil, are frequently used and may be helpful. But the overall gain might not be very great. The quality of life for those who are caring for someone with dementia can be enhanced by a variety of strategies. Treating associated symptoms of depression may benefit from cognitive and behavioral interventions.

One of the complications of dementia is behavioral and psychological symptoms. In addition to causing significant distress, the most prevalent symptoms—agitation, apathy, aggression, psychosis, hallucinations, and delusions—may be dangerous for patients and those who care for them. Unfortunately, medication is not always effective in treating several behavioral and psychological symptoms, including restlessness, obsessive-compulsive disorder, hoarding, inappropriate behavior (such as eating inappropriate objects or sexual disinhibition), wandering, and repetitive behavior. The term dementia—which the DSM-IV referred to as "dementia, delirium, amnestic and other cognitive disorders"—was superseded by the term neurocognitive disorder in the most recent edition of the Diagnostic and Statistical Manual of Mental Disorders (DSM-V). Learning and memory, language, complex attention, executive function, perceptual-motor, and social cognition are the six cognitive domains that are impacted by dementia. The neurocognitive disorder can be categorized as major or mild based on how severe the symptoms are. More specifically, individuals with mild neurocognitive disorder have modestly declined from prior performance levels in one or more domains of cognition. Major neurocognitive disorder, on the other hand, is identified when impairments in one or more domains impede an individual's ability to function independently in daily life.

2.1.1. Signs and Symptoms

The behavioral and psychological symptoms of dementia, commonly referred to as neuropsychiatric symptoms, are the indications and manifestations of dementia. Anger, restlessness, inappropriate conduct, sexual disinhibition, and physical or verbal aggression are examples of behavioral symptoms. These signs could be the consequence of deficits in cognitive inhibition. Apathy, anxiety, delusions, depression, and hallucinations—which are typically visual—are examples of psychological symptoms. Memory, visuospatial function (which affects perception and orientation), language, attention, and problem-solving are among the most frequently impacted areas. The rate of symptom progression varies amongst dementia subtypes and occurs on a continuum over multiple stages. The majority of dementia forms progress gradually, with some brain degeneration occurring long before symptoms appear. There are frequently additional conditions present, such as diabetes or high blood pressure, and occasionally there are as many as four of these conditions together.

Incontinence is also more common in those with dementia: compared to individuals of similar age, they are four times more likely to experience fecal incontinence and three times more likely to experience urinary incontinence.

Symptoms of dementia can differ greatly among individuals, impacting memory, attention, communication, reasoning, judgment, problem-solving, and visual perception. Possible signs of dementia include becoming disoriented in familiar surroundings, using unfamiliar words for common items, struggling to recall the names of loved ones, experiencing memory gaps, and difficulty completing tasks without assistance.

2.1.2. Subtypes of Dementia

Although the term "dementia" refers to a clinical syndrome of progressive cognitive decline, its subtypes are categorized based on the cause of the dementia. The following summarizes the four common types of dementia: AD, vascular dementia, Lewy body dementia, and frontotemporal dementia (Table 2.1).

Table 2.1. Diagnosis of Mild Cognitive Impairment (MCI) and Mild Dementia [1]

Criteria	MCI	Mild AD
Evidence of performance	Objective evidence of poorer performance in one or more cognitive domains greater than expected for the patients age and educational background	Objective evidence of poorer performance in more than one cognitive domain such as memory, language, visuospatial or executive function
Interference with daily activities	Limited interference with daily activity; however, complex functional tasks may be completed less efficiently, e.g., preparing meals, shopping alone for clothes and groceries, planning a day's activity, remembering appointments or paying bills	Significant interference in being able to function effectively at work or during usual activity; however, still able to carry out less complex activity, e.g., ADLs—bathing, dressing and grooming and IADLs—completing chores or attending social functions

[1] Concern about change in cognition, as compared with previous level based on information from the patient, clinician or corroborative informant. ADLs = Activities of Daily Living; IADLs = Instrumental Activities of Daily Living.

Source: Panegyres PK, Berry R, Burchell J. (2016). Early dementia screening. Diagnostics, 6(1), 6. https://doi.org/10.3390/diagnostics6010006.

2.1.2.1. Alzheimer's Disease

Of the neurodegenerative diseases that cause dementia, AD accounts for 60 to 80% of cases. The entorhinal cortex and the hippocampus are the first brain regions where beta-amyloid plaques and neurofibrillary tangles are thought to accumulate. This accumulation causes neuronal injury and, eventually, neuronal death. Memory loss and cognitive decline are the results of this reduction in cholinergic neurotransmission. More specifically, a decrease in the number of cholinergic neurons and a decrease in the activity of choline acetyltransferase, an enzyme involved in the synthesis of acetylcholine, are examples of neurotransmitter abnormalities. The symptoms of AD worsen as it spreads to other areas of the brain, where it causes neurons to gradually die. One factor that contributes to the development of AD is genetics. Early-onset AD, which is diagnosed in people between the ages of 30 and 60, is linked to autosomal dominant mutations in three genes: PSEN1, APP, and PSEN2. Late-onset AD is typically diagnosed in patients over the age of 60. It has been determined that apolipoprotein E is a genetic risk factor for late-onset AD.

Short-term memory loss is typically the initial symptom of AD, though it is usually undetectable at first. Multiple cognitive domains are affected by progressive deficits in cognitive function that build up over time. Cognitive and noncognitive symptoms of AD are distinguished for assessment and treatment. While the former are typically present for the duration of the illness, the latter are less predictable. More precisely, cognitive symptoms include disorientation (impaired sense of time, inability to recognize familiar faces), aphasia, agnosia, apraxia, memory loss (poor recall, losing objects), and impaired visuospatial and executive function. Noncognitive symptoms such as depression, psychotic symptoms (delusions, hallucinations), and behavioral symptoms (aggression, both verbal and physical), motor hyperactivity, uncooperativeness, wandering, repetitive behaviors, and combativeness are also possible in AD patients. Early issues with memory and visuospatial skills—such as getting lost in a familiar setting—are typically indicative of AD. As the illness worsens, personality changes and behavioral issues could appear.

Dementia ranging from moderate to severe can cause hallucinations. Patients may exhibit near mutism at the end of their condition when they are unable to sit up, hold their heads up, or follow objects with their eyes.

2.1.2.2. Vascular Dementia

The second most common type of dementia (20%) is vascular dementia. Vascular dementia, also known as multi-infarct dementia, is a condition where the brain's blood flow is blocked or reduced, leading to a lack of oxygen reaching the neurons. The most frequent cause of vascular dementia is stroke. Depending on the brain areas impacted and the extent of blood vessel damage, the symptoms can differ greatly. The most common symptoms following a large stroke are disorientation, confusion, difficulty speaking, trouble understanding speech, and vision loss. Vascular dementia may not impact memory, but an abrupt shift in executive function (e.g., reasoning, and thinking) may become apparent following a stroke. On the other hand, when damage mounts from several minor strokes, executive function declines more gradually. The co-occurrence of vascular dementia and AD is referred to as mixed dementia.

2.1.2.3. Lewy Body Dementia

Alpha-synuclein protein abnormal deposits, or "Lewy bodies," inside neurons are the cause of Lewy body dementia (LBD). It makes up between 5% and 15% of all dementia cases. The most notable characteristics of LBD are recurrent complex visual hallucinations, spontaneous parkinsonism, and fluctuating cognitive impairment with variations in attention and alertness. In LBD, varying mental status is present in between 30 and 89% of cases. Caregivers of patients with LBD may notice, in contrast to AD, periods of decreased attention, periods of improved memory, lethargy, daytime somnolence, prolonged periods of blank staring into space (episodes of blank staring with disengagement from the environment), and periods of improved memory. Moreover, in the early stages of LBD, rigidity, bradykinesia, and rapid eye movement (REM) sleep disorders are more frequently seen. Memory loss is more common in advanced LBD, despite the fact that it is typically reported in early AD. Parkinsonism develops in over 80% of people with LBD. The clinical presentation and the temporal course of the disease are taken into account when differentiating between Parkinson's disease dementia (PDD) and Lewy bodies disease (LBD). PDD patients exhibit parkinsonian symptoms at the time of dementia diagnosis, whereas patients with LBD have dementia beginning up to 12 months prior to parkinsonism. Furthermore, extrapyramidal symptoms linked to LBD are more frequently associated with gait difficulties and postural instability, whereas tremor is more frequently observed in PDD.

2.1.2.4. Frontotemporal Dementia

A general term for conditions affecting the frontal and temporal lobes of the brain, such as Pick's disease, is frontotemporal dementia (FTD). Compared to AD, FTD typically manifests at a younger age (40–75 years). Early in the course of the disease, personality changes and behavioral abnormalities are two of the main characteristics of FTD. The visuospatial function is typically unaffected, in contrast to AD.

2.1.3. Clinical Evaluation

In clinical settings, a thorough patient history, physical examination, cognitive evaluation, and laboratory testing are used to diagnose dementia and its subtypes. The diagnosis is established by neuroimaging techniques like computed tomography scans and magnetic resonance imaging. Since most cases of cognitive impairment are multifactorial, a thorough medical history is crucial. The clinician obtains information about the patient's medical history (cardiovascular disease, neurologic disease, history of head trauma or concussions), social history (current living arrangement, support network), functional status (basic activities of daily living), safety (driving, finances, ability to use appliances), and history of the present illness (details, timing and progression of complaints) from the patient and a trustworthy informant. Positive family history, recurrent head trauma, cardiometabolic factors (diabetes, hypertension, obesity, and dyslipidemia), atrial fibrillation, sleep apnea, and a history of depression are risk factors for dementia. The evaluation should include a review of the medications and the systems. Cognitive impairment can be caused by many conditions, such as delirium, atrial fibrillation, sleep apnea, depression, thyroid disease, vitamin B_{12} deficiency, and hypercalcemia. The latter differs from dementia in that it starts suddenly, progresses uneventfully, and affects attention rather than memory. The sedative effects of drugs like benzodiazepines, sedative hypnotics, anticholinergics, opioid analgesics, and antipsychotics are especially dangerous for elderly patients. For each patient with dementia symptoms, pharmacists should weigh the advantages of these drugs against their potential to exacerbate cognitive impairment, as medications may be reversible causes of cognitive impairment.

2.1.4. Assessment Scales

In the areas of cognition, function, behavior, quality of life, depression, caregiver burden, and illness severity, numerous assessment scales have been created for dementia. Table 2.2 provides examples of cognitive tests along with the kinds of symptoms they could be used to evaluate.

Table 2.2. Examples of Cognitive Assessment Tools

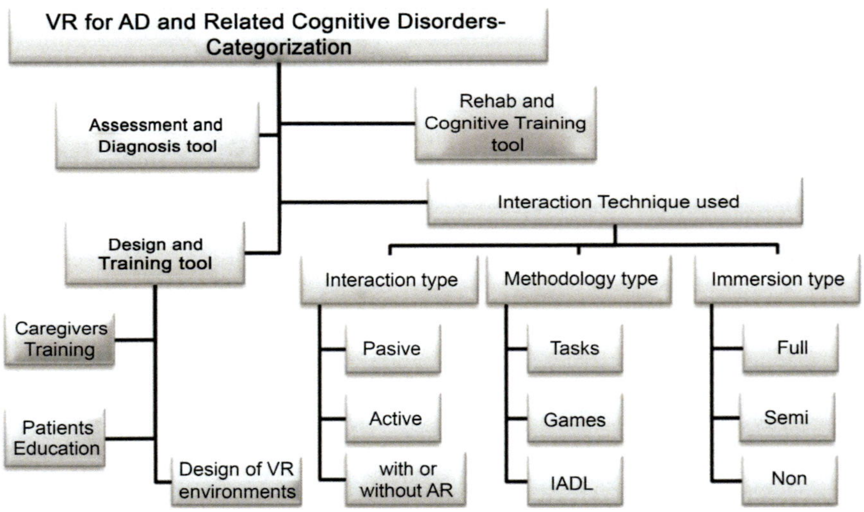

Source: Fernández Montenegro JM, Villarini B, Angelopoulou A, Kapetanios E, Garcia-Rodriguez J, & Argyriou V. (2020). A survey of Alzheimer's disease early diagnosis methods for cognitive assessment. Sensors, 20(24), 7292. https://doi.org/10.3390/s20247292.

Reports from patients, their caregivers, or observers can be used with these scales. Since cognitive impairment is the primary component in the diagnosis of dementia, short cognitive screening tools are frequently used in primary care to identify cognitive impairment.

Table 2.3. Cognitive Assessment Tools

CAI item	Cognitive domain
Item 1: Difficulty maintaining newly learned information in mind for brief periods (long enough to use)?	Working memory
Item 2: Difficulty performing "on the spot" mental manipulations or computations?	
Item 3: Problems sustaining concentration over time (without distraction)?	Attention/Concentration
Item 4: Difficulty focusing on select information (if there is not obvious distraction)?	
Item 5: Trouble learning and remembering verbal material?	Verbal learning and memory
Item 6: Difficulty recalling recent events?	
Item 7: Lack of flexibility in generating alternate plans when needed?	Reasoning and problem solving
Item 8: Problems in situations requiring judgment?	
Item 9: Performs tasks slowly?	Speed of processing
Item 10: Difficulty appreciating another person's intentions/point of view?	Social cognition
Global severity score	Global cognitive functioning
Global assessment of functioning score	

Source: Eilam-Stock T, Best P, Sherman K, Shaw MT, Ventura J, Krupp LB, & Charvet LE. (2021) An Interview-based assessment of the experience of cognitive impairment in multiple sclerosis: The cognitive assessment interview (CAI). Front. Neurol., 12, 637895. doi: 10.3389/fneur.2021.637895.

The MMSE is still the most researched instrument to date and is the most widely used cognitive screening tool in the world. The MMSE can be administered in 5 to 10 minutes, needs little clinical assessor training, and is available in multiple languages. It offers a comprehensive evaluation of many cognitive domains, including language and visual construction, orientation to time and place, word registration, calculation, attention, and concentration. With an MMSE score of 23 or less, cognitive impairment is indicated, and the test has high sensitivity and specificity. Nonetheless, interpretation needs to take the subject's educational background into account, as it has a significant impact on the score. Psychological Assessment Resources owns the copyright to the test and does not allow the MMSE to be reproduced in its entirety, which reduces the test's usefulness as a practice tool (Table 2.3).

The 10-point Abbreviated Mental Test Score evaluates a patient's orientation, focus, memory, and general knowledge. A score of 0 to 3 indicates severe cognitive impairment, 4 to 6 indicates moderate impairment and more than 6 indicates normal cognitive function. The test only takes five minutes to administer.

The MoCA was developed as an MCI screening tool for quick decisions. It takes 10 to 15 minutes to finish and assesses cognitive domains like conceptual thinking, calculations, orientation, executive functions, memory, language, attention and concentration, and visuoconstructional skills. Significant cognitive impairment is deemed to be indicated by a score of ≤25 out of 30. It has been demonstrated that the MoCA is more sensitive than the MMSE at distinguishing between mild dementia and normal cognitive function.

The Mini-Cog is a quick test that only takes three minutes to complete and is unaffected by a person's income or level of education. A 3-item word recall test comes first, and then there's a clock drawing test.

Patients are usually asked to draw a clock face with hands and numbers that indicate a predetermined time as part of the Clock Drawing Test. The exam's focus on the cognitive domains of executive functioning and visuoconstruction allowed it to be quickly developed as a dementia screening tool. A cutoff score of three yields the desired sensitivity (0.86) and specificity (0.96) according to the Shulman scoring system. To evaluate patients, this scale can be used alone or in conjunction with other screening instruments.

Designed for use in primary care, the General Practitioner assessment of Cognition (GPCOG) is a short dementia screening tool. It takes about six minutes and consists of an informant interview and patient examination. Cognitive impairment is indicated by a score of 10 or less.

The 7-minute screen, as its name suggests, consists of four tests that evaluate verbal frequency, memory, visuospatial skills, and visuoconstruction and orientation. It takes roughly 7 minutes to administer. The test shows competitive sensitivity and specificity in differentiating between dementia patients and healthy controls, and age, sex, or educational attainment have no bearing on the test's accuracy.

A 4-item measure called the Memory Impairment Screen was created to identify different forms of dementia in various contexts. The scale's ability to classify dementia has demonstrated good sensitivity and specificity. A dementia score of five or less is indicated.

Pharmacists need to learn how to use these evaluation tools so they can quickly and effectively provide patient care. When a patient has memory problems, the MMSE and the MoCA can be used to screen for cognitive impairment. In case cognitive impairment is suspected, patients may be directed to consult with their physicians for a comprehensive evaluation. By comparing scores obtained before and following the start of therapy, these instruments can also be used to track the effectiveness of pharmaceutical treatment. As part of patient counseling, the Mini-Cog, a 3-minute screening test that involves clock drawing and 3-word recall, can be used to identify cognitive impairments in older adults (McKhann et al., 1984; Knopman et al., 2001; Albert et al., 2011; Jack et al., 2011).

2.2. STAGES OF DEMENTIA

Dementia is classified as a progressive illness, meaning that it worsens with time. Dementia symptoms include memory loss along with diminished language, motor, and problem-solving abilities. A person who experiences this loss of cognitive function is unable to carry out everyday tasks on their own. Even though each person's journey is unique, it usually follows a predetermined path. Dementia progresses in seven stages, with each level bringing with it both new symptoms and a worsening of preexisting ones. Knowing the symptoms associated with each of the seven stages of dementia will help you decide when it's time to reevaluate your family member's care requirements. The Global Deterioration Scale is a comprehensive tool used by physicians and other health care providers to evaluate the seven stages of dementia in the elderly. Also referred to as the GDS, this reliable technique helps medical professionals and caregivers assess how quickly a senior patient's dementia is developing. It also assists caregivers and family members in understanding the symptoms associated with each of the seven stages of dementia.

Understanding the stages of dementia can assist caregivers in identifying the mental health status of a loved one by tracking and monitoring symptoms related to each stage.

The seven stages of dementia include:

- Stage 1: No cognitive impairment
- Stage 2: Very mild cognitive decline
- Stage 3: Mild cognitive decline
- Stage 4: Moderate cognitive decline
- Stage 5: Moderately severe cognitive decline
- Stage 6: Severe cognitive decline
- Stage 7: Very severe cognitive decline

The three progressive phases or levels of dementia are derived from the seven stages:

- **Early-Stage Dementia, Also Known as Pre-Dementia (Stages 1, 2, and 3):** A person can still live independently during this early stage, and they might not show any overt signs of memory loss or struggle to do daily chores. Mild dementia symptoms resemble aging-related forgetfulness episodes.
- **Moderate or Middle-Stage Dementia (Stages 4 and 5):** A person with moderate dementia symptoms has substantial behavioral and personality changes. A person suffering from middle-stage dementia will typically require full- or part-time care assistance with daily tasks. Signs of moderate-stage dementia include mood swings and a notable decline in cognitive function.
- **Severe or Late-Stage Dementia (Stages 6 and 7):** These last stages are linked to both a loss of physical abilities and severe cognitive impairment. Profound memory loss, incontinence, and the inability to move without assistance are examples of late dementia symptoms.

Certain dementias progress at different rates and vary from person to person, such as Alzheimer's, vascular, Lewy body, and frontotemporal dementia. Therefore, to promptly determine whether the dementia of your loved one has advanced, it's critical to comprehend the warning signs and symptoms at each stage.

- **Dementia Stage 1: No Cognitive Impairment:** Despite its peculiar sound, stage 1 dementia frequently presents as normal mental functioning in the absence of cognitive decline. Typically, a person in the initial three stages of dementia does not show enough symptoms to be given a diagnosis.

- Stages 1, 2, and 3 on the GDS are considered pre-dementia stages, even though there may be mild cognitive impairment present. It's crucial to remember that the brain is still changing in these early stages, which may ultimately result in a stage 4 dementia diagnosis.
- **Dementia Stage 2: Very Mild Cognitive Decline:** Stage 2 dementia includes simple memory mistakes like a loved one wondering, "Where did I put my keys?" or "What was that person's name?" This is a pre-dementia stage and does not yet warrant an official dementia diagnosis.

Age-related forgetfulness affects a large percentage of the elderly population, and caregivers or healthcare professionals might not even be aware of this mild impairment. This explains why the GDS refers to stage 2 as "age-associated memory impairment," indicating that many older adults will eventually develop symptoms similar to these. "About 40% of people aged 65 or older have age-associated memory impairment — in the United States, about 16 million people," said Professor Gary W. Small in research published by the British Medical Association. "Only about 1% of them will progress to dementia each year."

This indicates that a formal dementia diagnosis is not made for many individuals with pre-dementia stage 2. With the correct lifestyle adjustments that support their cognitive health, seniors can stay at this stage for an extended time, if not forever.

Stage 2 dementia symptoms include:

- Losing track of familiar objects
- Inability to recall names of friends, family members, and former acquaintances
- **Dementia Stage 3: Mild Cognitive Decline:** A person is said to have mild cognitive decline, also known as mild cognitive impairment (MCI), when memory and cognitive issues become more frequent and noticeable to caregivers and family members. Stage 3 dementia, also known as MCI, typically has little to no impact on daily functioning and may not yet be officially diagnosed as dementia.

The National Institute on Aging estimates that 10 to 20% of individuals 65 years of age or older with MCI will experience recognizable or diagnosable dementia within a year. But how quickly can this early stage of dementia progress to a dementia diagnosis in the elderly?

In order to support your brain health, it's critical to identify these stage 3 symptoms of MCI and seek medical advice as it may precede more severe dementia.

Stage 3 dementia symptoms include:

- Often forgetting to go to appointments or events
- Losing things often
- Getting lost while traveling
- Decreased work performance
- Difficulty finding the right words
- Verbal repetition
- Challenges with organization and concentration
- Trouble with complex tasks and problem-solving
- Problems with driving
- **Dementia Stage 4: Moderate Cognitive Decline:** In stage 4 of dementia, individuals display evident cognitive decline alongside noticeable personality changes,

including pronounced dementia symptoms and severe manifestations of stage 3. Typically, dementia is not diagnosed until stage 4 or later.

Stage 4 dementia is officially diagnosed by the GDS as "mild dementia," even though the medical community refers to this stage as "moderate cognitive decline." Doctors and caregivers will probably notice hallmark symptoms of worsening dementia at this point, such as language impairments and diminished problem-solving abilities.

Stage 4 dementia symptoms include:

- Social withdrawal
- Emotional moodiness
- Lack of responsiveness
- Reduced intellectual sharpness
- Trouble with routine tasks
- Forgetting recent events
- Denial of symptoms
- **Dementia Stage 5: Moderately Severe Cognitive Decline:** In the seven stages of dementia, this stage denotes the beginning of what many medical professionals refer to as middle-stage dementia, or simply "mid-stage." A person might then require the assistance of a caregiver to perform instrumental activities of daily living (IADLs) or normal activities of daily living (ADLs) like dressing or bathing.

Typically, stage five dementia patients go on for two to four years, but each person's progression is different.

Your loved one will probably need more intensive care and monitoring if they are in stage 5 dementia. They may not be able to recall the names of their grandchildren, their long-term address, or their high school graduation location, but they are likely aware of important details about themselves, such as their names and the names of their children.

Stage 5 dementia symptoms include:

- Pronounced memory loss, including personal details and current events
- Wandering
- Confusion and forgetfulness
- Disorientation and sundown syndrome
- Further reduced mental acuity and problem-solving ability
- **Dementia Stage 6: Severe Cognitive Decline:** When a person is in stage 6 dementia, they require assistance from a caregiver to carry out daily tasks like eating, using the restroom, and taking care of themselves. This stage of moderately severe dementia in seniors can make it difficult for them to sleep, socialize, or behave properly in public places.

As the symptoms of dementia worsen at stage 6, you might start to question if you need full-time care. By keeping track of symptoms, keeping an eye on your loved one's capacity to carry out ADLs and IADLs (instrumental activities of daily living), and investigating care options such as home care or memory care, you can remain prepared.

Stage 6 dementia symptoms include:

- Sleep difficulties
- Urinary or fecal incontinence
- Aggression and anxiety
- Personality changes including paranoia or delusions
- Inability to perform activities of daily living (ADLs)

- Pronounced memory loss
- Inability to recognize loved ones and caregivers
- **Dementia Stage 7: Very Severe Cognitive Decline:** When a person reaches stage 7, also known as end-stage dementia, their verbal and physical abilities shut down, making them barely responsive and incapable of taking care of themselves. Movement becomes severely impaired, all verbal ability is lost, and the body's organs start to fail.

Stage 7 dementia symptoms include:

- Inability to speak
- Inability to remember loved ones or caregivers
- Lack of physical ability to move without help
- Inability to chew or swallow
- Impaired bodily functions, including breathing, and organ failure
- Sleeping a lot
- Urinary and fecal incontinence (McKhann et al., 1984; Knopman et al., 2001; Albert et al., 2011; Jack et al., 2011)

2.3. ALZHEIMER'S DISEASE PROGRESSION

Over several years, Alzheimer's disease typically worsens gradually after developing slowly for a while. Alzheimer's eventually damages the majority of brain regions. The illness may have an impact on memory, thinking, judgment, language, problem-solving, personality, and movement. There are five stages associated with Alzheimer's disease. They include:

- Preclinical Alzheimer's disease;
- Mild cognitive impairment due to Alzheimer's disease;
- Mild dementia due to Alzheimer's disease;
- Moderate dementia due to Alzheimer's disease; and
- Severe dementia due to Alzheimer's disease.

The word "dementia" refers to a collection of symptoms that impair social and intellectual functioning to the point where they become disruptive to everyday life.

You can comprehend what might occur by knowing the five stages of Alzheimer's disease. It's crucial to understand, though, that these phases are merely broad generalizations. The illness is an ongoing condition. Everybody's experience with Alzheimer's and its symptoms is unique.

2.3.1. Preclinical Alzheimer's Disease

Alzheimer's disease starts much earlier than symptoms show up. Preclinical Alzheimer's disease is the term for this phase. It is typically only found in study environments. During this phase, neither you nor those around you will experience any symptoms.

Alzheimer's disease can linger in this stage for years or even decades. New brain imaging technologies can detect neurofibrillary tangles and amyloid plaques, even though you won't notice any changes. When tau proteins reorganize and form structures, tangles result. These are characteristics of Alzheimer's.

For clinical trials in particular, the capacity to recognize these early alterations is crucial. Trials are currently being conducted to see if treating individuals with preclinical Alzheimer's may postpone or reduce the onset of symptoms. As new therapies for Alzheimer's disease are developed, imaging technologies are also becoming increasingly important.

Alzheimer's disease biomarkers have been found in additional places. These can suggest a higher risk of illness and are present in blood samples. The diagnosis of Alzheimer's disease can be supported by these biomarkers, usually after the onset of symptoms.

Additionally, genetic testing can determine your increased risk of Alzheimer's disease, especially early-onset Alzheimer's disease. It is not advised for everyone to undergo these tests. You can talk to your doctor about whether genetic testing would be beneficial for you.

As new therapies for Alzheimer's disease are developed, newer imaging methods, biomarkers, and genetic testing will become increasingly significant.

2.3.2. Mild Cognitive Impairment (MCI) Due to Alzheimer's Disease

Mild cognitive impairment is characterized by modest alterations in thinking and memory. These modifications don't have a big enough impact on relationships or the workplace. Information that is typically easily remembered may escape the memory of those suffering from motor cognitive impairment (MCI). This could involve discussions, recent occurrences, or appointments.

Additionally, people with MCI may struggle to estimate how long a task will take. They might struggle to determine the quantity or sequence of steps required to finish a task. Making wise decisions can get more difficult.

Alzheimer's disease is not the only condition that causes mild cognitive impairment. A health care provider's professional judgment and examination of the patient's symptoms are often used to diagnose MCI. However, if required, the methods utilized to diagnose preclinical Alzheimer's disease can also be used to distinguish between Alzheimer's disease and other possible causes of MCI.

2.3.3. Mild Dementia Due to Alzheimer's Disease

When dementia is mild, Alzheimer's disease is frequently diagnosed. At this point, family members and medical professionals can see that the patient is experiencing severe memory and cognitive problems. Daily functioning is impacted by the symptoms.

In the mild dementia stage, people may experience:

- **Memory Loss of Recent Events**: Individuals may have a hard time remembering newly learned information. They may ask the same question over and over.
- **Trouble with Problem-Solving, Complex Tasks and Sound Judgments**: Planning a family event or balancing a checkbook may become overwhelming. Many people experience lapses in judgment, such as when making financial decisions.
- **Changes in Personality**: People may become subdued or withdrawn, especially in socially challenging situations. They may be irritable or angry when that's not typical for them. Reduced motivation to complete tasks also is common.
- **Trouble Organizing and Expressing Thoughts**: At this stage, people may not be able to find the right words to describe objects. They may have trouble clearly expressing ideas.

- **Getting Lost or Misplacing Belongings**: Individuals have increasing trouble finding their way around, even in familiar places. It's also common to lose or misplace things, including valuable items.

2.3.4. Moderate Dementia Due to Alzheimer's Disease

Individuals with Alzheimer's disease experience increased confusion and forgetfulness during the moderate dementia stage. They start to require more assistance with everyday tasks and self-care.

People with the moderate dementia stage of Alzheimer's disease may:

- **Show Increasingly Poor Judgment and Deepening Confusion:** People forget where they are, what day it is, or what season it is. They might mistake strangers for family or misidentify close friends as family.
- They might stray, maybe looking for more familiar surroundings. It is risky to leave them unsupervised because of these behaviors.
- **Experience Even Greater Memory Loss:** People may lose track of personal information like their address, phone number, or place of education. They retell their favorite tales or invent new ones to make up for lost time.
- **Need Help with Some Daily Activities:** They might require assistance dressing appropriately for the weather or the occasion. Individuals in this stage might also require help with other self-care tasks like bathing, grooming, and using the restroom. Some people may sometimes become uncontrollably bowel or bladder.
- **Undergo Significant Changes in Personality and Behavior:** People in the moderate stage of dementia frequently start to suspect things without any solid evidence. For instance, they could start to believe that their friends, relatives, or paid caregivers are embezzling money from them. They might also say that a spouse has had an affair. It's possible for others to perceive or hear unreal phenomena.

People frequently become agitated or restless, especially in the afternoon. Aggressive physical outbursts may occur in certain individuals.

2.3.5. Severe Dementia due to Alzheimer's Disease

Mental function continues to deteriorate in the advanced stages of the illness, known as severe dementia caused by Alzheimer's disease. The illness is also increasingly affecting one's ability to move and perform physical tasks.

In late-stage severe dementia due to Alzheimer's disease, people generally:

- **Lose the Ability to Communicate:** Individuals can no longer converse or speak in ways that make sense. They may only occasionally say words or phrases.
- **Require Daily Assistance with Personal Care:** This includes total assistance with eating, dressing, using the bathroom and all other daily self-care tasks.
- **Experience a Decline in Physical Abilities:** At this point, a person may lose their ability to walk

independently. Without assistance, they might not even be able to sit or hold their heads up. Reflexes may become abnormal and muscles stiffen. One eventually loses the capacity to control their bowel and bladder movements as well as their ability to swallow.

2.3.6. Rate of Progression Through Alzheimer's Disease Stages

Alzheimer's disease progression varies greatly in pace. People with Alzheimer's disease typically live for three to eleven years after being diagnosed. Some, however, live for 20 years or longer. The life expectancy may vary depending on the level of impairment at diagnosis. Alzheimer's disease progresses more quickly when vascular risk factors, like hypertension, are left untreated.

Because poor swallowing allows food or liquids to enter the lungs, where an infection can start, pneumonia is a common cause of death. Malnourishment, falls, dehydration, and other infections are among the other common causes of death (McKhann et al., 1984; Knopman et al., 2001; Albert et al., 2011; Jack et al., 2011).

2.4. THE DIAGNOSIS OF DEMENTIA DUE TO ALZHEIMER'S DISEASE

The Alzheimer's Disease and Related Disorders Association (ADRDA) and the National Institute of Neurological and Communicative Disorders and Stroke (NINCDS) organized a group in the fall of 1983 to define the clinical diagnosis of Alzheimer's disease (AD) and to develop criteria for it. The team completed a report that was released in July 1984, covering topics related to medical history, clinical examination, neuropsychological testing, and laboratory assessments. The report's criteria, also known as the NINCDS-ADRDA criteria, have been in place for more than 27 years and have proven to be highly effective. These criteria have demonstrated reliability in the diagnosis of probable AD, with a sensitivity of 81% and a specificity of 70% across over a dozen clinical-pathological studies. They have been extensively employed in clinical research and trials.

But after 27 years, these standards need to be updated. As a result, a workgroup was tasked by the Alzheimer's Association and the National Institute on Aging with updating the 1984 criteria for AD dementia.

The biology and clinical manifestations of AD are now much better understood. The features of the original criteria that required revision include the following:

- The fact that a wide range of clinical conditions can exhibit the histological pathology of AD (or surrogates for this pathology), including dementia, MCI, and cognitively normal people. For this reason, the term "AD patho-physiological process" is used to refer to both the neuropathological substrate and the antemortem biological alterations that occur before the postmortem neuropathological diagnosis of AD. The clinical syndrome that results from the AD pathophysiological process is referred to as AD dementia.
- Lack of recognition of characteristics that set apart other dementing conditions that affect people of a similar age but were not fully understood decades ago. Examples of dementias that have been thoroughly characterized include primary progressive aphasia,

vascular dementia, behavior variant frontotemporal dementia, and dementia with Lewy bodies.

- Decision-making processes do not incorporate the outcomes of CSF assays, positron emission tomography (PET) imaging, or magnetic resonance imaging. A more thorough approach to the diagnostic procedure must be used in conjunction with early attempts to use biomarkers in the diagnosis of AD dementia and MCI.
- The suggestion that memory loss is the main cognitive impairment present in every patient suffering from AD dementia. Experience has demonstrated that the pathophysiological process of AD manifests itself in a variety of nonamnestic ways. The two most prevalent ones are the syndromes of logopenic-primary progressive aphasia and posterior cortical atrophy.
- Lack of knowledge regarding AD's genetic makeup. An early onset, autosomal dominantly inherited AD is caused by mutations in three genes: presenilin 1, presenilin 2, and amyloid precursor protein.
- Proposed age cutoffs for the diagnosis of AD dementia. Work over the past decades has established that AD dementia in those aged, 40 years, although rare, does not differ in its pathophysiology from older persons. AD dementia in persons aged.90 years is also part of that same spectrum as that of younger persons, even though clinical–pathological correlations are attenuated.
- Extreme heterogeneity of the "Possible" AD dementia category, including a group of patients who would now be diagnosed as "Mild cognitive impairment (MCI)."

2.4.1. Criteria for All-Cause Dementia: Core Clinical Criteria

Here, we list fundamental clinical standards that should be applied in every clinical context. We will first go over the requirements for dementia with all-cause dementia because there are numerous causes of dementia.

From the mildest to the most severe stages of dementia, the diagnosis of dementia is meant to cover the whole spectrum of severity. The workgroup was not responsible for the dementia severity staging methodology. Dementia is diagnosed when there are cognitive or behavioral (neuropsychiatric) symptoms that:

- Interfere with the ability to function at work or at usual activities; and
- Represent a decline from previous levels of functioning and performing; and
- Are not explained by delirium or major psychiatric disorder;
- A combination of (1) obtaining a patient's and an informed informant's history and (2) conducting an objective cognitive assessment, such as a "bedside" mental status examination or neuropsychological testing, is used to identify and diagnose cognitive impairment. When a reliable diagnosis cannot be made with a routine history and bedside mental status examination,

neuropsychological testing ought to be carried out.

- At least two of the following domains are involved in the cognitive or behavioral impairment:
- Impaired ability to acquire and remember new information-- symptoms include repetitive questions or conversations, misplacing personal belongings, forgetting events or appointments, and getting lost on a familiar route.
- Impaired reasoning and handling of complex tasks, poor judgment--symptoms include: poor understanding of safety risks, inability to manage finances, poor decision-making ability, and inability to plan complex or sequential activities.
- Impaired visuospatial abilities-- symptoms include inability to recognize faces or common objects or to find objects in direct view despite good acuity, inability to operate simple implements, or orient clothing to the body.
- Impaired language functions (speaking, reading, writing) -- symptoms include: difficulty thinking of common words while speaking, hesitations; speech, spelling, and writing errors.
- Changes in personality, behavior, or comportment-- symptoms include: uncharacteristic mood fluctuations such as agitation, impaired motivation, initiative, apathy, loss of drive, social withdrawal, decreased interest in previous activities, loss of empathy, compulsive or obsessive behaviors, and socially unacceptable behaviors.

Determining whether or not there is a notable disruption in one's capacity to perform daily tasks or function at work is the first step in differentiating dementia from motor cognitive impairment (MCI). This is fundamentally a clinical decision made by an experienced clinician based on the particular circumstances of the patient and the patient's and an informed informant's account of daily activities.

2.4.2. Proposed Classification Criteria for AD Dementia

We propose the following terminology for classifying individuals with dementia caused by AD: (1) Probable AD dementia, (2) Possible AD dementia, and (3) Probable or possible AD dementia with evidence of the AD pathophysiological process. The first two are intended for use in all clinical settings. The third is currently intended for research purposes.

2.4.3. Probable AD Dementia: Core Clinical Criteria

2.4.3.1. Probable AD Dementia is Diagnosed When the Patient

1. Meets criteria for dementia described earlier in the text, and in addition, has the following characteristics:
    - Insidious onset. Symptoms have a gradual onset over months to years, not sudden over hours or days;
    - Clear-cut history of worsening of cognition by report or observation; and
    - The initial and most prominent cognitive deficits are evident on history and examination in one of the following categories.

a. **Amnestic Presentation:** This is the most typical syndromic presentation of dementia caused by AD. Deficits in learning and recall of recently learned material should be among the impairments. Cognitive dysfunction should also be evident in at least one additional cognitive domain.

b. Non-Amnestic presentations:

- **Language Presentation:** The most prominent deficits are in word-finding, but deficits in other cognitive domains should be present.
- **Visuospatial Presentation:** The most prominent deficits are in spatial cognition, including object agnosia, impaired face recognition, simultanagnosia, and alexia. Deficits in other cognitive domains should be present.
- **Executive Dysfunction:** The most prominent deficits are impaired reasoning, judgment, and problem-solving. Deficits in other cognitive domains should be present.

- The diagnosis of probable AD dementia should not be applied when there is evidence of (a) substantial concomitant cerebrovascular disease, defined by a history of a stroke temporally related to the onset or worsening of cognitive impairment; or the presence of multiple or extensive infarcts or severe white matter hyperintensity burden; or (b) core features of Dementia with Lewy bodies other than dementia itself; or (c) prominent features of behavioral variant frontotemporal dementia; or (d) prominent features of semantic variant primary progressive aphasia or nonfluent/agrammatic variant primary progressive aphasia; or (e) evidence for another concurrent, active neurological disease, or a non-neurological medical comorbidity or use of medication that could have a substantial effect on cognition.

2.4.3.2. Probable AD Dementia with the Increased Level of Certainty

- **Probable AD Dementia with Documented Decline:** Documented cognitive decline raises the likelihood that the condition represents an active, evolving pathologic process in people who meet the essential clinical criteria for probable AD dementia, but it does not prove that AD pathophysiology is the cause of the decline.

Evidence of progressive cognitive decline on subsequent evaluations based on information from informants and cognitive testing in the context of either formal neuropsychological evaluation or standardized mental status examinations is what is referred to as probable AD dementia with documented decline. Evidence of a causative genetic mutation (in APP, PSEN1, or PSEN2) increases the certainty that the condition is caused by AD pathology in individuals who meet the core clinical criteria for probable AD dementia. This condition is known as probable AD dementia in a carrier of a causative AD genetic mutation. The workgroup concluded that the 34 allele of the apolipoprotein E gene was not specific enough to be categorized as such.

2.4.4. Possible AD Dementia: Core Clinical Criteria

- **Atypical Course:** Atypical course either exhibits a sudden onset of cognitive impairment or lacks objective cognitive documentation of progressive decline, but it still satisfies the core clinical criteria for AD dementia in terms of the nature of the cognitive deficits.

- **Etiologically Mixed Presentation:** The etiologically mixed presentation of AD dementia satisfies all core clinical criteria for the disease, but it also exhibits some of the following: (a) concomitant cerebrovascular disease, which is defined as a history of stroke that occurred within a certain time frame of the onset or worsening of cognitive impairment; (b) features of dementia with Lewy bodies other than dementia itself; or (c) evidence for another neurological disease or a non-neurological medical comorbidity; or medication use that could have a significant impact on cognition.

2.4.5. Probable AD Dementia with Evidence of the AD Pathophysiological Process

Based on the biology they measure, the major AD biomarkers that have been extensively studied to date can be divided into two classes. Two biomarkers for brain amyloid-beta (Aβ) protein deposition are positive PET amyloid imaging and low CSF Aβ. Biomarkers of downstream neuronal degeneration or injury comprise the second category. The three main biomarkers in this category are disproportionate atrophy on structural magnetic resonance imaging in the medial parietal cortex, basal and lateral temporal lobe, and medial and total tau in the CSF, as well as phosphorylated tau (p-tau). Additionally, there is decreased ^{18}fluorodeoxyglucose (FDG) uptake on PET in the temporo-parietal cortex. In this study, total tau and p-tau are treated similarly, though p-tau might be more specific for AD than other dementing conditions.

Evidence from biomarkers may strengthen the belief that the AD pathophysiological process forms the basis of the clinical dementia syndrome in individuals who satisfy the core clinical criteria for probable AD dementia. However, at this time, we do not support the routine use of AD biomarker tests for diagnostic purposes. This limitation can be attributed to multiple factors: (1) the diagnosis accuracy and utility of the core clinical criteria are very good in the majority of patients; (2) further research is needed to ensure that criteria involving the use of biomarkers have been appropriately designed; (3) there is limited standardization of biomarkers across different locales; and (4) access to biomarkers is restricted to varying degrees in community settings. Currently, there are three situations in which the use of biomarkers to increase certainty of the pathophysiological process of AD may be helpful: clinical trials, investigational studies, and optional clinical tools that a clinician may choose to use when available and judged suitable.

2.4.6. Possible AD Dementia with Evidence of the AD Pathophysiological Process

Those who fit the neuropathological criteria for AD or who have biomarker evidence of the AD pathophysiological process but do not fit the clinical criteria for a non-AD dementia fall into this category. Examples would be people who have a positive AD biomarker study, or who are found to meet the pathological criteria for AD at autopsy, but who do not meet the clinical criteria for dementia with Lewy bodies or for a subtype of frontotemporal lobar degeneration. The biomarker table shows that for a person who exhibits a nonAD phenotype clinically to meet the criteria for potential AD, both categories of biomarkers need to be positive. This is a cautious approach that might be modified as more knowledge about the long-term effects of various combinations of biomarker findings becomes available. There may be more than one pathophysiological condition despite a diagnosis of probable AD dementia with evidence of the AD pathophysiological process.

2.4.7. Considerations Related to the Incorporation of Biomarkers into AD Dementia Criteria

A range of biological and clinical phenomena include AD dementia. In essence, AD dementia is a clinical diagnosis. The core clinical diagnosis of AD dementia must be met before an AD dementia diagnosis with biomarker support can be made.

CSF biomarkers by definition require a quantitative interpretation about normative standards. It is possible to interpret imaging biomarkers qualitatively or quantitatively. Biomarker results are frequently obviously normal or abnormal. In these situations, a qualitative analysis of a biomarker test will clearly identify "positive" results that strongly suggest the existence of the underlying pathophysiological process causing AD, or negative results that strongly suggest the absence of the pathophysiological process causing AD. On the other hand, unclear or indeterminate results may occasionally be obtained. This is unavoidable since all biomarkers are continuous measurements and continuous biological phenomena must have cutoff values applied to receive the diagnostic labels "positive" or "negative." There are advanced quantitative and objective image analysis techniques available, but there are currently no recognized guidelines for the quantitative analysis of AD imaging tests. Diagnostic imaging standard clinical practice is qualitative in nature. As a result, standards unique to the local laboratory must be used for imaging biomarker quantification. This also applies to CSF biomarkers, albeit with more developed efforts toward standardization than with imaging tests. Techniques for quantitative analysis are still evolving and will do so for some time to come. Thus, until standardization is completely achieved, the practical application of biomarkers must adhere to best-practice guidelines within laboratory-specific contexts.

There is a known sequence of events whereby downstream neuronal injury biomarkers become abnormal later on, after abnormal Aβ pathophysiological processes. This could suggest that Aβ biomarkers should be ranked higher in a hierarchy than downstream neuronal injury biomarkers when it comes to diagnostics. Nevertheless, there is currently insufficient evidence to support the use of such a hierarchical scheme for AD dementia. It is inevitable that different combinations of test results may occur due to the multitude of distinct AD biomarkers. Individual cases may present, for instance, with a positive tau measure and a negative neuronal injury biomarker, or a positive FDG PET and a negative neuronal injury biomarker, and so forth. There is currently not enough information available to suggest a plan that balances all possible combinations of biomarkers.

2.4.8. Pathophysiologically Proved AD Dementia

If the patient satisfies the previously described clinical and cognitive criteria for AD dementia and the neuropathological examination, utilizing widely accepted criteria, indicates the presence of AD pathology, the diagnosis of pathophysiologically proven AD dementia would apply (McKhann et al., 1984; Knopman et al., 2001; Albert et al., 2011; Jack et al., 2011).

2.5. DEMENTIA CAREGIVING

The care of those suffering from dementia has increased in popularity as populations age. There are two types of caregiving for the elderly: formal and informal. While informal care entails the assistance of friends, family, and the local community, formal care entails the services of medical and community partners. Spouses or adult children are typically the primary caregivers in mild-to-medium cases of dementia. Whether at home or in a long-term care facility, additional medical attention in the form of nursing and other supportive care may be needed over time. Empirical data supports the notion that case management enhances both the quality of care provided to dementia patients and the caregiver experience. In the medium run, case management may also lower overall expenses and institutional care. In the United States, millions of people care for friends or family members who have dementia, including Alzheimer's disease.

2.5.1. Family Caregivers

Family caregivers are playing a bigger and bigger role in healthcare; providing care in the comforts of one's own home can prevent or delay the onset of certain symptoms as well as reduce the need for more expensive and specialized care. Home-based care, however, could come at a very high financial and psychological cost. Family caregivers spend an average of 47 hours a week with an afflicted loved one, especially if they are unable to be left alone, and frequently forfeit pay and time from their jobs to do so. The direct and indirect costs of caring for an Alzheimer's patient in the US averaged $77,500 annually, according to a 2006 survey of long-term care insurance holders.

Caregivers are at a higher risk of experiencing depression, anxiety, and potential physical health issues. Research conducted in the UK found that nearly 2 out of 3 caregivers of individuals with dementia reported feelings of loneliness. The majority of caregivers in the study were family members or friends.

According to research, African Americans will experience more negative life changes and health outcomes as a result of providing care, as well as a greater burden when it comes to managing Alzheimer's disease. Compared to other ethnic groups, African Americans have a twice-higher diagnosis rate for dementia, and because providing care has a detrimental effect on their health and well-being, caregivers frequently become secondary patients. Furthermore, 60% of caregivers for Alzheimer's disease and dementia who are 55 years of age or older are typically female, according to the Alzheimer's Association and NAC/AARP. The aforementioned data highlights the disproportionate impact of Alzheimer's disease and other dementias on African Americans.

Furthermore, there is a tendency for the Hispanic population to have a higher prevalence of caregiver burden. Caregiving in Hispanic/Latino families can vary greatly from that of other populations for a variety of reasons. Most women in their 40s who care for an elderly parent-in-law or other family members are Hispanic/Latina family caregivers. Although their caregiving situations are frequently very intense, they are less likely than other populations to use professional caregiving services. A study found that while 51% of non-Hispanic/Latino caregivers faced similarly difficult circumstances, 63% of Hispanic/Latino caregivers described their situations as high-burden. Moreover, a significant proportion of Hispanic/Latino caregivers reported inadequate support, which puts them at an increased risk of burnout and distress. Additionally, the needs of Hispanic/Latino caregivers are not adequately addressed in the studies that are currently available.

In addition to ambiguous loss and anticipatory grief, research indicates that African American caregivers are less likely than their Caucasian counterparts to seek treatment for depression and grief. Furthermore, since stress is a known causative factor for Alzheimer's disease, physiological changes like elevated levels of cortisol, the body's primary stress hormone, contribute to impaired cognitive function and perpetuate the issue within the African American community.

Family caregivers play a critical role in caring for patients with dementia both at home and within nursing or residential aged care facilities. However, caregivers in nursing homes may lack the necessary tools and guidance to effectively manage the complex needs of dementia patients, including behavioral and psychological symptoms and medication use. It is important for nurses to educate caregivers on proper care techniques to ensure the patients receive the attention they require.

2.5.2. Caregiver Burden and Respite Care

Numerous mental and physical difficulties that come with providing dementia care can result in caregiver burden. The term "caregiver burden" describes the financial, social, emotional, physical, and other difficulties faced by those who provide care for a loved one who has dementia, such as Alzheimer's disease.

A wide range of emotions, such as stress, anxiety, depression, guilt, and grief, are frequently experienced by caregivers. It can be extremely upsetting and stressful to watch a loved one's cognitive and functional abilities deteriorate. It can be physically taxing to care for someone who has Alzheimer's, particularly as the illness worsens and the patient needs help with everyday tasks like eating, dressing, taking a shower, and using the restroom. Lifting or helping a loved one can cause physical strain, fatigue, and sleep disturbances in caregivers. Providing care can come at a high cost, which includes paying for medical attention, prescription drugs, in-home care, assisted living facilities, and other associated expenses. To provide care, caregivers might have to cut back on their work hours or quit their jobs completely, which would result in a loss of income and financial stress. Caregivers may find it more difficult to maintain relationships, pursue personal interests, and participate in social activities due to their caregiving responsibilities. Caregivers frequently experience social isolation and loneliness, which can worsen depressive and stressful symptoms. Many caregivers don't receive enough support from friends, family, medical professionals, and local resources. Feeling misunderstood or abandoned can exacerbate caregiving difficulties and heighten feelings of burden.

Depending on the needs of everyone involved, respite care can take place in a variety of settings and is intended to provide caregivers with a break or some relief. Adult daycare centers, assisted living facilities, and private homes all provide respite care services. Because there haven't been enough studies conducted in the US on caregiver burden and the value of respite, there isn't enough information available about the possible advantages or disadvantages of these interventions.

Positive effects of providing respite care to friends or family members tending to a loved one with dementia include lowered stress levels, more time for leisure, socialization, and concentration on personal tasks. While early use of in-home help services can delay institutionalization, respite care offered by a nursing home (or other similar facility) may increase the patient's chance of being transferred into an institution.

2.5.3. Environmental Design

When creating designs for aging in place, architects can take into account how the built environment affects senior functioning and wellbeing and design secure and engaging spaces for those with dementia. A person suffering from dementia must live in a very specific environment. Nurses ought to assist in creating a healthy environment for dementia patients. Patients may experience emotional neglect if the nurses' mood is one of frustration and negativity. An environment that is chaotic and hostile may result from nursing home managers' lack of understanding regarding how to care for their patients who have dementia. An environment that is engaging, stimulating, and conducive to relaxation is ideal. As a result, there may be less stress for the residents and the nurses. Stress levels are lower for nurses who work in a tranquil setting. Individuals with dementia should live in environments that support their participation in life, not just as observers, and that offer opportunities for independence. Their surroundings ought to permit them to maintain their individuality. It is significant and important to include items that are personal to them and act as reminders of who they are. They should also be able to have privacy in this private setting if necessary. To lessen the chance of falling or getting hurt, the areas should also have good lighting and few objects on the ground.

The setting where people with dementia consume their food ought to be friendly and encourage interaction with others. As an example, industrial designer Sha Yao's tableware, which has features that address cognitive, motor, and physical impairments that frequently arise in addition to a colorful and unique design that stimulates people with dementia, can be helpful. Other items made specifically to help individuals with dementia can also be beneficial.

Things to do for people with dementia would be:

- Try to keep a routine, such as bathing, dressing, and eating, at the same time each day.
- Help the person write down to-do lists, appointments, and events in a notebook or calendar.
- Plan activities that the person enjoys and try to do them at the same time each day.
- Consider a system or reminders for helping those who must take medications regularly.
- When dressing or bathing, allow the person to do as much as possible.
- Buy loose-fitting, comfortable, easy-to-use clothing, such as clothes with elastic waistbands, fabric fasteners, or large zipper pulls, instead of shoelaces, buttons, or buckles.
- Use a sturdy shower chair to support an unsteady person and to prevent falls. You can buy shower chairs at drug stores and medical supply stores.
- Be gentle and respectful. Tell the person what you are going to do, step by step, while you help them bathe or get dressed.
- Serve meals in a consistent, familiar place, and give the person enough time to eat.

2.5.4. Communicating

Because individuals with dementia quickly lose their ability to speak or interact in any other way and appear to be unable to comprehend what is being said to them, caring for someone with dementia can be particularly difficult. It can be frustrating for the nurse to work with dementia patients who have difficulty expressing their needs. The communication barrier between nurses and dementia patients may make it difficult for the former to establish a rapport. The social interactions that a dementia patient has determine how they feel, and this barrier may cause them to feel neglected. When a patient has dementia, nurses experience suffering and a sense of powerlessness. The goal of care approaches referred to as comfort-centered care or patient-centered care is to address the communication gap that exists between the patient and the caregiver. Not just dementia patients, but all patient populations are referred to by these terms.

Nontraditional forms of communication are used to communicate with dementia patients who have lost the ability to communicate in traditional ways. Caregivers can gain a better understanding of their patients by observing their body language, facial expressions, and eye movements. Since dementia affects people differently, it might be necessary to develop a special communication style. In their conversations with patients, nurses must employ therapeutic communication. Nurses can use therapeutic lying as a tactic to reassure patients that everything is well, provided that the patient is not in danger. Trying to put yourself in the other person's shoes is a useful tactic. Referred to as gentle deception, joining them on their journey, or therapeutic fabrication at times. This is frequently difficult since caregivers have never felt comfortable "lying" to their loved ones. Families and professional caregivers need to understand that listening to them in their reality is more important than lying. They may not always speak, but that does not always mean they don't want to engage with the world around them.

2.5.5. Memory Strategies

Studies on Alzheimer's patients have shown that emotional memory can be improved; this suggests that emotional memory enhancement could be used to help Alzheimer's patients on a daily basis. According to one study, when objects are given as birthday presents, Alzheimer's patients remember them much better.

- **Assistive Technology:** There is insufficient high-quality evidence to say whether assistive technology helps dementia patients manage their memory problems. Therefore, it is currently unknown if assistive technology can help with memory issues.

2.5.6. Psychological and Psychosocial Therapies

Providing individually designed activities to residents of long-term care facilities who have dementia may aid in the management of difficult behavior. There is no proof to back up the claim that activities are better when they cater to each person's unique interests. Simultaneously, a program demonstrated that basic actions such as engaging in conversation about one's hobbies can enhance the quality of life for dementia patients residing in assisted living facilities. The program demonstrated how these easy steps helped residents feel less agitated and depressed. Additionally, they required fewer GP visits and hospital stays, which further reduced the program's cost.

2.5.7. Nursing

A considerable proportion of patients with dementia who are admitted to acute care facilities have hip fractures. Nurses are therefore in great demand to provide care for this population. It can be difficult to determine whether an elderly person who is cognitively impaired is in pain. It's not uncommon to overlook nursing care when tending to dementia patients. Depending on the patient's age and dementia stage, some nurses may give other patients priority care. Inadequate care may result in problems like incontinence, infections, and falls. A common definition of pain is a subjective experience that the patient best understands. As a result, nurses frequently rely on patients' verbal declarations to determine whether they are in pain. This population's lower verbal skills can make it more likely that they will not accurately assess someone's needs, including whether they are in pain. According to research, the biggest obstacle to providing care for the elderly is patients' inability to express themselves.

The number of dementia patients in hospital settings is expected to rise as the population continues to age. To ensure that elderly patients suffering from dementia are not denied adequate pain recognition, nurses should incorporate common sense into their assessments. It has been demonstrated that reading body language can help ease discomfort. Getting to know the patient better through the perspectives of family members is another strategy to enhance perceptions of pain. Linking typical behaviors is facilitated by getting additional details about the patient from family members. Research on dementia patients in the acute care setting is still lacking, despite the fact that some of these pain-relieving techniques are helpful. Regretfully, a lot of nurses lack the necessary training to care for patients who have dementia. Although their facilities offer a variety of programs for nurses to participate in, slightly less than half of them feel comfortable applying what they have learned to patients. This raises the possibility of stress for both patients and nurses.

But generally speaking, individuals with dementia may find the strange surroundings and everyday routines of the acute care setting especially taxing. In addition to the physical problem that prompted the admission, being away from family and familiar surroundings exacerbates feelings of anxiety, bewilderment, and distress. Effective pain management is impacted by communication problems, which also have an impact on nutrition, hydration, and all other facets of physical and emotional care. Even though these difficulties have been known for a while, the COVID-19 pandemic has made them even more of a problem. Person-centered care can help those providing care for individuals with dementia in an acute care setting by easing some of the unfamiliar stress they may be experiencing. Adopting hospital-wide protocols is necessary to implement best practices in dementia care. Enhancing the quality of dementia care in the acute-care setting has been demonstrated by increases in workforce capacity, physical environments that facilitate social interaction and activities, inclusive caregiver policies, and knowledge-sharing cultures.

2.5.8. Incontinence Care

Compared to people of similar ages, those with dementia are four times more likely to experience fecal incontinence and three times more likely to experience urinary incontinence. This may significantly affect the dignity and standard of living of dementia patients as well as those who care for them.

In general, incontinence is stigmatized and not well understood. In addition, professionals are not well-versed in the topic of incontinence in dementia patients. Inadequate management of incontinence can have detrimental effects on the physical, psychological, social, and economic well-being of individuals with dementia who live in their homes as well as their unpaid carers.

According to guidelines, treatment should always take precedence over containment because catheterization and pads can be uncomfortable and have a negative impact on the person's dignity. But individuals with dementia have different continence issues than those without, and the care plan should consider the various viewpoints of both the patient and their carers. The Continence Care Framework is one set of guidelines for the needs of individuals with complex medical conditions in terms of continence care.

2.5.8.1. At Home

A research project examined ways to enhance in-home care for individuals with dementia. The importance of early clinical assessment (instead of using pads), promoting continence through a healthy diet, exercise, and hand hygiene, encouraging and assisting with toilet use, and sensitively managing incontinence to protect the person's dignity were identified as the top priorities for action. This could come at a price, though, as caring for a family member with dementia frequently requires the caregiver to give up personal obligations, which can result in stress and burden for them.

Giving at-home care to a loved one suffering from dementia is extremely important, but equally important is providing the caregiver with the same caliber of care. One-quarter of dementia caregivers are members of the sandwich generation, and 80% of dementia patients are cared for at home. Many at-home caregivers are unaware of the physically, emotionally, and mentally taxing nature of caregiver stress. Managing unpredictability, feeling undervalued, juggling multiple roles, feeling isolated from family and friends, and changing previous relationship roles are a few challenges. Poor eating habits, inactivity, lack of sleep, neglecting to rest when sick, and skipping or postponing self-care appointments are among the common habits that home caregivers develop. To lessen stress, increase happiness, and vitality, lessen anxiety and burnout, and foster stronger interpersonal bonds, caregivers must practice self-care.

2.5.8.2. In Care Homes

Fecal incontinence rates among dementia patients in assisted living facilities range from 30% to 50%. Urinary incontinence and this typically coexist, though about 30% of residents in assisted living facilities only experience urine incontinence. Individualized continence care should aim to promote personal dignity, according to UK research. The affected person's preferences and personal history should be considered when implementing new measures. Moving around and eating a healthy diet can help, and using prompts to use the restroom is preferable to using pads. Staff need practical training and an understanding of how dementia affects continence in order to support and encourage toilet use.

2.5.8.3. In Hospitals

The management of continence in a hospital setting is frequently subpar. This may result in increased infection risk, worse clinical outcomes for dementia patients, and the emergence of fecal and urine incontinence. Following a clinical evaluation, a customized plan for continence should be developed, taking into account both modifiable causes and contributing variables. Individuals suffering from dementia also face communication difficulties in addition to continence issues. Employees must pay attention to the unique verbal and nonverbal cues of the affected individuals as they may find it difficult to communicate their needs related to continence. The language used should respect dignity and shouldn't cause embarrassment. An ethnographic study in the UK pointed out the existence of "pad culture," which means that the main care strategy was the use of continence pads even in cases where people were continent. This approach was primarily motivated by concerns about falls and safety, which kept people in bed and discouraged independence. This kind of caring frequently results in dehumanizing circumstances and words being spoken (McKhann et al., 1984; Knopman et al., 2001; Albert et al., 2011; Jack et al., 2011).

A Closer Look

A Closer Look into Challenging Behavior in Dementia

Difficult behaviors resulting from a complex combination of memory issues, communication difficulties, and emotional distress are frequently identified as signs and symptoms of dementia. These actions may endanger both the person and the people around them. To address these behaviors, one must comprehend the underlying causes of them and develop a customized strategy that takes into account the particular needs and experiences of each person.

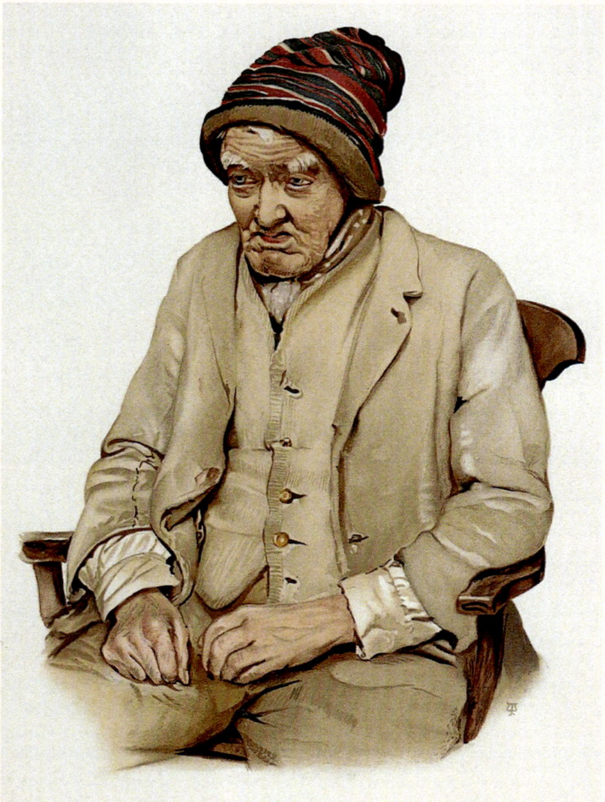

By https://wellcomeimages.org/indexplus/obf_images/48/f4/16baadbd8b96c9a3d9c07c67c55c.jpgGallery: https://wellcomeimages.org/indexplus/image/L0026689.htmlWellcome Collection gallery (2018-03-23): https://wellcomecollection.org/works/zj5vgsbz CC-BY-4.0, CC BY 4.0, https://commons.wikimedia.org/w/index.php?curid=36013071.

- **Aggression and Agitation:** In dementia, agitation and aggression are common behavioral patterns that cause distress. Verbal outbursts, physical restlessness, and emotional distress are all possible signs of dementia. These actions are frequently the consequence of the confusion and annoyance that people with dementia feel as a result of their memory loss and cognitive issues. By creating calming surroundings for individuals with dementia and using skillful communication methods, caregivers can support their ability to maintain composure.

- **Wandering:** A common form of challenging behavior in dementia is wandering, which involves aimless movement and puts a person's safety at serious risk. This type of behavior is frequently the result of confusion, restlessness, or the need to satisfy particular needs. Being lost can result in confusion, mishaps, and heightened anxiety among caregivers. Safe spaces, interesting activities, and wholesome routines are examples of preventive strategies for individuals with dementia who are at risk of wandering.
- **Sundowning:** Sundowning, a term used to describe cognitive and behavioral difficulties in the late afternoon and evening, is a phenomenon observed in people with dementia, especially Alzheimer's disease. This includes signs and symptoms like anxiety, restlessness, mood swings, and confusion. Sundowning can be brought on by many things, including fatigue, sensory overload, and disturbed circadian rhythms, though its precise etiology is still unknown. Sundowning presents challenges for the person and increases stress for those who are caring for them.
- **Repetitive Behaviors:** One of the most prevalent signs of dementia and Alzheimer's disease is repetitive behavior. These behaviors include a variety of actions such as pacing, hand wringing, asking the same questions over and over, talking incoherently, or performing simple tasks repeatedly. Both the dementia patient and their carers may find them upsetting. The person's inability to properly express their needs or feelings as a result of cognitive decline leads to repetitive behaviors.
- **Delusions and Hallucinatio**ns: Hallucinations and delusions are common symptoms of dementia, particularly Alzheimer's disease and Lewy body dementia. Delusions are deeply held, false beliefs that are usually grandiose or paranoid. On the other hand, hallucinations are experiences in which one hears or sees things that are not there. For those who have dementia, these symptoms can be extremely upsetting, and they can also be difficult for caregivers (McKhann et al., 1984; Knopman et al., 2001; Albert et al., 2011; Jack et al., 2011).

Summary

- Dementia is a syndrome associated with many neurodegenerative diseases (most commonly Alzheimer's), which is characterized by a general decline in cognitive abilities that impacts a person's ability to perform everyday activities.
- A diagnosis of dementia requires the observation of a change from a person's usual mental functioning and a greater cognitive decline than what is caused by normal aging.
- Several diseases and injuries to the brain such as a stroke can give rise to dementia. However, the most common cause is Alzheimer's disease, a neurodegenerative disorder.
- The signs and symptoms of dementia are termed as the neuropsychiatric symptoms, also known as the behavioral and psychological symptoms of dementia.
- AD is the most common neurodegenerative disease responsible for dementia, comprising 60% to 80% of cases.
- In clinical practice, the diagnosis of dementia and its subtype is based on detailed patient history, physical examination, cognitive assessment and laboratory testing. Neuroimaging tools, such as magnetic resonance imaging or computed tomography scans, establish the diagnosis.
- Many types of assessment scales have been developed for dementia in the domains of cognition, function, behavior, quality of life, depression, caregiver burden and severity of illness.
- There are seven stages of dementia, and each progressive level comes with both new symptoms and a worsening of existing symptoms. Understanding the seven dementia stages and related symptoms will help you determine when it's time to reassess your family member's care needs.
- People with mild cognitive impairment have mild changes in their memory and thinking ability. These changes aren't significant enough to affect work or relationships.
- During the moderate dementia stage of Alzheimer's disease, people grow more confused and forgetful. They begin to need more help with daily activities and self-care.
- The major AD biomarkers that have been widely investigated at this time may be broken into two classes based on the biology that they measure.
- AD dementia is part of a continuum of clinical and biological phenomena. AD dementia is fundamentally a clinical diagnosis. To make a diagnosis of AD dementia with biomarker support, the core clinical diagnosis of AD dementia must first be satisfied.
- The role of family caregivers is becoming increasingly important; care in the familiar surroundings of the home may delay the onset of some symptoms and postpone or eliminate the need for more professional and costly levels of care.
- Caring for someone with dementia is especially challenging because dementia patients soon lose the ability to speak or otherwise communicate and seem unable to understand what's said to them.

References

1. Albert, M. S., DeKosky, S. T., Dickson, D., Dubois, B., Feldman, H. H., Fox, N. C., et al. (2011). The diagnosis of mild cognitive impairment due to Alzheimer's disease: Recommendations from the national institute on aging-Alzheimer's association workgroups on diagnostic guidelines for Alzheimer's disease. *Alzheimer's & Dementia, 7*, 270–279. https://doi.org/10.1016/j.jalz.2011.03.008.
2. Alladi, S., Xuereb, J., Bak, T., Nestor, P., Knibb, J., Patterson, K., et al. (2007). Focal cortical presentations of Alzheimer's disease. *Brain, 130*, 2636–2645. https://doi.org/10.1093/brain/awm213.
3. Bertram, L., & Tanzi, R. E. (2008). Thirty years of Alzheimer's disease genetics: The implications of systematic meta-analyses. *Nature Reviews Neuroscience, 9*, 768–778. https://doi.org/10.1038/nrn2494.
4. Chang, F., Patel, T., & Schulz, M. E. (2015). The "rising tide" of dementia in Canada: What does it mean for pharmacists and the people they care for? *Canadian Pharmacists Journal (Ottawa), 148*(4), 193–199. https://doi.org/10.1177/1715163515588106.
5. Chételat, G., Villemagne, V. L., Bourgeat, P., Pike, K. E., Jones, G., Ames, D., et al. (2010). Relationship between atrophy and beta-amyloid deposition in Alzheimer's disease. *Annals of Neurology, 67*, 317–324. https://doi.org/10.1002/ana.21955.
6. Dolan, D., Troncoso, J., Resnick, S. M., Crain, B. J., Zonderman, A. B., & O'Brien, R. J. (2010). Age, Alzheimer's disease, and dementia in the Baltimore Longitudinal Study of Aging. *Brain, 133*, 2225–2231. https://doi.org/10.1093/brain/awq164.
7. Dubois, B., Feldman, H. H., Jacova, C., DeKosky, S. T., Barberger-Gateau, P., Cummings, J., et al. (2007). Research criteria for the diagnosis of Alzheimer's disease: Revising the NINCDS-ADRDA criteria. *Lancet Neurology, 6*, 734–746. https://doi.org/10.1016/S1474-4422(07)70178-3.
8. Fagan, A. M., Head, D., Shah, A. R., Marcus, D., Mintun, M., & Morris, J. C., et al. (2009). Decreased cerebrospinal fluid Aβ42 correlates with brain atrophy in cognitively normal elderly. *Annals of Neurology, 65*, 176–183. https://doi.org/10.1002/ana.21559.
9. Gorno-Tempini, M. L., Hillis, A. E., Weintraub, S., Kertesz, A., Mendez, M., Cappa, S. F., et al. (2011). Classification of primary progressive aphasia and its variants. *Neurology, 76*, 1006–1014. https://doi.org/10.1212/WNL.0b013e31821103e6.
10. Hampel, H., Burger, K., Teipel, S. J., Bokde, A. L., Zetterberg, H., & Blennow, K. (2008). Core candidate neurochemical and imaging biomarkers of Alzheimer's disease. *Alzheimer's & Dementia, 4*, 38–48. https://doi.org/10.1016/j.jalz.2007.10.003.
11. Hyman, B. T., & Trojanowski, J. Q. (1997). Consensus recommendations for the postmortem diagnosis of Alzheimer's disease from the national institute on aging and the Reagan institute working group on diagnostic criteria for the neuropathological assessment of Alzheimer's disease. *Journal of Neuropathology & Experimental Neurology, 56*, 1095–1097. https://doi.org/10.1097/00005072-199710000-00002.
12. Jack, C. R., Jr., Albert, M. S., Knopman, D. S., McKhann, G. M., Sperling, R. A., Carrillo, M. C., et al. (2011). Introduction to the recommendations from the national institute on aging-Alzheimer's association workgroups on diagnostic guidelines for Alzheimer's disease. *Alzheimer's & Dementia, 7*, 257–262. https://doi.org/10.1016/j.jalz.2011.03.004.

13. Jack, C. R., Jr., Knopman, D. S., Jagust, W. J., Shaw, L. M., Aisen, P. S., Weiner, M. W., et al. (2010). Hypothetical model of dynamic biomarkers of the Alzheimer's pathological cascade. *Lancet Neurology, 9*, 119–128. https://doi.org/10.1016/S1474-4422(09)70299-6.

14. Jack, C. R., Jr., Lowe, V. J., Senjem, M. L., Weigand, S. D., Kemp, B. J., Shiung, M. M., et al. (2008). 11C PiB and structural MRI provide complementary information in imaging of Alzheimer's disease and amnestic mild cognitive impairment. *Brain, 131*, 665–680. https://doi.org/10.1093/brain/awm316.

15. Knopman, D. S., DeKosky, S. T., Cummings, J. L., Chuit, H., Corey-Bloom, J., Relkin, N., et al. (2001). Practice parameter: Diagnosis of dementia (an evidence-based review). *Neurology, 56*, 1143–1153. https://doi.org/10.1212/WNL.56.9.1143.

16. Lleo, A., Berezovska, O., Growdon, J. H., & Hyman, B. T. (2004). Clinical, pathological, and biochemical spectrum of Alzheimer's disease associated with PS-1 mutations. *American Journal of Geriatric Psychiatry, 12*, 146–156. https://doi.org/10.1097/00019442-200403000-00002.

17. Mayeux, R., Saunders, A. M., Shea, S., Mirra, S., Evans, D., Roses, A. D., et al. (1998). Utility of the apolipoprotein E genotype in the diagnosis of Alzheimer's disease. *New England Journal of Medicine, 338*, 506–511. https://doi.org/10.1056/NEJM199802193380704.

18. McKeith, I. G., Dickson, D. W., Lowe, J., Emre, M., O'Brien, J. T., Feldman, H., et al. (2005). Diagnosis and management of dementia with Lewy bodies: Third report of the DLB Consortium. *Neurology, 65*, 1863–1872. https://doi.org/10.1212/01.wnl.0000187889.17253.b1.

19. McKhann, G. M., Albert, M. S., Grossman, M., Miller, B., Dickson, D., & Trojanowski, J. Q. (2001). Clinical and pathological diagnosis of frontotemporal dementia: Report of the Work Group on Frontotemporal Dementia and Pick's Disease. *Archives of Neurology, 58*, 1803–1809. https://doi.org/10.1001/archneur.58.11.1803.

20. McKhann, G., Drachman, D., Folstein, M., Katzman, R., Price, D., & Stadlan, E. M. (1984). Clinical diagnosis of Alzheimer's disease: Report of the NINCDS-ADRDA Work Group under the auspices of department of health and human services task force on Alzheimer's Disease. *Neurology, 34*, 939–944. https://doi.org/10.1212/WNL.34.7.939.

21. Neary, D., Snowden, J. S., Gustafson, L., Passant, U., Stuss, D., Black, S., et al. (1998). Frontotemporal lobar degeneration: A consensus on clinical diagnostic criteria. *Neurology, 51*, 1546–1554. https://doi.org/10.1212/WNL.51.6.1546.

22. Rabinovici, G. D., Jagust, W. J., Furst, A. J., Ogar, J. M., Racine, C. A., Mormino, E. C., et al. (2008). Aβ amyloid and glucose metabolism in three variants of primary progressive aphasia. *Annals of Neurology, 64*, 388–401. https://doi.org/10.1002/ana.21451.

23. Rascovsky, K., Hodges, J. R., Kipps, C. M., Johnson, J. K., Seeley, W. W., Mendez, M. F., et al. (2007). Diagnostic criteria for the behavioral variant of frontotemporal dementia (bvFTD): Current limitations and future directions. *Alzheimer Disease & Associated Disorders, 21*, S14–S18. https://doi.org/10.1097/WAD.0b013e31815c3449.

24. Roman, G. C., Tatemichi, T. K., Erkinjuntti, T., Cummings, J. L., Masdeu, J. C., Garcia, J. H., et al. (1993). Vascular dementia: Diagnostic criteria for research studies: Report of the NINDS-AIREN International Workshop. *Neurology, 43*, 250–260. https://doi.org/10.1212/WNL.43.2.250.

25. Sperling, R. A., Aisen, P. S., Beckett, L. A., Bennett, D. A., Craft, S., Fagan, A. M., et al. (2011). Towards defining the preclinical stages of Alzheimer's disease: Recommendations from the National Institute on Aging-Alzheimer's Association workgroups on diagnostic guidelines for Alzheimer's disease. *Alzheimer's & Dementia, 7*, 280–292. https://doi.org/10.1016/j.jalz.2011.03.003.

Chapter 3

THE PREVALENCE OF ALZHEIMER'S DISEASE

Contents

Introduction ... 71
3.1. Prevalence of Ad in the United States ... 73
3.2. Worldwide Prevalence Rates of Ad and Dementia ... 79
3.3. Methodological Issues in Prevalence Studies ... 84
3.4. Prevalence Rates by Sex ... 92
3.5. Prevalence by Race Or Ethnicity ... 93
3.6. Looking To The Future ... 98
Summary ... 103
References ... 103

INTRODUCTION

Up to 24 million people worldwide are thought to be affected by dementia, and until at least 2040, this number is expected to double every 20 years. The number of people at risk will rise along with the global population's aging, especially among the elderly. The most common cause of dementia that starts with memory impairment is Alzheimer's disease. Alzheimer's disease is characterized by neuropathological features such as diffuse and neuritic extracellular amyloid plaques in the brain, which are often encircled by intraneuronal neurofibrillary tangles and dystrophic neurites. Alzheimer's disease has no known cause, although environmental and genetic factors probably play a role.

Orientation and Directional Terms

Term	Definition	Illustration
Dystrophic neurites	Dystrophic neurites (DNs) are abnormal neuronal processes characterized microscopically by aberrant sprouting, dystrophic expansion, and accumulation of various cellular organelles and cytoskeletal/signaling proteins.	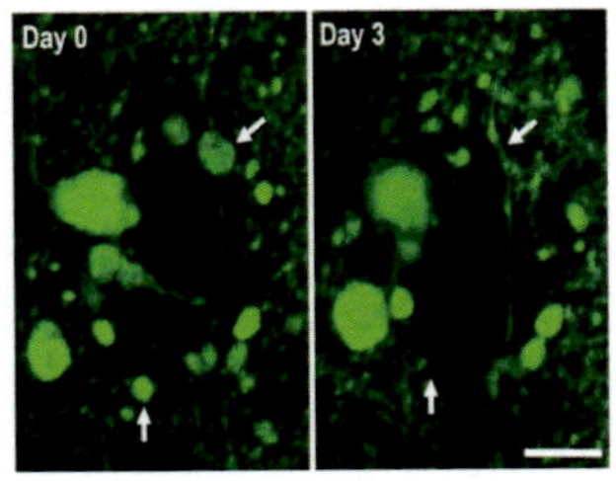
Neurofibrillary tangles	Neurofibrillary tangles (NFTs) are intracellular aggregates of hyperphosphorylated tau protein that are most commonly known as a primary biomarker of Alzheimer's disease. Their presence is also found in numerous other diseases known as tauopathies. Little is known about their exact relationship to the different pathologies.	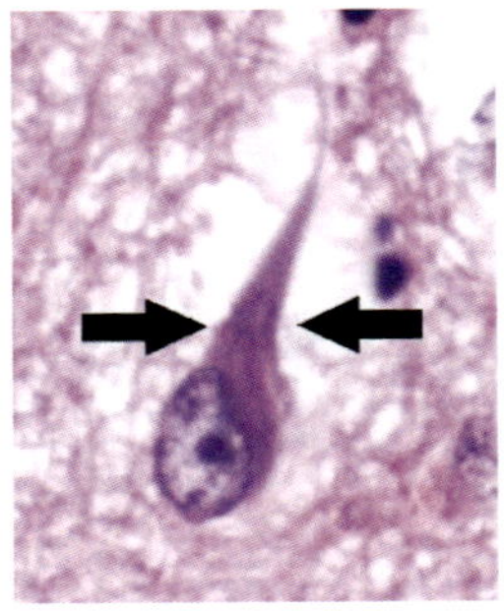
Cognitive testing	Cognitive testing is used if a person shows signs of a problem with memory, thinking, or other brain functions. The tests show if a person has a problem that requires more testing. Cognitive testing is often used to screen older adults for a condition called mild cognitive impairment (MCI).	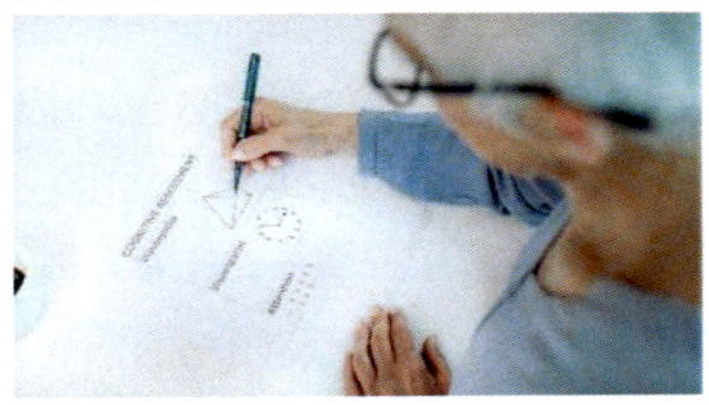
Subjective cognitive decline	Subjective cognitive decline (SCD) is defined as self-perceived cognitive decline among cognitively normal individuals.	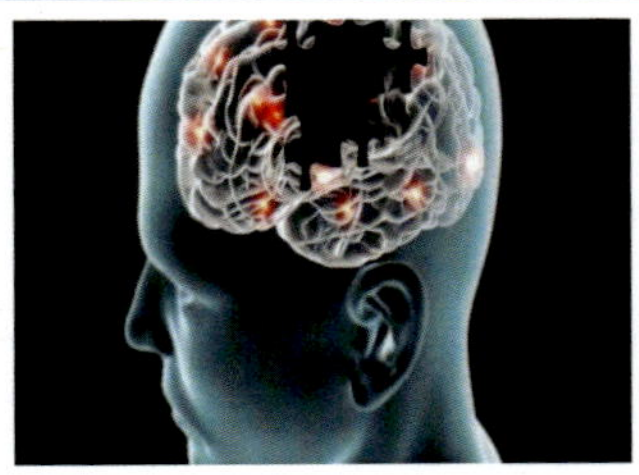

3.1. PREVALENCE OF AD IN THE UNITED STATES

In 2023, there will be 60.7 million Americans 65 years of age and older who have Alzheimer's dementia. Of them, 73% are 75 years of age or older (Figure 3.1).

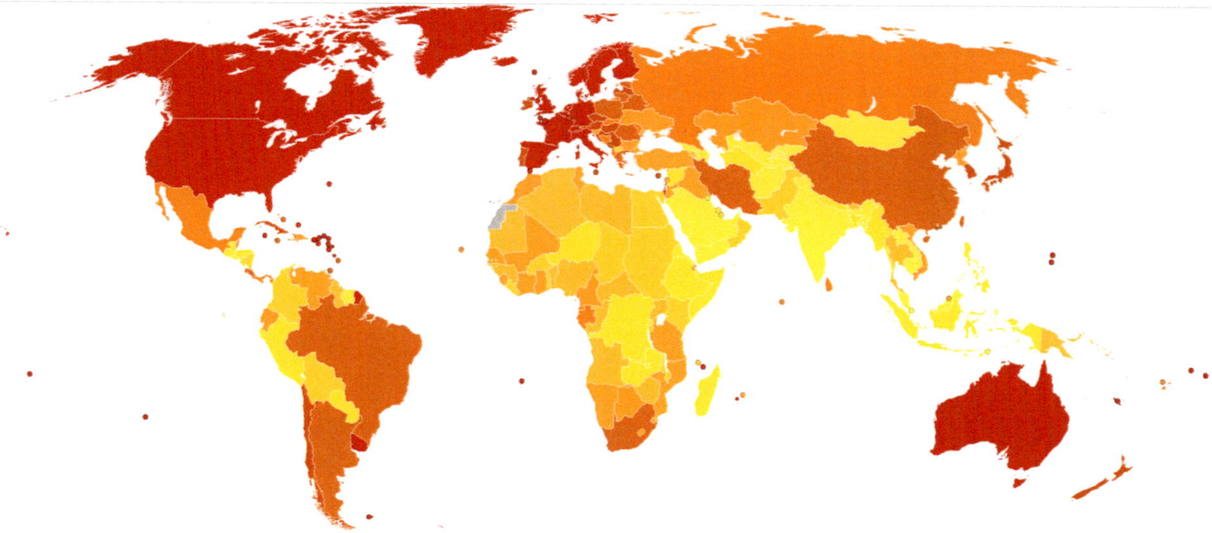

Figure 3.1. *Deaths per million persons in 2012 due to dementias including Alzheimer's disease 0–4 5–8 9–10 11–13 14–17 18–24 25–45 46–114 115–375 376–1266.*

Source: By Chris55 – Data from World Health Organization Estimated Deaths 2012 Vector map from BlankMap-World6, compact.svg by Canuckguy et al., CC BY-SA 4.0, https://commons.wikimedia.org/w/index.php?curid=50319537.

Of the total U.S. Population:

- Approximately 10% of individuals 65 years of age and above have Alzheimer's dementia.
- The prevalence of Alzheimer's dementia rises with age: 5% of those 65 to 74 years old, 13% of those 75 to 84 years old, and 33% of those 85 years of age and above have the disease. Alzheimer's dementia can also strike those under the age of 65. Although there are few studies on the prevalence of younger-onset dementia in the US, experts estimate that roughly 110 out of every 100,000 persons in the 30- to 64-year-old age range, or roughly 200,000 Americans overall, have the condition.

The estimated number of people age 65 and older with Alzheimer's dementia comes from an updated study using the latest data from the 2023 population projections from the U.S. Census Bureau and the Chicago Health and Aging Project (CHAP), a population-based study of chronic health conditions of older people. While CHAP does not provide national estimates of the prevalence of all dementias, other population-based studies, such as the Health and Retirement Study (HRS), which uses a nationally representative sample of older adults, do. According to recently released data from HRS's Harmonized Cognitive Assessment Protocol (HCAP), 10% of Americans 65 and older suffered from dementia in 2016 (Ferri et al., 2005; Thies & Bleiler, 2011).

3.1.1. Prevalence Estimates

The numbers for prevalence are derived from estimates of the number of Americans living with Alzheimer's dementia (prevalence) and the rate at which the illness is developing in new cases (incidence). A single longitudinal study that involved participants who were systematically evaluated and then re-evaluated regularly yielded the estimate of 6.7 million older adults who have Alzheimer's dementia. Participants who displayed the clinical symptoms of Alzheimer's were classified as having Alzheimer's dementia. This method's main benefit is that it aims to include every person affected by the illness rather than depending on the medical community's diagnosis of Alzheimer's patients, which has led to a significant underdiagnosis of the disease. The disadvantage is that the longitudinal study is located in a single, small geographic area and may not be nationally representative (although the modeling estimates attempt to account for the demographics of the entire U.S. population). Future iterations of this report may incorporate data from several longitudinal studies with varying symptom-based diagnostic criteria; as a result, prevalence estimates may differ from those presented here.

The majority of current studies on the prevalence of Alzheimer's dementia rely on the presence of clinical symptoms to diagnose a person as having the disease; they do not take into account the alterations in the brain thought to be the cause of Alzheimer's disease at any stage of the illness. Estimates of prevalence may take these alterations in the brain into account as data sources, techniques, and scientific understanding advance. There are several reasons why this addition might result in significantly different prevalence estimates, some of which are covered below.

- **Prevalence Estimates of Dementia Due to Alzheimer's Disease Based on Biomarkers and Dementia Symptoms:** First, the 6.7 million number reported here is probably not representative of the prevalence of dementia caused by Alzheimer's disease, which is estimated based on changes in the Alzheimer's brain as well as overt clinical dementia symptoms. This is due to research using biomarkers to show that some people who are diagnosed with Alzheimer's dementia based only on symptoms actually do not have the disease's biological brain alterations; instead, their dementia is brought on by a different condition. According to autopsies and clinical trials, 15–30% of people who fit the symptoms-based criteria for clinical Alzheimer's dementia did not exhibit brain abnormalities associated with the disease. Accordingly, these studies suggest that estimates of the prevalence of Alzheimer's disease using biomarkers may be as much as 30% lower than current estimates when compared to prevalence estimates based only on symptoms. According to this estimate, 4.7 million Americans 65 years of age and older will have dementia as a result of Alzheimer's disease in 2023.
- **Prevalence Estimates of Alzheimer's Disease Based on Biomarkers and Any Cognitive Symptoms (Mild to Severe):** Second, we will be able to estimate the number of people with Alzheimer's disease (not just dementia caused by Alzheimer's disease) as measurements of the disease's brain changes become

more widely available in studies. This estimate would take into account those who are in the early stages of cognitive impairment, meaning they have Alzheimer's-related brain changes but not the overt symptoms of dementia that make it difficult for them to perform daily tasks. For many years, it has been understood that all dementia patients go through a prelude phase known as mild cognitive impairment (MCI). It is now feasible to identify the patients who have been diagnosed with MCI and determine whether or not their condition is caused by Alzheimer's disease thanks to the development of biomarkers that identify the brain abnormalities thought to characterize the disease. People with MCI brought on by Alzheimer's disease will be counted in prevalence estimates of the number of Americans with Alzheimer's disease, which will make them more than those with Alzheimer's dementia as biomarker-based diagnoses become more widespread. Using the best available data, the information presented in this section estimates that 5 to 7 million Americans 65 years of age and older have MCI as a result of Alzheimer's disease. This would equate to roughly 10 to 12 million older Americans with Alzheimer's disease and some kind of cognitive symptoms in 2023 when combined with the approximately 4.7 million Americans 65 and older who have dementia due to Alzheimer's disease based on Alzheimer's brain changes. Given that MCI can occur years before dementia does and that it can afflict people under the age of 65, it is possible that there are more than 5 to 7 million people with MCI related to Alzheimer's disease across all age groups.

- **Prevalence of Alzheimer's Disease Across the Entire Cognitive Spectrum:** Lastly, before cognitive symptoms of either MCI or dementia appear, the National Institute on Aging – Alzheimer's Association (NIA-AA) believes that Alzheimer's disease is in its early and silent (i.e., "preclinical") stage. Estimates of the population's preclinical Alzheimer's disease prevalence are beginning to emerge, though more research is needed on this topic. To validate preclinical Alzheimer's and figure out how to measure it with biomarkers that uniquely identify Alzheimer's disease from other diseases that cause dementia, more research is required. Additionally, we must learn more about whether individuals in this preclinical stage accurately reflect those who may eventually develop dementia as a result of Alzheimer's disease. When there is clear evidence linking biomarkers to the preclinical stage and when biomarker-based diagnoses are included in epidemiological studies, an estimate of the prevalence of Alzheimer's disease that encompasses people at every stage of the disease's progression (i.e., greater than any estimates, including those with biomarker-confirmed Alzheimer's dementia, MCI brought on by Alzheimer's disease, and biomarker-confirmed preclinical Alzheimer's disease.

- **Future Facts and Figures Prevalence Estimates:** This includes the best estimate of the prevalence of MCI caused by Alzheimer's disease as well as the estimated prevalence of people with Alzheimer's dementia, which is currently estimated to be 60.7 million Americans based solely on clinical symptoms. The estimated prevalence of people with Alzheimer's disease will be reported to represent both those in the dementia phase and those in the MCI phase of the disease when biomarker-based prevalence estimates become available. Prevalence estimates of the preclinical stage of Alzheimer's disease will not be included in Facts and Figures until two things have occurred: (1) there is strong evidence linking biomarkers in this silent stage to the development of MCI as a result of Alzheimer's disease and (2) prevalence studies have attempted to estimate the population in this stage. Furthermore, estimates of the prevalence of dementia from all causes may be included in future reports, as warranted by the evidence and epidemiological data. It should be noted that estimates of the prevalence of Alzheimer's dementia based on symptoms and Alzheimer's disease based on biomarkers are predicted to rise in the future due to an increase in the percentage of Americans 65 and older, who are most at risk of developing cognitive symptoms as well as the underlying disease.

3.1.2. Mild Cognitive Impairment (MCI) Due to Alzheimer's Disease

Because population-based prevalence measures of MCI and Alzheimer's biomarkers are needed, and because research on this topic is still in its early stages, it is currently difficult to estimate the number and proportion of older adults with MCI as a result of Alzheimer's disease. Moreover, the level of biomarker burden that indicates the presence of Alzheimer's disease and the threshold of cognitive impairment necessary for an MCI diagnosis vary amongst studies. However, by combining several data sources, we can infer an approximate estimate of this prevalence. Approximately 17% of adults 65 years of age and older had MCI, according to a systematic review of over 30 studies on the condition. More recently, the HRS HCAP study estimated that 22% of adults 65 years of age and older had MCI. According to research evaluating PET scan biomarkers for Alzheimer's disease, roughly 50% of MCI patients have brain abnormalities associated with the disease. Consequently, 5 to 7 million older Americans, or approximately 8–11% of the 62 million Americans who will be 65 and older in 2023, may have MCI as a result of Alzheimer's disease. More precise age-specific estimates and population-based studies utilizing biomarkers are required to validate this approximate prevalence estimate.

Table 3.1. Subgroup Analysis of the Prevalence of Mild Cognitive Impairment

Subgroups	Categories	No. of Studies	Event	Total	Prevalence (%)	95% CI (%)	I^2 (%)	*P* Value Within Subgroup	*Q* (*P* Value Across Subgroups)
Region	Europe & Central Asia	29	12,867	55,259	19.7	14.9–24.5	99.5	<0.001	0.35 (0.840)
	North America	14	69,857	315,901	20.7	16.7–24.8	99.8	<0.001	–
	East Asia & Pacific	8	762	4557	18.2	10.7–25.8	98.1	<0.001	–
Countries by income	Upper middle income	8	885	4631	26.4	12.7–40.0	99.5	<0.001	0.75 (0.388)
	High income	45	82,798	371,408	20.3	17.7–22.8	99.6	<0.001	–
Sample method	Random	16	4144	18,926	19.3	15.8–22.7	96.9	<0.001	3.83 (0.147)
	Convenience	31	77,684	347,134	23.4	20.1–26.8	99.8	<0.001	–
	Cluster	3	1289	6764	14.7	1.4–28.0	99.5	<0.001	–
Screening scale	CAREDiag	2	478	2166	28.7	12.5–44.9	94.2	<0.001	16.51 (0.011)
	CPS	9	23,265	149,679	14.7	13.0–16.3	97.1	<0.001	–
	GCS	4	7173	20,337	32.4	15.5–49.4	99.9	<0.001	–
	MMSE	25	3216	16,897	19.5	15.7–23.4	98.0	<0.001	–
	MoCA	2	229	751	49.8	0–123.4	99.9	<0.001	–
	Pfeiffer test	3	117	599	18.8	6.8–30.8	93.7	<0.001	–
	SPMSQ	3	116	1182	9.6	3.6–15.6	90.5	<0.001	–
Age group (years)	70–74	2	42	581	18.2	0–45.1	90.1	0.001	2.84 (0.417)
	75–79	7	524	3587	15.0	7.4–22.6	97.8	<0.001	–
	80–84	16	2645	13,633	21.7	17.0–26.4	98.2	<0.001	–
	85–89	15	24,494	146,490	17.9	15.6–20.2	98.1	<0.001	–

Survey starting year	Before 2000	4	7082	25,816	34.9	9.5–60.2	99.9	<0.001	4.85 (0.304)
	2000–2004	2	2915	17,132	11.6	0.30–23.0	99.2	<0.001	–
	2005–2009	9	19,126	120,602	17.0	13.3–20.8	98.1	<0.001	–
	2010–2014	12	51,085	194,489	19.9	17.2–22.5	96.4	<0.001	–
	2015–2019	7	873	5600	16.8	10.0–23.5	98.3	<0.001	–

CAREDiag the care dementia diagnostic scale, CPS minimum data Set 2.0-cognitive performance Scale, GCS Gottfries cognitive scale, MMSE mini-mental state examination, MoCA Montreal cognitive assessment, SPSMQ short portable mental status questionnaire.

Source: Chen, P., Cai, H., Bai, W. et al. Global prevalence of mild cognitive impairment among older adults living in nursing homes: a meta-analysis and systematic review of epidemiological surveys. Transl. Psychiatry, 13, 88 (2023). https://doi.org/10.1038/s41398-023-02361-1.

3.1.3. Underdiagnosis of Alzheimer's and Other Dementias in the Primary Care Setting

Every participant in a prevalence study, like CHAP and the Aging, Demographics and Memory Study (ADAMS), is evaluated for dementia. However, a significant percentage of people who would fit the diagnostic criteria for Alzheimer's and other dementias are not given a dementia diagnosis by a doctor outside of research settings. Additionally, only roughly 50% of Medicare enrollees with an Alzheimer's or other dementia diagnosis in their Medicare billing records report having been informed of the diagnosis. A substantial percentage of Americans with Alzheimer's may not be aware that they have the disease because Alzheimer's dementia is frequently underdiagnosed and, if it is, people often seem to be unaware of their diagnosis.

3.1.3.1. Prevalence of Subjective Cognitive Decline

One of the first indicators of Alzheimer's disease is experiencing increasing or more frequent problems with thinking or memory (also known as subjective cognitive decline). This can help identify individuals who are more likely to develop MCI as well as other dementias or Alzheimer's. Subjective cognitive decline is the term used to describe a person's subjective perception—unaffected by cognitive testing, a doctor's diagnosis, or other observers—that their memory or other thinking skills are deteriorating. Although many people who experience subjective cognitive decline go on to develop dementia or MCI, this is not always the case. Subjective cognitive decline frequently calls for medical intervention, and a correct diagnosis can help separate experiences associated with an increased risk of Alzheimer's disease from those that have other contributing factors, such as other underlying medical conditions. According to one study, people who over time consistently reported subjective cognitive decline that concerned them were more likely to acquire Alzheimer's dementia. 10% of Americans 45 and older reported subjective cognitive decline, according to the Behavioral Risk Factor Surveillance System survey, a large nationwide survey that asks questions about subjective cognitive decline. However, 54% of those who reported subjective cognitive decline had not sought medical advice. People who are worried about memory loss and other cognitive declines ought to speak with a medical professional (Ferri et al., 2005; Thies & Bleiler, 2011).

3.2. WORLDWIDE PREVALENCE RATES OF AD AND DEMENTIA

Globally, dementia prevalence appears to be influenced by cultural and socioeconomic variations across national boundaries. It's interesting to note that developed nations appear to have a higher prevalence of dementia overall and AD in particular than developing ones (Table 3.2). According to a review on the worldwide burden of dementia, exposure to cerebrovascular risk factors such as smoking, obesity, diabetes, and hypertension varies between developed and developing nations, which explains why dementia is more common in developed nations.

Table 3.2. Worldwide Estimate for the Absolute Number of Cases of Dementia According to the Delphi Consensus Study

	Absolute Number of People Over 60 Years Old Who Have Dementia (Millions)		
	2001	2020	2040
Western Europe	4.9	6.9	9.9
Eastern Europe low adult mortality	1.0	1.6	2.8
Eastern Europe high adult mortality	1.8	2.3	3.2
North America	3.4	5.1	9.2
Latin America	1.8	4.1	9.1
North Africa and Middle Eastern Crescent	1.0	1.9	4.7
Developed Western Pacific	1.5	2.9	4.3
China and the developing Western Pacific	6.0	11.7	26.1
Indonesia, Thailand, and Sri Lanka	0.6	1.3	2.7
India and South Asia	1.8	3.6	7.5
Africa	0.5	0.9	1.6
Total	24.3	42.3	81.1

Source: Liara Rizzi, Idiane Rosset, Matheus Roriz-Cruz, (2014). "Global epidemiology of dementia: Alzheimer's and vascular types." BioMed Research International, 2014, Article ID 908915, 8. https://doi.org/10.1155/2014/908915.

As of 2001, 60.1% of dementia patients lived in developing nations; by 2040, this percentage is predicted to increase to 71.2%. The aging population shift is happening quickly, particularly in China, India, and Latin America, where dementia is quickly rising to the top of the public health agenda.

The Delphi Consensus Study discovered that the prevalence of dementia was highest in the Americas and lowest in less developed regions of the world, such as Africa and the Middle East, despite the paucity of epidemiological data regarding the prevalence of dementia and its subtypes. By 2040, the prevalence of dementia in Latin America will resemble that of North America. Japan has the lowest rates of dementia overall and Alzheimer's disease specifically among developed nations. Also, the prevalence of dementia was comparatively consistent across Eastern European nations.

3.2.1. European Studies

In 11 cohorts, a collaborative study of population-based cohorts in Europe found a total of 2346 cases of mild to severe dementia. Age-standardized prevalence was 1.6% for VAD, 4.4% for AD, and 6.4% for dementia (all causes).

According to a study on incidence rates in the UK, the incidence of vascular dementia (VaD) was 0.99/1000 (95% CI 0.96–1.02) and the incidence of AD was 1.59/1000 person-years (95% CI 1.55–1.62). Women were more likely than men to experience AD, but not VaD. However, they discovered that demented individuals with heart conditions might be assigned a VaD diagnosis rather than an AD one. According to the ILSA Study, the average incidence rates per 1000 person-years in Italy were 3.30 for VaD, 6.55 for AD, and 12.47 for overall dementia. They did discover, however, that women are more likely than men to develop AD, while men are more likely to develop VaD.

3.2.2. North American Studies

0Five and a half million Americans, or one in nine people 65 years of age or older (11%), are thought to have Alzheimer's disease. The majority of these people are women, most likely due to the fact that women typically outlive men. Already ranking fifth among Americans over 65, AD is the sixth most common cause of death in the United States. According to the Aging Demographics and Memory Study (ADAMS), 14% of Americans over 71 suffer from dementia. In the coming years, the number of people living with AD will be impacted by sharp increases in the population over 85 across all racial and ethnic groupings. The number of AD patients in the USA is expected to rise by 50% by 2030 and could nearly triple by 2050. In 2013, about 450,000 older Americans with AD passed away; the majority of these deaths were caused by AD complications. Data reveal that older black Americans are twice as likely as older white Americans to have Alzheimer's disease (AD) and other dementias, highlighting racial disparities in this nation.

3.2.3. Latin American Studies

Dementia prevalence in Latin America is nearly identical to that of North America. This phenomenon could be caused by the unique combination of high vascular risk profile and low average educational attainment found in older Latin American populations. As the Delphi Consensus Study revealed, the most impoverished parts of Latin America had a higher prevalence of dementia than other developed parts of the world after the age of 75. The prevalence of dementia (15.7%) was twice as high as that of literate people (7.16%) and the rate of illiteracy among older Latin Americans was 9.3%. This phenomenon aims to explain the relationship between decreased cognitive reserve and low educational attainment.

Therefore, it is important to recognize the potential link between socioeconomic deprivation and an increased risk of cerebrovascular disease. By 2040, there will be twice as many dementia sufferers in Latin America (9.1 million) as there are in North America (9.2 million).

3.2.4. Asian Studies

With over 60% of the population living in the Asia-Pacific region, the prevalence of dementia is rising rapidly. Compared to Asia's low-income nations, dementia appears to be more common in developed nations like Japan and Korea. According to a Japanese study, the prevalence of dementia in people over 65 is 11%, while a Korean study found that the prevalence is 6.3%. Excluding extremely mild cases, the Seoul study, another Korean study, revealed that the prevalence of dementia was roughly 5.3% for total dementia and 4.3% for AD. Significant differences exist in the prevalence of dementia among various ethnic groups residing in the same nation, such as Singapore, which is arguably the most multicultural country in Asia. According to a Singaporean study, the frequency of vascular risk factors had no bearing on the low standardized dementia prevalence among ethnic Chinese (2.5% among the elderly) as opposed to ethnic Malays (4.0% among the elderly). It is still up for debate whether or not these differences are caused by distinct lifestyle choices or genetics.

3.2.4.1. Chinese Studies

Widespread population aging is taking place in the nation with the largest population in the world. 10% of Chinese citizens were 60 years of age or older in 2000, and by 2050, one in four Chinese citizens will be over the age of 65. Studies conducted in China indicate that the prevalence of dementia overall is lower there than in Western nations and among Caucasian populations (an average 3% in various studies). According to a meta-analysis, the prevalence of AD was 1.9% and the prevalence of VaD was 0.9% in people 60 years of age or older. Greater prevalence rates were found in provinces close to the east coast and in major cities. Currently, it is estimated that 8.4 million older adults in Taiwan, Hong Kong, and mainland China suffer from dementia.

Similar to Japan several decades prior, VaD is more prevalent than AD in China. On the other hand, research from Southern China has already indicated that AD is starting to outnumber VaD in prevalence. In the adult population, the prevalence of AD was 2.0% in Southern China and 1.2% in Northern China in 2004. On the other hand, the prevalence of VaD was 0.11% and 0.66%, respectively. Since 1990, AD has become more prevalent than VaD in China. On the other hand, data from other surveys shows that the current prevalence of dementia subtypes is comparable to that of developed, western nations.

3.2.4.2. Japanese Studies

Japan appears to have the lowest rates of dementia overall and Alzheimer's disease specifically among developed nations. In the past, VaD predominated in Japan more than AD. The Hisayama Study identified risk factors and dementia incidence specific to the Japanese population. Between 1985 and 1992, the age-adjusted total incidence of dementia (per 1000 person-years) was 19.3 for men and 20.9 for women. In contrast to AD, where corresponding rates were 5.1 for men and 10.9 for women, vascular dementia had corresponding rates of 12.2 for men and 9.0 for women. Age was a significant risk factor for AD, while systolic blood pressure, alcohol consumption, and prior stroke episodes were independent risk factors for VaD, according to multivariate analysis.

Recent data from a prospective 17-year follow-up survey with the same community revealed that the following incidences (per 1000 person-years) were found: overall dementia (32.3), AD

(14.6), VaD (9.5), dementia of Lewy bodies (1.4), mixed type (3.8), and other types (3.1). Age-related increases in the incidence of AD, mixed-type dementia, and other dementias were noted, especially beyond the age of 85. However, dementia associated with Lewy bodies did not exhibit this trend.

Over the previous 20 years, there has been a generalized increase in the age-adjusted prevalence of dementia and AD in the Japanese population, along with a decline in the ratio of VaD to AD. These trends are secular in nature. Examining correlations between blood pressure and dementia, it was found that elevated midlife and late-life hypertension levels significantly increased the age- and sex-adjusted incidence of VaD; however, this did not happen for AD. Midlife hypertension, independent of late-life blood pressure levels, was substantially linked to an increased risk of VaD. Indeed, the best blood component to predict incident dementia is midlife systolic blood pressure. Therefore, the decreased prevalence of VaD in Japan may have been primarily caused by improved hypertension control. On the other hand, the main causes of the rising prevalence of AD in Japan were most likely the aging population and the westernization of lifestyle.

The VaD/AD prevalence ratio dropped from 2:1 to 1:1 during the previous three decades. Modifications in the way of life, such as cutting back on salt and managing hypertension, appear to be the primary reasons for the decline in the prevalence of VaD and stroke. But longer life spans and a more westernized lifestyle, including food, may also have played a role in the rise in AD prevalence in this nation, which in turn may have decreased the VaD/AD ratio. This theory is consistent with the vascular hypothesis for AD, which postulates that the risk of AD may be higher than the risk of VaD itself due to vascular risk factors other than hypertension. In line with this, compared to Japanese residing in Japan and Americans residing in the United States, elderly Japanese immigrants in Hawaii and California typically have an intermediate risk profile for both AD and VaD.

Cross-Cultural Studies of Japan. According to data from the Honolulu-Asian Aging Study, the prevalence of AD is higher among Japanese residents of the United States than it is in Japan. Hawaii's dementia prevalence was comparable to that of Caucasian American populations, and the subtype distribution of dementia was strikingly similar to that of North American and European Caucasian populations. An intriguing survey linked dietary factors to the higher prevalence of dementia among Japanese-Brazilians from Okinawa when compared to the Japanese population residing in Okinawa. Dementia was more common among immigrants due to the dietary habits of Japanese immigrants in Brazil, which were marked by a high intake of meat and little fish.

Studies comparing eastern and western nations particularly highlight the differences in the prevalence rates of dementia subtypes. However, methodological variations across studies may account for at least some of this large variation. For example, among various Japanese population samples aged 65 or over, the prevalence of dementia varies from 3.8% to 11%. In addition, the AD/VaD ratio varied between 2.1% and 4.1% in these populations. Therefore, the actual differences in overall dementia prevalence among Asian populations, even between them and western countries, are probably lower than believed, given the challenges associated with establishing diagnostic thresholds for dementia and incomplete population mean age adjustments.

3.2.5. African Studies

In Africa today, the absolute number of people living longer is rising rapidly, and dementia is typically written off as a normal aspect of aging. Furthermore, there has been a substantial increase in dementia-related morbidity and health care costs linked to delayed diagnosis and a lack of accurate information about the disease. Many factors, including disparate survival rates, case concealment, aversion to seeking medical attention, limited access to healthcare facilities, and inadequate case-finding methods, may contribute to the challenge of obtaining and organizing accurate rates in Africa.

According to a systematic analysis conducted in Africa, 2.4% (2.76 million people) of those over 50 have dementia overall, with the majority of those affected (76%) residing in Sub-Saharan Africa. It is the only place on Earth where an increase in the number of wretched people is predicted in the coming years, and it also has the highest disease burden worldwide. The highest overall prevalence was found in females 80 years of age or older (19.7%), with little regional variation. The most common cause of dementia was Alzheimer's disease (57.1%), followed by vasculitis (26.9%).

In a study done in Sub-Saharan Africa, the 10/66 diagnostic criteria—which is intended for use in low- and middle-income countries—was used to compare the prevalence rates of dementia with those obtained using the DSM-IV criteria. According to the findings, the age-standardized prevalence of clinical DSM-IV dementia was approximately 6.4%, and the prevalence of 10/66 dementia was approximately 21.6%. There was an educational bias in the diagnostic tool that led to the correlation between dementia using the 10/66 criteria and educational level in that area. The DSM-IV criteria served as an international benchmark for the diagnosis of dementia in this instance.

In two culturally distinct but genetically related communities of elderly Yoruba people who live in communities—one in Ibadan, Nigeria, and the other among African Americans in Indianapolis, Indiana—the incidence rates of Alzheimer's disease were compared as part of the Indianapolis-Ibadan Dementia Project. The findings demonstrated that native Yoruba people had age-standardized yearly incidence rates for both total dementia and Alzheimer's disease that were significantly lower than those of African Americans (2.3% and 8.3%, respectively). Notably, the higher prevalence of AD (4.9%) in the aforementioned African-American community was primarily responsible for the increased prevalence of dementia (6.0%), while the prevalence of other causes of dementia (1.1%) increased less. This includes VaD. Similar to Japan, the United States had a higher proportion of Alzheimer's disease (3.2:1.0) compared to other causes of dementia (1.6:1.0) in Nigeria. Although there were significant differences in dementia prevalence rates depending on the diagnostic system used, the ecological studies mentioned above provide stronger evidence for the significance of environmental factors than ethnic factors in determining dementia prevalence.

It's interesting to note that, despite having a superior educational system, the USA had a higher prevalence of dementia in the Nigeria-USA study. While these findings may suggest that other environmental factors, such as diet and physical activity, may be even more significant risk factors for dementia than a low educational background, they do not necessarily refute the education-related "cognitive reserve" hypothesis in dementia (Ferri et al., 2005; Thies & Bleiler, 2011).

3.2.6. Middle East

Few Middle Eastern epidemiological studies on AD and VaD have been published; those that have come from Israel have been the majority. In Wadi Ara, Israel, a survey conducted among the most illiterate elderly population revealed that over 25% of them had an AD diagnosis. Among those with mild cognitive impairment, the annual incidence of AD was 4.4%. VaD accounted for roughly 22% of dementia cases and was highly correlated with both hypertension and illiteracy. The high prevalence rates of dementia made these findings special. According to a study, Wadi Ara had an exceptionally high prevalence of both AD and cognitive impairment, but a low conversion rate from AD to cognitive impairment. In comparison to developed nations, where the proportionate increase in dementia cases is expected to be around 100%, the number of dementia cases in this region and North Africa is expected to increase by roughly 300% by 2040.

While the prevalence of dementia, especially AD, is rising quickly in both developed and developing nations, there are significant regional variations. According to the Delphi Consensus Study, dementia was more common in the Americas and less common in less developed parts of the world like the Middle East and Africa. It appears to be fairly uniform in Eastern European nations, falling somewhere between Japan and the United States. This variation can be partly explained by the fact that studies' methods, particularly their diagnostic criteria, vary widely. Even when focusing solely on senior populations, heterogeneity may arise from differing mean population ages. Higher percentages of oldest-old people and lower percentages of youngest-old people are typically found in nations with longer life expectancies than in those with shorter life expectancies. Many epidemiological studies on dementia did not perform standardized age adjustment. Nevertheless, there are still minor but significant differences in the age-adjusted prevalence of dementia across the globe, even after taking these potential sources of bias into account.

It is also absolutely necessary to employ a standardized international epidemiological method worldwide to compare the actual prevalence of VaD and AD across various global regions. The majority of the variations in dementia prevalence across the various regions can be explained by differences in nutrition and physical activity on the one hand, and educational attainment on the other, in addition to unequal methodologies and life expectancies. Furthermore, even though education level guards against dementia, a higher prevalence of the disease appears to be correlated with increased cardiovascular risk factors such as diabetes, obesity, dyslipidemia, and hypertension in developed nations.

However, developing nations where hypertension is the main issue appear to have a disproportionately high VaD prevalence. Even though the prevalence of obesity continues to rise, development, whether in western or eastern countries, increased the prevention, treatment, and control of hypertension (theory of morbidity compression). The prevalence of AD rises along with the high life expectancy and socioeconomic development, which raises the AD/VaD rate. Whether for AD or VaD, the best way to date to put public policies into place to lessen the burden of dementia on societies is to improve adult and child education and promote healthy environments and lifestyles, such as regular exercise and a balanced diet (Ferri et al., 2005; Thies & Bleiler, 2011).

3.3. METHODOLOGICAL ISSUES IN PREVALENCE STUDIES

Correlates of cognitive function, cognitive decline, and dementia are found in epidemiologic research on cognitive aging. It is common to overlook the importance of precisely defining the scientific question and determining whether it is causal or predictive as a necessary first step in carrying out efficient research. Causal questions are addressed by research on the etiology of dementia or the assessment of potential preventive or therapeutic interventions. Predictive studies are crucial for predicting future trends in the public health burden of dementia and the outcomes of individual patients. They are intended to estimate prevalence or identify high-risk individuals. Predictive studies have different analytical concerns than studies meant to bolster causal inferences.

Although it is common for statistical analysis to be used as a means of supplying evidence to support causal inferences, observational research is frequently criticized for concluding without supporting data. Intervention trials are usually fielded only after substantial observational research, even though evidence from RCTs may ultimately be necessary to draw firm conclusions for many treatments. The purpose of gathering this observational data should be to shed light on causal relationships and direct the planning of (future) trials.

3.3.1. Selection Into the Analysis Sample

In dementia research, selection problems stem from differences in participant survival, attrition, and enrollment, which can be caused by differences in participant survival or refusal to participate up until the point of study initiation. Effect estimates may be skewed by any of these procedures. When selection processes are connected to both cognitive status and the exposure of interest (or their determinants), erroneous associations may arise between the putative risk factor and dementia or cognitive decline. The bias isn't always in favor of the null (i.e., which would typically hide an association) and occasionally change the direction of the association (i.e., producing the appearance of harmful exposures as protective or harmful exposures as protective). Dementia and impaired cognition have widely crippling effects, which creates the conditions for selection bias in long-term dementia studies. People with impaired cognition are also more likely to get sick, die, or drop out of the study. If attrition is also correlated with the risk factor under investigation, selection bias is probably going to occur. For instance, there are significant risks of morbidity and mortality associated with race, socioeconomic status, chronic disease, and unhealthy behaviors. To address potential selection bias, a variety of strategies are used, but the effectiveness of these strategies is rarely assessed. Even the possibility of significant bias resulting from "ignoring the selection process," which is arguably the most popular tactic in the applied literature, is rarely formally measured, though certain instances imply that it might be sizable. Including selective attrition in the Chicago Health and Aging Project raised the estimated correlations between smoking and cognitive decline by 56–86%. The purpose of MELODEM guidelines is to offer data to assess if a selection is likely to introduce a significant bias.

Table 3.3. Risk-of-Bias Assessment of RCTs Using the ROB-2 Tool. Traffic Light Plot of Study-by-Study Bias Assessment. Weighted Summary Plot of the Overall Type of bias Encountered in All Studies Performance (i.e., Providing A Precise Estimate of the Effect of Interest) in Dementia Research

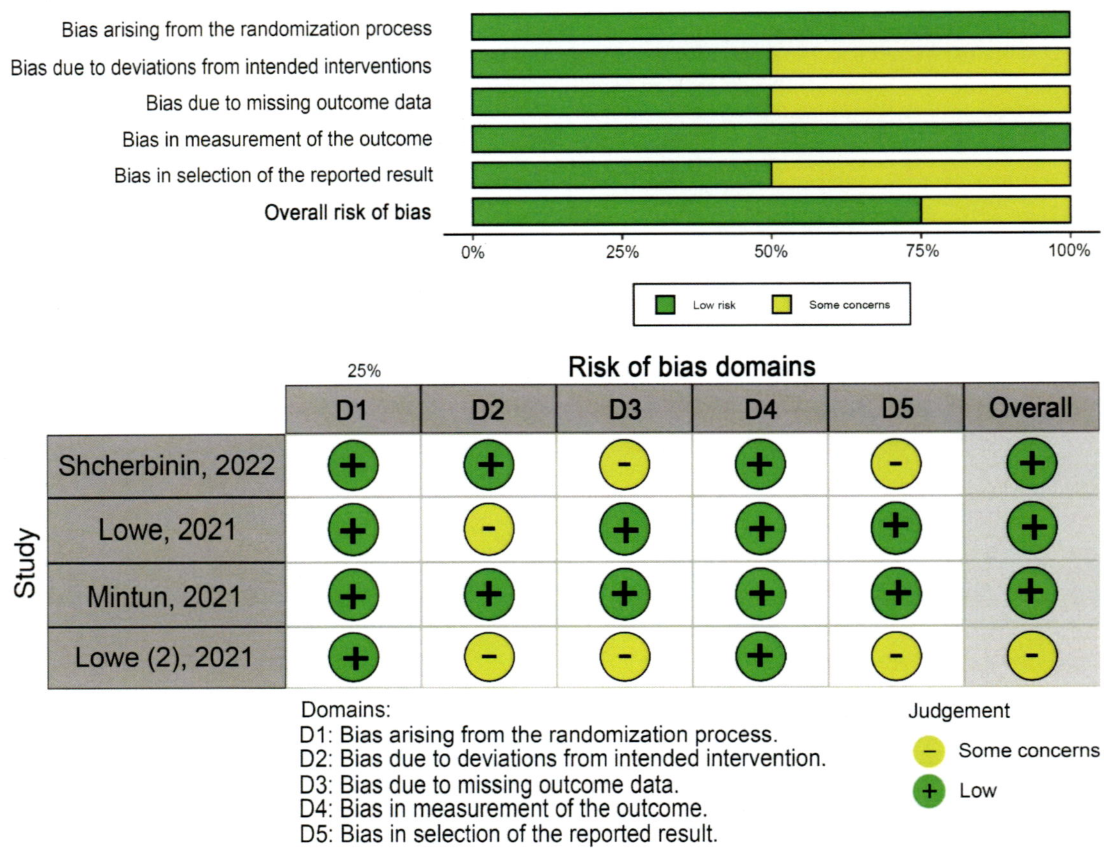

Source: Rashad A, Rasool A, Shaheryar M, Sarfraz A, Sarfraz Z, Robles-Velasco K, & Cherrez-Ojeda I, (2023). Donanemab for Alzheimer's disease: A systematic review of clinical trials. Healthcare, 11(1), 32. https://doi.org/10.3390/healthcare11010032.

A large number of older participants may "drop out" of the study or decide not to participate in it for the duration of the longitudinal follow-up. Several analytical techniques can offer objective effect estimates if drop-out is dependent on measured parameters (a "missing at random" mechanism); however, bias correction is difficult to achieve if drop-out is dependent on unknown or unmeasured parameters. Sensitivity analyzes in this case can shed light on how solid the results are.

Another important source of censoring in longitudinal studies is mortality. In the context of survival, many strategies deemed suitable for managing dropout-related attrition are more debatable, and there isn't currently agreement on the best strategies. While those who leave a study are considered to have "missing" cognitive function, those who pass away are better characterized as having "undefined" cognitive function. According to this conceptualization, individuals whose survival depends on exposure ought to be left out of the population that we attempt to estimate effects for. For instance, by accelerating the death rate from other causes, smoking may be associated with a decreased diagnosis rate of dementia. Therefore, defining the scientifically relevant question with clarity is crucial when discussing selective survival. This includes identifying the parameter to be estimated, the target audience for the estimate, and the analysis techniques that align with the estimate.

Interval censoring is introduced by truncating follow-up by death in dementia cohort studies because dementia diagnosis can only be made at periodic follow-up visits. For participants who did not have dementia at their final visit before passing away, the dementia status at death is therefore unknown. When there is a competing risk of death, interval censoring can lead to an underestimation of dementia incidence and change the estimated effects of exposures. For instance, in the French PAQUID cohort, the protective effect of high education against the risk of dementia was overestimated by 36% in men when interval censoring was not taken into consideration. This was probably because while having more education indicates a higher chance of developing dementia, it also indicates a higher risk of passing away sooner after diagnosis.

When participants are chosen for a study based on factors such as exposure to interest and results (or factors influencing those outcomes), bias may also result from the selection process. Either because individuals with certain dementia risk factors consistently decline study participation or because these individuals are unlikely to live to the enrollment age, similar biases may arise. Imagine a fictitious research that enlists participants in the age of 70 to examine the impact of smoking on AD. If smoking and APOE-ε4 status have a synergistic effect on mortality, meaning they work together rather than multiplying each other, then the surviving 70-year-old smokers will have a lower APOE-ε4 prevalence than the surviving 70-year-old nonsmokers. The study might mix up the effects of smoking and APOE-ε4. Pre-enrollment selective mortality is especially likely to occur in population-based studies involving older adults: individuals who were exposed to harmful risk factors might only have made it to enrollment age by a genotype that allows for exceptionally efficient detoxification or exceptional cognitive ability. The potential for selective enrollment to undermine internal validity and generalizability is sometimes overlooked, although challenges resulting from this practice are widely acknowledged.

Estimates of the effects may be somewhat "muted" by each of these selection procedures. For instance, in older samples, the correlation between smoking and AD gradually diminishes or even turns protective. When participant age increases, similar muting effects are seen for several other risk factors. Additionally, selection may lead to erroneous variations in effect estimates amongst subgroups. While problems with selective survival and attrition impact both observational studies and randomized controlled trials (RCTs), selective enrollment does not undermine the internal validity of RCTs, even though it might lessen the generalizability that comes with randomization.

3.3.2. Measurement Validity and Reliability

The disjunction between disease pathophysiology and clinical and research measures, resulting from imperfect validity and reliability, poses measurement challenges in the field of dementia research. For instance, results on neuropsychological tests may not accurately represent the brain's biological capabilities and functioning. Measures of the effects, severity, and progression of dementia, such as functional dependency, neuropsychiatric symptoms, and behavioral patterns, present similar measurement challenges. It is crucial to distinguish between the trajectories of cognitive symptoms and neuropathologic processes in the brain to identify particular disease-causing pathways and potential interactions with other closely related outcomes.

If a measurement tool evaluates the phenomenon of interest, it is said to be valid. While alternative measurements can be evaluated for validity using gold standard measures, dementia research frequently lacks a definitive gold standard. Estimates of disparities and risk factor effects may be skewed because measures that are appropriate for one group of people may not be appropriate for another. For instance, historically, African Americans have had less access to education than White Americans, which has resulted in systematic disparities in older adults' literacy levels. The racial differences in dementia risk seem to be influenced by these literacy differences. Finding reliable biomarkers for dementia is important, but many approaches run the risk of circular reasoning—that is, using biomarkers to support clinical diagnoses and clinical diagnoses to support biomarkers—rather than using the latter approach. In fact, even the phenotype of interest is frequently disputed, and a variety of underlying pathologies may be included in many common definitions of disease.

Table 3.4. Bias

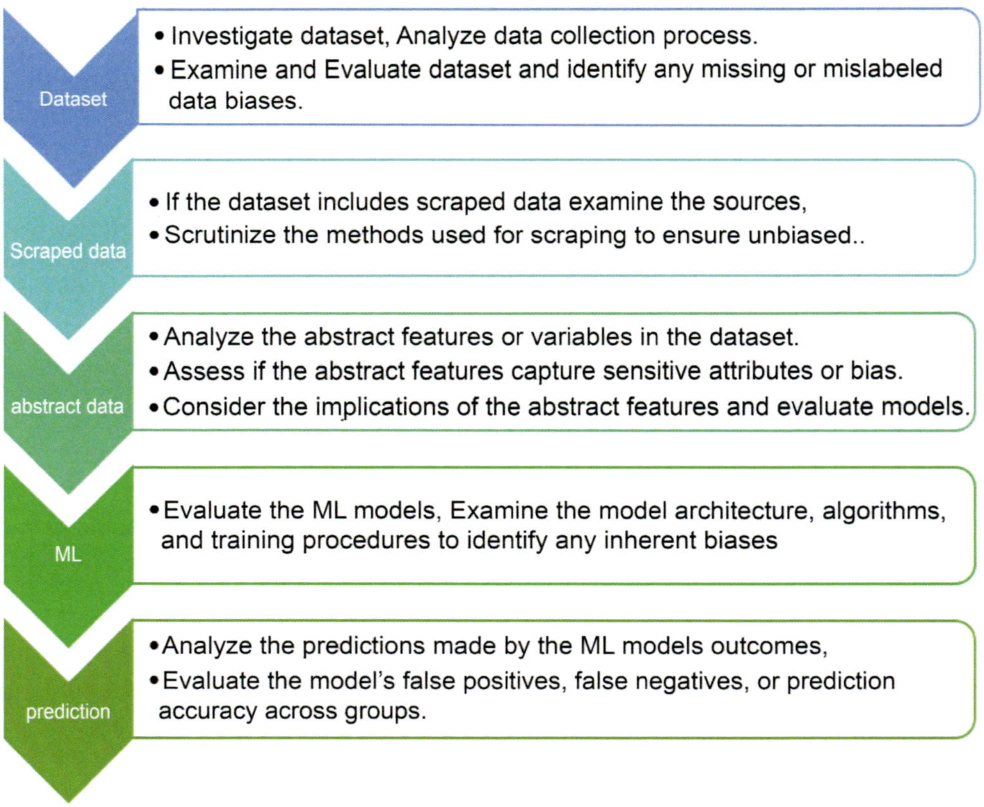

Source: Siddique S, Haque MA, George R, Gupta KD, Gupta D, Faruk MJH, (2024). Survey on machine learning biases and mitigation techniques. Digital, 4(1), 1–68. https://doi.org/10.3390/digital4010001.

In contrast to the portion attributable to measurement error—random fluctuations in the measurement that do not reflect changes in the underlying construct—reliability is the proportion of variability in a measure explained by the construct of interest. Significant unreliability exists in almost all neuropsychological tests, which lowers statistical power and increases the risk of regression to the mean.

Because practice effects can be large enough to offset several years of cognitive decline in elderly adults, practice or retest effects resulting from changes in familiarity with the testing procedure, use of strategies, or recall of test-specific content can also impede the detection of cognitive decline. As a result, practice-related gains in test performance may make it impossible to identify cognitive declines resulting from early dementia. Practice effects may cause underestimations of dementia incidence and rate as well as inaccurate conclusions about the causes of cognitive decline if practice effect magnitude varies with background characteristics. There is still debate over statistical methods for managing practice effects.

The assumption made by the majority of popular analytical techniques that a 1-point difference in a test score has the same substantive meaning at the high and low ends of the scale presents another measurement challenge. But a drop from 25 to 24 on the Mini-Mental State Examination (MMSE) might not be the same as a drop from 20 to 19. Extreme examples of this uneven interval scaling include floors and ceilings. In cross-sectional analyzes, ceilings and floors reduce effect estimates; however, in longitudinal analyzes, they may increase or decrease effect estimates. An extensive simulation study demonstrated that type 1 errors (i.e., errors related to the effects of a risk factor on cognitive slope) can be significantly inflated when unequal interval scaling of psychometric tests is not taken into account (i.e., spurious associations) if baseline cognitive level is also predicted by the risk factor.

3.3.3. Alternative Timescales and Specification of Longitudinal Models

In longitudinal studies, the definition of the timescale(s) and functions of within-person change can have a significant impact on reproducibility and outcomes. Due to the strong correlation between dementia and aging, researching dementia risk or associated binary outcomes is best done within the context of age. This also holds true for research on time-invariant exposures (genetics or gender) in cognitive aging studies. That being said, studies frequently focus on time-varying exposures that are only measured once (e.g., diet, diabetes, and therapy) and consequently at various stages of life. In this case, it might be more appropriate to use the timescale as the time since exposure measurement, which is typically enrollment. When concentrating on particular stages of cognitive aging, such as the terminal decline or prodromal phase of dementia, reverse time (e.g., years before diagnosis or passing away) might also be instructive. Reverse time biases estimated longitudinal changes because it naturally selects participants who developed the outcome.

As a result, studying cognitive change with age mixes two processes: within-person change with age (usually of main interest) and between-person age differences that are also influenced by birth cohort. This is because the majority of observational studies on cognition recruit participants over a wide age range. When examining cognitive decline with aging, it is only appropriate to ignore age differences at baseline if all individuals "converge" onto the same age trajectory, regardless of their birth cohort, if someone entering at age 85 is anticipated to possess the same level of cognitive function as someone entering at age 65 and being followed for 20 years. This might not be feasible. For instance, due to significant cohort differences in educational attainment, between-person age effects for women in the Whitehall cohorts overestimated the rate of cognitive decline when compared to within-person effects. It is simple to separate the two timescales involved in the "convergence" problem: a longitudinal timescale (e.g., age at enrollment or the present) for within-person variations and a cross-sectional timeline (e.g., age at enrollment) to account for variations in individual age.

It is not anticipated that average annual changes in cognition will be constant across all age groups; in fact, cognitive decline may quicken with age. Linear approximations may be sufficient in studies with brief follow-ups, but linearity is rarely true in studies with longer follow-ups, age-heterogeneous samples, or pathologic events. Polynomial cognitive trajectories, biphasic trajectories with change points, and nonparametric estimation of cognitive trajectories are some methods to explain this heterogeneity (Ferri et al., 2005; Thies & Bleiler, 2011).

3.3.4. Time-Varying Exposure/ Time-Varying Confounding

At least 20 years before a clinical dementia diagnosis is made, pathologic brain alterations are visible. The timing of exposure can have an impact on cognitive outcomes, and exposures that affect pathogenesis, disease progression, and/or function maintenance may have different timing implications. Clinical judgments and preventative measures that target established risk factors depend on research identifying pertinent etiologic periods. For instance, higher blood pressure in middle age does not always indicate a higher risk of dementia; elevated blood pressure in later life does. The reason for this discrepancy is unknown, but treatment recommendations for hypertension should take an individual's age and pre-existing morbidities into account when preventing dementia. Regarding the impact of hormone therapy on dementia, a "critical window" theory has been put forth, which states that starting treatment during the perimenopausal stage has advantages and starting later has disadvantages. A recent systematic review found very few studies that answer this question specifically. Cohorts with very long follow-up are useful for assessing etiologic periods because they offer exposure measures at various ages. It takes caution to quantify how an exposure's effects on dementia change with exposure age because different approaches to the analysis of time-varying exposure data can produce results that differ significantly in terms of magnitude and, more importantly, in terms of interpretation. While age-specific differences in risk factor-dementia associations could indicate pertinent etiologic windows, they could also indicate reverse causation or variations in measurement error between age-specific exposures. Repeated measures of exposure can be combined (e.g., averaged) to obtain more accurate exposure estimates when cumulative effects of long-term exposure, rather than variation in exposure or point in time exposure effects, are hypothesized.

Confounding factors can change over time, just like exposures can. The fact that different studies measure exposures and potential confounders differently and at different times makes the situation more difficult. As with time-varying exposure data analysis, extra caution is needed to account for confounding when exposures and confounders change over time, particularly when confounders may also function as potential mediators.

3.3.5. High-Dimensional Data

The emergence of high-dimensional data and the multiplicity of data sources have the potential to significantly accelerate dementia research, but only if they are properly utilized. Among the many new opportunities and challenges that arise are administrative databases, omics data, brain imaging data (positron emission tomography and magnetic resonance imaging), biomarker panels that evaluate gene expression, and metabolic pathways. New technologies will yield data on a multitude of biomarkers that could help us differentiate between more specific dementia phenotypes. However, to fully utilize these data, we need robust measurement tools.

Statistical analyzes of high-dimensional data present some challenges, even in cases where the number of observations is substantially greater than that usually found in research cohorts. Big data may in some cases exacerbate issues with measurement validity and selection bias, and they do not always provide a solution to the well-known internal and external validity problems in epidemiologic studies. For instance, it is well known that underdiagnosis contributes to the significant underrepresentation of dementia in many US administrative databases. Underdiagnosis rates can vary depending on background variables such as demographics. Obese people had a third lower risk of developing dementia than their peers of normal weight, according to a provocative and unexpected finding recently released from a UK administrative database with nearly 2 million individuals ages ≥40 years and over 45,000 incident dementia cases. The large sample size yielded extremely accurate effect estimates, but it also came with many trade-offs that could have led to biases, like limited confounder control based on variables listed in the database and the possibility of misclassifying the results.

New global initiatives to combine data from various dementia cohorts are creating distinctive and exciting databases: the European Medical Information Framework-AD is a collaboration between academic institutions, pharmaceutical companies, and medical informatics experts that aims to identify preclinical biomarkers of Alzheimer's disease. Even with large sample sizes, the results won't be meaningful until harmonized exposure, biomarker, and outcome measures can be determined. Organizing these initiatives is a significant task. The goal of the Integrated Analysis of Longitudinal Studies of Aging collaboration is to improve the reproducibility and harmonization of data from international longitudinal studies that examine the relationship between aging and changes in health, well-being, and cognition.

4Many statistical tests and comparisons are produced by high-dimensional data analysis, and these tests and comparisons may be addressed by different statistical corrections (such as family-wise error and false discovery). Potential "overfitting" is a related problem, which occurs when a statistical model describes noise or random error rather than the underlying relationship. In this situation, dimension reduction techniques (like Lasso or partial least-squares methods) can be applied either before or during supervised analyzes. In order to better understand dementia etiology, the challenges here are to both account for the high dimensionality in models (multiple testing and overfitting) and to extract meaningful information from these data.

Improved hypothesis-driven research, such as assessing predetermined social, behavioral, or clinical dementia determinants, as well as agnostic search carried out in the lack of well-defined hypotheses, may be made possible by new data sources. Type 1 error issues make unbiased search techniques difficult, but this is a crucial area for the field. Assessing the interplay between risk factors and pathologic processes may present new opportunities as biomarkers become more widely available in large data sets. For instance, based on the degree of underlying neuropathology, researchers might be able to model whether behavioral or genetic risk factors have a different effect on cognitive symptoms. Crucially, careful mediation models to dissect direct, indirect, and interactive pathways will be required because many risk factors—though not all—will directly impact neuropathology (Ferri et al., 2005; Thies & Bleiler, 2011).

3.4. PREVALENCE RATES BY SEX

Other groups may be at varying risk of developing Alzheimer's and other dementias due to shared social identities and characteristics. Members of sexual and gender minority (SGM) groups are included in this. SGM encompasses people who identify as gender nonbinary, transgender, or lesbian, gay, or bisexual (sexual minorities), as well as people whose gender expression, gender identity, or reproductive development deviates from conventional, societal, cultural, or physiological norms (gender minorities).

Due to their widespread exposure to institutionalized discrimination, marginalization, disadvantage, and/or exclusion from social institutions and businesses, older SGM adults may be at least partially at risk for dementia. Until recently, little was known about the dementia risks associated with self-identifying as SGM, including whether SGM older adults are more likely to develop dementia than non-SGM older adults. These endeavors include Alzheimer's research. There haven't been many studies aimed at answering this question, but an increasing amount of preliminary data points to this possibility. Adults residing in any of the 25 U.S. states, compared to older adults who are not SGM, SGM older adults reported having more cognitive issues. While a third study found that the risk of dementia and mild cognitive impairment was similar for people in same-sex relationships and those in other-sex relationships, two population-based studies found higher rates of cognitive impairment among older adults who were SGM than among non-SGM older adults. Transgender adults may have an increased risk of dementia, according to two studies. According to one study of Medicare beneficiaries, the prevalence of dementia in transgender adults 65 years of age and older was estimated to be 18%, while it was only 12% in cisgender (non-transgender) adults. Transgender adults were found to have a higher likelihood than cisgender adults of having an Alzheimer's or other dementia diagnosis in their electronic medical records, according to a second study of adults in Florida.

To determine whether dementia risk varies among older SGM adults and to determine the causes of any such variation, more research is required. According to research, SGM older adults may be more susceptible to dementias like Alzheimer's due to stressors like marginalization and discrimination. These pressures may have an adverse effect on their physical and mental well-being. According to one study, older SGM adults with depression had a higher risk of dementia than their non-SGM counterparts. Disparities in other health-related factors that increase the risk of Alzheimer's and other dementias are also experienced by SGM older adults. When compared to older adults who are not SGM, these include higher rates of alcohol and tobacco use, obesity, and other cardiovascular risk factors. Furthermore, due in part to obstacles like discrimination and heterosexist attitudes in healthcare settings, SGM older adults have lower rates of receiving preventive health screenings and health care access. Finally, since HIV/

AIDS was first identified, the SGM population, especially gay and bisexual men and transgender individuals, has been associated with the disease's history, burden of illness, mortality rate, and social stigma. These days, HIV/AIDS is a chronic illness that is effectively treated with medication, and many patients with the disease live longer into old age. Apart from the potential impact of this past on the previously mentioned social stressors and health care accessibility, dementia is also at risk due to HIV/AIDS. Gay, bisexual, and transgender persons have a higher prevalence of HIV/AIDS than non-SGM older adults, which increases their risk of developing dementia as a result of the virus.

The idea that historically marginalized groups are rarely homogeneous in terms of their identities and experiences is becoming more widely acknowledged. These groups can be classified by gender, sexual orientation, race/ethnicity, or other characteristics. Belonging to more than one of these groups may have a particularly significant impact on health, including the risk of dementia, as these identities and experiences intersect. The development of more insightful dementia research and more efficient and compassionate dementia care in these communities depend on the adoption of this "intersectionality" paradigm. Research and care initiatives should take into account the potential intersections and influences of gender, race, ethnicity, class, sexual orientation, and HIV status on dementia (Ferri et al., 2005; Thies & Bleiler, 2011).

3.5. PREVALENCE BY RACE OR ETHNICITY

The available data on Alzheimer's disease and related dementias indicates that racial and ethnic groups differ significantly in terms of the disease's prevalence, incidence, course of treatment, and mortality. Significant variations also exist in terms of service utilization, clinical trial participation, and illness-related expenses. From an ethical and policy standpoint, disparities in diagnosis and treatment rates, as well as in service utilization, among racial and ethnic groups should raise concerns. In a perfect world, a person's race or ethnic background would not affect their access to services or the burden of disease. Minorities will account for a larger share of the elderly population as the population ages and their share of Alzheimer's patients rises. It is predicted that the percentage of White people 85 years of age and older—the age group most likely to have Alzheimer's disease—will drop from 90% in 2010 to 81% in 2050. It is predicted that by 2050, the percentage of non-Hispanic White people aged 85 and over will drop from 85% in 2010 to 67%. The percentage of Hispanic people 85 years of age and older is expected to rise from 5% to 15% over the same time period.

3.5.1. Ethnic Comparisons Within the United States

Within the U. S. Alzheimer's disease and other dementias are disproportionately more common in non-Hispanic Black and Hispanic older adults than in White older adults. According to data from the CHAP study, compared to 10% of White older adults, 19% of Black and 14% of Hispanic adults 65 and older have Alzheimer's dementia. Black older adults are roughly twice as likely as White older adults to have Alzheimer's or other dementias, according to the majority of other prevalence studies. While some studies have found similar prevalences among Hispanic and White older adults, others suggest that Hispanic older adults are approximately 1.5 times more likely than White older adults to have Alzheimer's or other dementias. The Hispanic population is made up of a wide range of groups with varying cultural backgrounds and health profiles. Research suggests that the prevalence of various Hispanic ethnic groups may vary (for instance, Mexican Americans versus Caribbean

Americans). The increased occurrence of Alzheimer's dementia in Black and Hispanic communities compared to White communities is likely a result of a higher prevalence of dementia in these populations. Race is not determined by genetics, and genetic factors do not fully explain the disparities in dementia rates among different racial groups. While some studies suggest that certain genetic risk factors may have varying effects on Alzheimer's risk based on race, these differences are not significant enough to explain the overall disparities. Race is a social construct that has been used historically by those in power to justify control over others and does not have a biological basis.

The disparities between older Black and Hispanic populations and older White populations in life experiences, socioeconomic indicators, and ultimately health conditions are most likely the cause of the differences in risk for Alzheimer's and other dementias among racial and ethnic groups. These disparities are the result of their historical and ongoing marginalization in the United States. These include the structural racism in laws and practices. The quality of schools in a community, the places where people can live, and their exposure to dangerous pollutants and toxicants are all impacted by structural racism. It also affects exposure to violence, employment opportunities, occupational safety, the ability to pass wealth down to future generations, and how the legal system handles cases.

The risk of dementia may be directly impacted in historically marginalized and socially disadvantaged racial and ethnic groups by the cumulative stress caused by the effects of structural racism and the resulting differences in social and physical environment. Furthermore, structural racism causes racial and ethnic disparities in a wide range of health outcomes, such as diabetes and cardiovascular disease, which are linked to a higher risk of dementia for historically marginalized racial and ethnic groups. A large portion of the increased risk of dementia among Black and Hispanic populations is thought to be explained by these medical conditions, which disproportionately affect these populations. Numerous studies indicate that when thorough analyzes take socioeconomic and health-related variables into account, racial and ethnic disparities in dementia risk do not hold true.

Over the course of a person's life, the effects of structural racism on health and dementia risk may cascade and intensify. For instance, some research suggests that Black Americans' later cognitive health may suffer as a result of early experiences with residential schools and school segregation. This suggests that to account for the various environmental and sociopolitical factors that may increase the risk of Alzheimer's and other dementias in disproportionately affected populations, health disparities research must incorporate life course perspectives and the knowledge of race equity scholars. Numerous social factors that affect differences in the course of Alzheimer's disease may also have an impact on the timing and outcome of a dementia diagnosis. There is proof that older Black and Hispanic adults are more likely than older White adults to have missed or delayed diagnoses of Alzheimer's disease and other dementias. It has been estimated that 10.3% of White older adults, 12.2% of Hispanic older adults, and 13.8% of Black older adults have been diagnosed with Alzheimer's disease or another dementia based on data from Medicare beneficiaries 65 and older. While these percentages show that older adults of color face a higher burden of dementia than older adults of color, prevalence studies that identify all cases of dementia, regardless of health care utilization, suggest that these percentages should be much higher. There are comparatively few population-based cohort studies examining the national prevalence of dementias other than Alzheimer's and Black and Hispanic in racial and ethnic groups. Dementia incidence, as measured by the first dementia diagnosis found in members' medical records, was found to be highest among African American older adults (the term used in the study for those who self-reported as Black or African-American); intermediate among Latino older adults (the term used in the study for those who self-reported as Latino or Hispanic); lowest among Asian American older adults. This information was derived from an examination of the electronic medical records of members of a large health plan in California. Although there was variation among Asian American subgroups in a follow-up study using the same cohort, the incidence of dementia was lower in every subgroup than in the White population. According to a recent systematic review of the literature, the only Asian American subgroup with accurate prevalence data was Japanese Americans, who also had the lowest dementia prevalence of any ethnic group. The effects of Alzheimer's disease on persons of Middle Eastern and North African descent, individuals who identify as members of multiple racial or ethnic groups, and origin subgroups within racial or ethnic groups are not well understood. Conclusions about the prevalence of Alzheimer's and other dementias in various racial and ethnic groups and subgroups need to be drawn from more research, particularly from community-based cohorts and studies that concentrate on racial/ethnic groups that have historically not been included in Alzheimer's research.

3.5.2. South America

The racial, ethnic, cultural, and socioeconomic diversity of South America offers a great opportunity to assess biological and environmental risk factors for cognitive decline and Alzheimer's in the elderly; further research is needed in this area, though, to match the epidemiological data from other areas. According to a study conducted in Chile, 5.98% of seniors 65 years of age and older had dementia, with 60% of these cases fitting the criteria for Alzheimer's disease. The prevalence of dementia appears to be similar in Brazil to that of white Americans and Europe, with illiterates having the highest rates. Other South American nations seem to have dementia and cognitive impairment rates that are similar to those in Europe and the US.

3.5.3. Africa

"No authentic case of AD has been reported in an indigenous black African," according to several studies. These researchers reported not finding any cases of severe dementia in a door-to-door survey of 1,122 people in Ibadan, Nigeria, who were over 40 (or 32% over 65). They discovered that although 31.6% of the sample had cognitive impairment, they were still able to perform their functional tasks. The same research team discovered that none of the 198 brains examined during an autopsy showed pathological alterations similar to AD. Vascular dementia was found to be prevalent among the senior clinical patients in this region.

The goal of the study on the epidemiology of dementia among community-dwelling African Americans in Indianapolis and Yoruba people in Ibadan was to capitalize on the fact that, although African Americans are primarily descended from West African blacks, they live in very different environments than Nigerians and are thus probably exposed to different environmental risk factors. A total of 2,494 Nigerians and 2,212 African-American elders were evaluated. Each population underwent door-to-door screening, though it's unclear how precisely the American sample was classified as "African American.." According to WHO guidelines, diagnoses were made using the

NINCDS-ADRDA criteria for AD and the DSM-II-R and ICD-10 criteria for dementia. In community-dwelling Yoruba elders in Ibadan, age-adjusted prevalence rates for dementia (2.29%) and AD (1.41%) were significantly lower than rates for dementia (8.24%) and AD (6.24%) among African Americans. Age-standardized yearly incidence rates of dementia (1.35%) and AD (1.15%) in Ibadan were substantially lower than those of African Americans in Indiana (3.24%) and (2.52%) for dementia. Researchers in the Indianapolis-Ibadan study proposed many potential reasons for lower rates among older Nigerians, including differential mortality (people in Nigeria who would eventually develop AD may pass away at a younger age); the population's comparatively younger age distribution; the lack of environmental factors that could raise the risk of AD; and different diagnostic standards for functional decline. A recent study indicates that this is not the case among East Africans, contrary to the study's suggestion that Nigerians may have a lower rate of amyloid deposition than African Americans.

3.5.4. Asia

It has generally been observed that while the overall rates of dementia in older adults from Asian and European backgrounds are similar, the distribution of dementia subtypes varies. In particular, preliminary research suggests that vascular dementia (VAD) may be more common in Asian populations, while AD is more common in most European studies. At first, it was thought that the Japanese had a significantly higher prevalence of VAD and a significantly lower prevalence of AD. More recent research, however, has indicated a rise in AD and a decline in the prevalence of VAD. This shifting pattern of dementia diagnosis could be the result of improved control over cardiovascular risk factors leading to a decrease in the prevalence of VAD, or it could be the result of the Westernization of risk factors such as a diet high in fat and cholesterol leading to an increase in the prevalence of AD.

An intriguing study calculated the dementia prevalence among Japanese immigrants to Brazil before World War II. On the Japanese mainland, dementia prevalence was previously estimated to be around 8%. The Cognitive Abilities Screening Instrument was used to measure cognitive ability and the DSM-IV criteria were used to make the dementia diagnosis. The general prevalence of dementia (7.8%) and the distribution of dementia types (half of the cases were AD, and the other half were VAD) were found to be the same for Japanese immigrants as for the Japanese population living on the mainland or native Brazilians. This study refutes the idea that environmental factors have an impact on the prevalence or subtype of dementia, at least later in life.

In a study involving 5,055 senior citizens in Shanghai, China, 4.6% of people 65 years of age and older had dementia, with 65% of them having a clinical diagnosis of AD. Of the sample, roughly 47% had no formal education, and another 29% had less than seven years of schooling. A Chinese version of the MMSE was used to screen participants, with cutoffs based on educational attainment. The Chinese versions of the Fuld Object Memory Test, a Verbal Fluency Test, and the Digit Span and Block Design subtests from the Wechsler Adult Intelligence Scale-Revised (WAIS-R) were also given to those who scored below the cutoffs.

3.5.5. Europe

Data from 23 population-based prevalence studies (collected by the EURODEM Prevalence Research Group) from various European countries were combined in a study. The studies used the NINCDS-ADRDA criteria for AD and the DSM-III or comparable criteria to diagnose dementia. The prevalence rates were age-specific and varied from 0.3% in the 60–69 age group to 10.8% in the 80–89 age group. In an additional study conducted in Gothenburg, Sweden residents between the ages of 85 and 88 who were not demented found that the incidence of AD was 36.3% per 1,000 per year. It seems that among Swedish seniors 85 years of age and older, the incidence and prevalence of vascular dementia are higher than that of AD.

According to the Liverpool Health and Ethnicity Project, the prevalence of dementia was similar to that of white people (2–9%) among a sample of 418 English-speaking elderly people with African, Caribbean, Chinese, Asian, and Middle Eastern ancestry. But in the same study, the researchers also discovered that there was a higher prevalence of dementia (21–27%) among non-English speaking individuals with similar ethnic backgrounds. According to the study, the bias in the orientation test items was the cause of these higher rates. The exact date of their birth, their address, and the name of the prime minister were less likely to be known by non-English speakers than by English speakers, but there was no difference between them on any other test item.

3.5.6. Israel

The researchers discovered that there were no ethnic differences in survival, but the age- and sex-adjusted incidence of AD was higher in people born in Europe or America (2.9% per 100,000 population) than in people born in Africa or Asia (1.4 per 100,000). This information was gleaned from an analysis of the Israeli National Neurologic Disease Register and clinical records of hospital patients.

A brief cognitive screening test, which did not require reading or writing, and a 5-point rating scale of cognitive and daily functioning were given to 1,399 Ashkelon, Israel, residents who were 75 years of age and older. Of the participants, half were of African or Asian descent, and the other half were of European or American descent. Dementia frequency rose with age, and rates were higher in women, illiterate people, and people who were born in Asia or Africa. The researchers hypothesized that the most likely cause of these gender and ethnic group differences was a low level of education. In the Arab neighborhood of Wadi-Ara in northeastern Israel, the prevalence of AD was also investigated among the total population of 823 elders 60 years of age and above. 96% of the female participants and 42% of the male participants were illiterate. An Arabic-speaking neurologist who identified dementia using DSM-IV criteria and AD using NINCDS-ADRDA criteria examined each participant. 2.5% of that population was diagnosed with AD, and among those who were 80 years of age and older, the frequency of dementia increased from 6% to 49%.

3.5.7. Native Indians

In order to compare dementia rates among elderly residents of a rural area of northern India with those of elders living in the Monongahela Valley in Pennsylvania, the Indo-US Cross-National Dementia Epidemiology project (MoVIES project) was established. In a community survey of 5,126 residents of Ballabgarh, India, the group first reported an overall prevalence rate of 1.36% for all dementias and a prevalence rate of 1.07%for AD (meeting NINCDS-ADRDA criteria) among those 65 and older. Incidence rates for AD were among the lowest ever recorded, according to a recent report: 3.24 per 1,000 person-years for those 65 and older, and 1.74 for those 55 and older. Compared with seniors in the Monongahela Valley, these rates were noticeably lower. Similar to the Indianapolis/Ibadan study, the researchers hypothesized that low incidence rates might be explained by shorter follow-up periods, shorter life expectancies, or short survival rates with AD. Notably, the team discovered no correlation between literacy level and dementia incidence or prevalence.

3.6. LOOKING TO THE FUTURE

Approximately 5 million new cases of dementia are diagnosed annually, affecting over 25 million people worldwide, the majority of whom have Alzheimer's disease (AD). It is projected that the number of dementia cases will double every 20 years.

3.6.1. Continued Population Aging

The baby-boom generation, the largest demographic group in American history, began to reach retirement age in 2011. As of 2030, the portion of the U.S. The number of Americans 65 and older is expected to have increased significantly, accounting for 74 million of the country's total population (up from 18% in 2023).

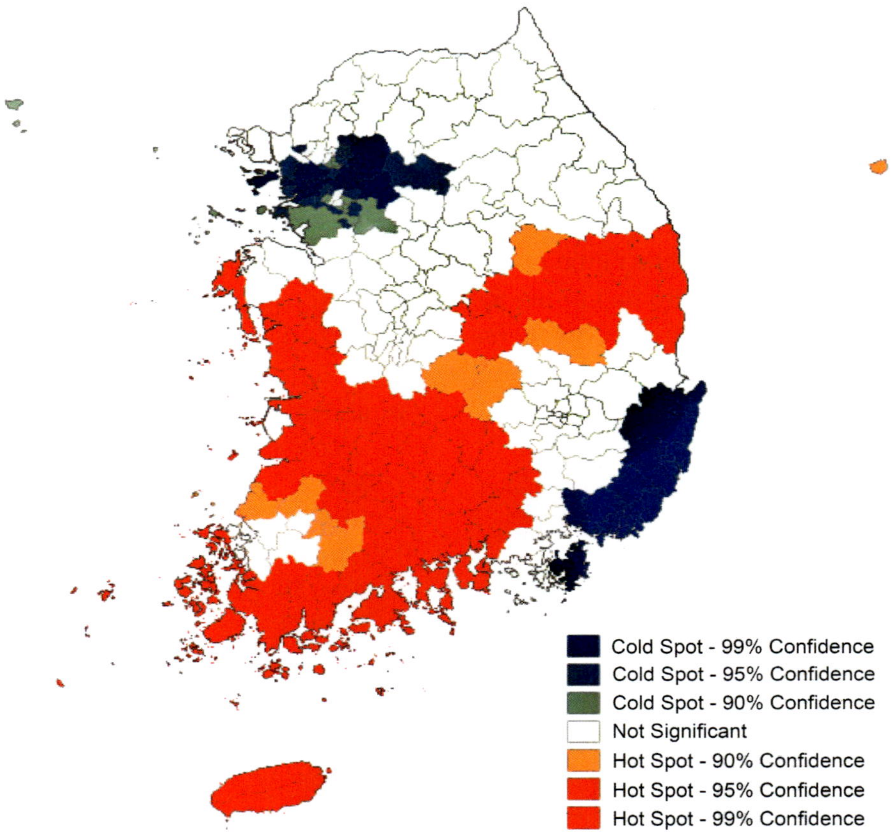

Figure 3.2. *Hot spot distribution of dementia prevalence in Korea.*

Source: Lim J, Park J-H, (2022). A predictive model of regional dementia prevalence using geographic weighted regression analysis. Journal of Personalized Medicine, 12(9), 1388. https://doi.org/10.3390/jpm12091388.

Furthermore, due to improvements in mortality at older ages and a projected decline in fertility, the population of older adults is expected to continue to grow relative to that of people 64 and younger, a trend known as population aging. Since 1960, fertility—or the average number of children born to each woman in the US—has declined. The population's proportion of older adults will increase as fewer babies are born annually. Since growing older is the main risk factor for Alzheimer's dementia, the number of new and existing cases of the disease will increase along with the number and proportion of older Americans, as Figure 3.2 illustrates.

- According to projections, there will be 7.2 million individuals aged 65 and above living with Alzheimer's dementia by 2025, which represents a 7% increase from the 6.7 million individuals affected in 2023.
- If there are no breakthroughs in medicine to stop, slow down, or cure Alzheimer's disease, the number of people 65 and older who have the dementia is expected to reach 13.08 million by 2060.

3.6.2. Growth of the Age 85 and Older Population

The aging of the sizable baby-boom cohort is predicted to cause a sharp increase in the number of Americans in their 80s, 90s, and beyond. The proportion of Americans 85 and older will rise as a result of this. It is anticipated that between now and 2050, this age group will make up a growing percentage of the U. S. population 65 years of age and above will increase from 11% in 2023 to 22% in 2050. As a result, there will be an extra 12 million people who are 85 years of age or older, who are most at risk of getting Alzheimer's disease.

- About 24.4 million Alzheimer's patients are expected to be 85 years of age or older in 2023, making up 33% of the total population with the disease.
- 67 million adults 85 years of age and older are predicted to have Alzheimer's dementia by 2060, making up roughly half (48%) of all individuals 65 and older who have the disease.

3.6.3. Increased Diversity of Older Adults

Estimates for older adults between 2018 and 2040 indicate increases in the American Indian population of 75%, the Black population of 88%, the Asian population of 113%, and the Hispanic population of 175%.

Furthermore, compared to earlier generations of women, women 65 years of age and older will be among the first to have worked outside the home on a large scale, and they will have completed more years of formal education. Concurrently, these female generations reached adulthood amid a decline in the fertility rate, leading to a reduction in the size of families. In the coming decades, it will become more evident how these social and economic experiences affect women's resilience and Alzheimer's risk.

It is uncertain what changes in dementia incidence and prevalence will result from the diverse life experiences of future older adult populations, both in terms of population-level changes and within racial/ethnic, socioeconomic, and sex/gender groups. In the upcoming decades, a birth cohort perspective—which takes into account how a specific group of people has experienced various life stages in specific years—will become more and more significant in helping us understand the resilience and risk factors that may be particular to the populations most at risk for dementia (Ferri et al., 2005; Thies & Bleiler, 2011).

A Closer Look

Mortality From Alzheimer's Disease in the United States: Data for 2000 and 2010

Alzheimer's disease was identified as a contributing factor in 26,488 deaths and the underlying cause of 83,494 deaths in 2010. Over the past 30 years, there has been a steady rise in the death rate from Alzheimer's disease. In the US, Alzheimer's disease ranks fifth among causes of death for those over 65 and sixth among all causes of death. In the US, the estimated number of people with Alzheimer's is 544 million. In 2012, the estimated cost of health care for individuals suffering from Alzheimer's disease and other dementias was $200 billion, with Medicare and Medicaid bearing the brunt of 140 billion of those costs. By 2050, the estimated cost of care is projected to reach $11 trillion.

Geographical location, age, sex, race, and Hispanic origin all affect the mortality rate from Alzheimer's disease. Based on information from the National Vital Statistics System for the years 2000 through 2010, which is the most recent year for which comprehensive data are available, this report provides mortality data related to Alzheimer's disease.

- **Alzheimer's Disease Mortality Increased Compared with Selected Major Causes of Death:** Over the past 10 years, Alzheimer's disease cases have increased when compared to other specific causes. While death rates from other major causes of death declined, the age-adjusted death rate from Alzheimer's disease increased by 39% between 2000 and 2010. Stroke (36%), heart disease (31%), and Cancer (32%) showed the biggest declines in death rates among the chosen major causes of death.
- **Alzheimer's Disease Mortality Risk Increased Most for the Oldest Age Groups:** The age-related increase in the risk of dying from Alzheimer's disease is substantial. In 2010, the risk of dying from Alzheimer's disease was 50 times higher in the 85+ age group than in the 65–74 age group. In a similar vein, the risk of dying from Alzheimer's disease was five times higher for those 85 years of age and older than for those 75–84 years of age.

Between 2000 and 2010, age-specific death rates from Alzheimer's disease increased by 6% for those 65 to 74 years of age, 32% for those 75 to 84 years of age, and 48% for those 85 years of age and older.

- **Alzheimer's Disease Mortality is Highest for the Non-Hispanic White Population and for Women:** Compared to non-Hispanic Black people, the age-adjusted death rate from Alzheimer's disease in the non-Hispanic White population was 26% higher in 2010. Comparably, the non-Hispanic white population's age-adjusted death rate is 43% greater than that of the population of Hispanic origin. In general, women had a 30% higher risk than men (21.0) of passing away from Alzheimer's disease (27.3 per 100,000 population). The highest death rate from Alzheimer's disease was seen in non-Hispanic white women, then non-Hispanic black women. Similarly, non-Hispanic white men had the highest age-adjusted death rates among men (22.0), followed by non-Hispanic black men (18.2). Hispanic women (19.5) and men (16.6) had the lowest rates of Alzheimer's disease-related deaths.

- **Alzheimer's Disease Death Rates Varied Widely Across the States:** There is no discernible regional trend in the age-adjusted death rates from Alzheimer's disease across the states. North Dakota (37.2), Tennessee (38.5), and Washington (43.6) had the highest age-adjusted death rates in 2010. Overall, 31 states had rates above the U.S. rate (25.1), whereas 19 states and the District of Columbia had rates lower than the U.S. rate.

2010 saw an increase in Alzheimer's disease-related deaths across the majority of age, sex, race, and Hispanic origin groups. Preliminary data indicates that 84,691 deaths in 2011 were thought to be related to Alzheimer's disease. At the moment, Alzheimer's disease ranks as the sixth most common cause of death in the US. Between 2000 and 2010, the age-adjusted death rate increased by 39%, from 18.1 in 2000 to 25.1. Alzheimer's disease claims more lives in women than in men, and it also affects non-Hispanic Whites more often than it does Non-Hispanic Blacks and People of Hispanic Origin. While all of the groups under discussion saw continuous increases in the mortality rate from Alzheimer's disease, there were notable variations in Alzheimer's mortality among the various racial and ethnic groups (Ferri et al., 2005; Thies & Bleiler, 2011).

Summary

- An estimated 6.7 million Americans age 65 and older are living with Alzheimer's dementia in 2023. 73% are age 75 or older.
- The number and proportion of older adults who have MCI due to Alzheimer's disease is currently difficult to estimate because they require population-based prevalence measures of MCI and Alzheimer's biomarkers, and this line of research is in its infancy. Furthermore, there is variation across studies in both the threshold of cognitive impairment required for an MCI diagnosis and the level of biomarker burden that defines the presence of Alzheimer's disease.
- The distribution of dementia around the world seems to vary according to cultural and socioeconomic differences among nations.
- A collaborative study of European population-based cohorts identified a total of 2346 cases of mild to severe dementia in 11 cohorts. Age-standardized prevalence was 6.4% for dementia (all causes), 4.4% for AD, and 1.6% for VaD.
- The burden of dementia is increasing exponentially, especially in the Asia-Pacific region, where more than 60% of the population resides. The prevalence of dementia seems to be higher in developed countries, like Japan and Korea, than in countries with low incomes in Asia.
- A systematic analysis in Africa estimated the overall prevalence of dementia in people older than 50 years in about 2.4% (2.76 million people), the majority of them living in Sub-Saharan Africa (76%).
- Epidemiologic research in cognitive aging identifies correlates of cognitive performance, cognitive decline, and dementia. A critical first step in conducting effective research is often taken for granted: clearly defining the scientific question and distinguishing whether this question is causal or predictive.
- Disparities across racial and ethnic groups in diagnosis and treatment rates and in the use of services are concerns from an ethical and policy perspective.
- The group of older adults who will be at risk for Alzheimer's in the coming years will be socially, culturally and economically different from previous groups of older U.S. adults. For example, between 2018 and 2040, projections for older adults show increases in the American Indian population of 75%, in the Black population of 88%, in the Asian population of 113% and in the Hispanic population of 175%.

References

1. Bennett, D. (2001). Public health importance of vascular dementia and Alzheimer's disease with cerebrovascular disease. *International Journal of Clinical Practice, Supplement, 120*, 41–48.
2. Etgen, T., Sander, D., Bickel, H., & Förstl, H. (2011). Mild cognitive impairment and dementia: The importance of modifiable risk factors. *Deutsches Ärzteblatt International, 108*, 743. https://doi.org/10.3238/arztebl.2011.0743.

3. Ferri, C. P., Prince, M., Brayne, C., et al. (2005). Global prevalence of dementia: A Delphi consensus study. *The Lancet, 366*(9503), 2112–2117. https://doi.org/10.1016/S0140-6736(05)67889-0.

4. Forette, F., & Boller, F. (1991). Hypertension and the risk of dementia in the elderly. *The American Journal of Medicine, 90*(3) Supplement 1S1-S116, DOI:https://doi.org/10.1016/0002-9343(91)90430-6 .

5. Harnack, L. J., Jeffery, R. W., & Boutelle, K. N. (2000). Temporal trends in energy intake in the United States: An ecologic perspective. *American Journal of Clinical Nutrition, 71*(6), 1478–1484. https://doi.org/10.1093/ajcn/71.6.1478.

6. Hendrie, H. C., Murrell, J., Gao, S., Unverzagt, F. W., Ogunniyi, A., & Hall, K. S. (2006). International studies in dementia with particular emphasis on populations of African origin. *Alzheimer's Disease and Associated Disorders, 20*(2), S42–S46. https://doi.org/10.1097/01.wad.0000213863.35605.3f.

7. Hillman, C. H., Erickson, K. I., & Kramer, A. F. (2008). Be smart, exercise your heart: Exercise effects on brain and cognition. *Nature Reviews Neuroscience, 9*(1), 58–65. https://doi.org/10.1038/nrn2298.

8. Horton, R. (2012). GBD 2010: Understanding disease, injury, and risk. *The Lancet, 380*(9859), 2053–2054. https://doi.org/10.1016/S0140-6736(12)62133-3.

9. Hoyert, D. L., & Xu, J. Q. (2012). Deaths: Preliminary data for 2011. *National Vital Statistics Reports, 61*(6), 1–51. Hyattsville, MD: National Center for Health Statistics.

10. Kalaria, R. N., Maestre, G. E., Arizaga, R., et al. (2008). Alzheimer's disease and vascular dementia in developing countries: Prevalence, management, and risk factors. *The Lancet Neurology, 7*(9), 812–826. https://doi.org/10.1016/S1474-4422(08)70169-8.

11. Knuth, A. G., & Hallal, P. C. (2009). Temporal trends in physical activity: A systematic review. *Journal of Physical Activity and Health, 6*(5), 548–559. https://doi.org/10.1123/jpah.6.5.548.

12. Kochanek, K. D., Xu, J. Q., Murphy, S. L., Miniño, A. M., & Kung, H. (2011). Deaths: Final data for 2009. *National Vital Statistics Reports, 60*(3), 1–116. Hyattsville, MD: National Center for Health Statistics.

13. Mayeda, E. R., et al. (2016). Inequalities in dementia incidence between six racial and ethnic groups over 14 years. *Alzheimer's & Dementia, 12*, 216–224. https://doi.org/10.1016/j.jalz.2015.12.007.

14. Mehta, K. M., et al. (2017). Systematic review of dementia prevalence and incidence in United States race/ethnic populations. *Alzheimer's & Dementia, 13*, 72–83. https://doi.org/10.1016/j.jalz.2016.06.2360.

15. Petersen, R. C., Doody, R., Kurz, A., Mohs, R. C., Morris, J. C., Rabins, P. V., et al. (2001). Current concepts in mild cognitive impairment. *Archives of Neurology, 58*, 1985–1992. https://doi.org/10.1001/archneur.58.12.1985.

16. Román, G. (2001). Diagnosis of vascular dementia and Alzheimer's disease. *International Journal of Clinical Practice, Supplement, 120*, 9–13.

17. Stites, S. D., et al. (2022). Establishing a framework for gathering structural and social determinants of health in Alzheimer's disease research centers. *The Gerontologist, 62*, 694–703. https://doi.org/10.1093/geront/gnab182.

18. Suh, G.-H., & Shah, A. (2001). A review of the epidemiological transition in dementia—Cross-national comparisons of the indices related to Alzheimer's disease and vascular dementia. *Acta Psychiatrica Scandinavica, 104*(1), 4–11. https://doi.org/10.1034/j.1600-0447.2001.104001004.x.

19. Thies, W., & Bleiler, L. (2011). 2011 Alzheimer's disease facts and figures. *Alzheimer's & Dementia, 7*(2), 208–244. https://doi.org/10.1016/j.jalz.2011.02.004.

20. Thun, M. J., Carter, B. D., Feskanich, D., et al. (2013). 50-year trends in smoking-related mortality in the United States. *New England Journal of Medicine, 368*(4), 351–364. https://doi.org/10.1056/NEJMsa1211127.

Chapter 4

EPIDEMIOLOGY OF ALZHEIMER'S DISEASE

Contents

Introduction 108
4.1. Epidemiology of Alzheimer's Disease: Occurrence, Determinants, and Strategies.. 110
4.2. Epidemiology of Alzheimer's Disease Modifiable Risk Factors and Prevention 124
4.3. Analytic Epidemiology of Alzheimer's Disease 134
Summary 146
References 146

INTRODUCTION

Alzheimer's disease is a neurodegenerative disorder that progresses over time and poses a major global public health challenge because of its high prevalence, impact on individuals and families, and cost of healthcare. Understanding the trends, contributing factors, and effects of Alzheimer's disease in different populations is made possible through the use of epidemiology. Alzheimer's disease is the most common cause of dementia, accounting for 60–70% of cases, according to epidemiological studies. Alzheimer's disease is more common as people age, with those over 65 having the highest rates of occurrence. Though less common, early-onset Alzheimer's can also strike people under the age of 65. Epidemiological research has identified several risk factors, such as genetics, age, and lifestyle choices. The main risk factor is advanced age, as the prevalence of Alzheimer's doubles every five years after 65. Early-onset familial Alzheimer's disease is linked to genetic factors, specifically mutations in genes like presenilin 1 (PSEN1), presenilin 2 (PSEN2), and the amyloid precursor protein (APP). Furthermore, the apolipoprotein E (APOE) gene has been linked to an increased risk of late-onset Alzheimer's disease; the ε4 allele of APOE appears to be protective, while the ε2 allele may be protective.

Apart from genetics, modifiable risk factors have been found by epidemiological studies to potentially play a role in the development of Alzheimer's disease. Heart-related risk factors include high blood pressure, diabetes, obesity, smoking, and other lifestyle factors like social isolation, physical inactivity, and cognitive inactivity. It may be possible to prevent or postpone the onset of Alzheimer's disease by addressing these risk factors through lifestyle changes and public health initiatives. Alzheimer's patients' relatives, carers, and the healthcare system are all impacted by the disease. The aging population and changing demographics are expected to drive a significant increase in the global prevalence of Alzheimer's disease in the upcoming decades, according to epidemiological projections. The development of strategies for early detection, diagnosis, and management of Alzheimer's disease, as well as support services for caregivers, is imperative in light of the significant challenges this demographic transition presents to healthcare systems. Furthering our knowledge of the natural history of Alzheimer's disease, finding biomarkers for early detection and diagnosis, and assessing potential interventions to stop or slow the disease's progression are all made possible by epidemiological research. Among the main epidemiological techniques used to clarify the intricate interactions between genetic, environmental, and lifestyle factors in the genesis and progression of Alzheimer's disease are longitudinal cohort studies, population-based surveys, and clinical trials.

Orientation and Directional Terms:

Term	Definition	Illustration
Dementia	A specific disease but is rather a general term for the impaired ability to remember, think, or make decisions that interferes with doing everyday activities.	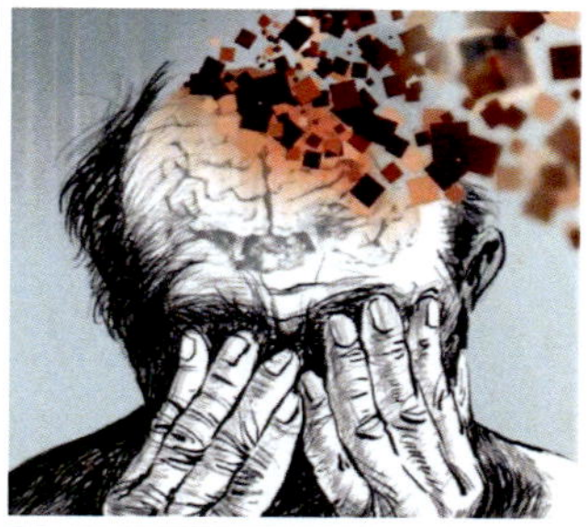
Cerebrovascular disease	A group of conditions that affect blood flow and the blood vessels in the brain. Problems with blood flow may occur from blood vessels narrowing (stenosis), clot formation (thrombosis), artery blockage (embolism), or blood vessel rupture (hemorrhage).	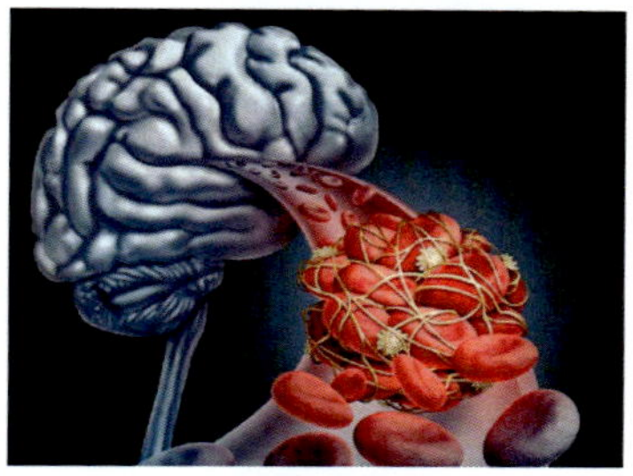
Cognitive function	A broad term that refers to mental processes involved in the acquisition of knowledge, manipulation of information, and reasoning.	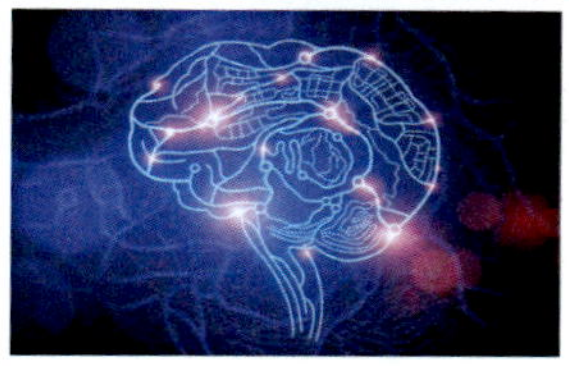
Gender difference	The distinctions between individuals based on their gender identity, which is typically categorized as male, female, or non-binary. These differences can manifest in various aspects of life, including behavior, cognition, emotions, and social roles.	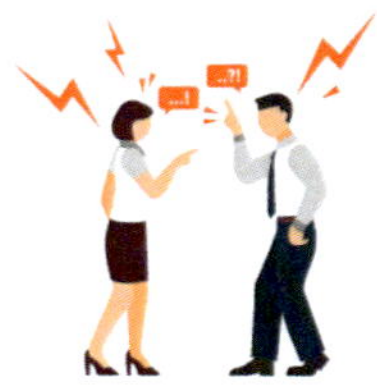
Neuroimaging	Neuroimaging is the use of quantitative techniques to study the structure and function of the central nervous system, developed as an objective way of scientifically studying the healthy human brain in a non-invasive manner.	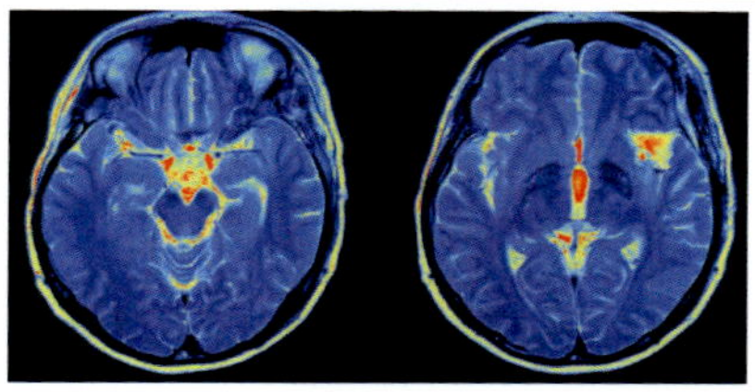

4.1. EPIDEMIOLOGY OF ALZHEIMER'S DISEASE: OCCURRENCE, DETERMINANTS, AND STRATEGIES

When dementia strikes an elderly person, Alzheimer's disease is the most common cause. The prevalence ratios (cases per 100 people 65 years of age and older) that are currently available vary from 0 points6 in China to 5 points8 in Scotland. Various case ascertainment techniques and definitions of the disease being studied may have an impact on this variability. Age-specific prevalence ratios were consistently higher in women than in men in many of the studies, and all of the studies demonstrated an exponential increase in prevalence ratios with age. The incidence rates of Alzheimer's disease rise exponentially with age and are higher in women, in line with the prevalence pattern. In the 40–60-year-old age group, the rate is estimated to be around 0.01 per 1000, and in subjects 75 years of age and older, it rises to 10 per 1000. Our understanding of the risk factors for Alzheimer's disease is primarily based on data from case-control studies. In case-control studies, Alzheimer's disease was found to be associated with a prior head trauma and a family history of dementia. Genetic studies that revealed a genetic defect localized on chromosome 21 in certain families with a high incidence of Alzheimer's disease also provided evidence for the involvement of genetic factors in the etiology of the disease. Smoking and aluminum exposure have also been linked to Alzheimer's disease in case-control studies. More research is necessary to fully understand these and other proposed risk factors (Harvey, Fox, Rossor, 1999; Kalaria et al., 2008; Xu, Ferrari, & Wang, 2013).

4.1.1. Global Aging

The phenomenon of population aging has spread globally. Over 2 million senior citizens, or those 65 and over, lived in 26 countries in 1990; by 2030, projections show that 34 more countries will have joined the group. The world's population of people 65 years of age or older was estimated to be 420 million in 2000. By 2030, that number is expected to rise to nearly 1 billion, with an increase in the percentage of elderly people from 7 to 12%. The number of elderly people will nearly triple in developing nations from 249 million in 2000 to an estimated 690 million in 2030, representing the biggest increase in the world. The percentage of the global aging population that lives in developing regions will rise from 59 to 71%. The elderly population will gradually age in developed nations, where there has already been a noticeable rise in the number of people over 65. The "demographic transition," which is characterized by a decline in mortality and subsequently in fertility, is the underlying process of global population aging. The age distribution of the population has changed in most parts of the world due to a combination of declining fertility and increasing life expectancy, which has caused a relative shift in weight from younger to older age groups.

As aging societies become more common, both developed and developing nations will have to deal with the challenge of managing a high frequency of chronic conditions like dementia. These illnesses lower the well-being of those who are affected and their families, making it more difficult for elderly people to live their best lives in the community. Furthermore, the entire society is responsible for covering the high costs of healthcare-associated with these conditions. As a result, the global trend of population aging has a significant effect on public health, healthcare financing, and delivery systems globally. As the population ages, dementia has emerged as a significant issue for public health and elder care.

4.1.2. Dementia and Alzheimer's Disease

A clinical syndrome known as dementia is typified by the emergence of several cognitive impairments severe enough to impede day-to-day functioning, including social and professional functioning. Memory impairment is one of the cognitive deficits, along with at least one other cognitive domain such as aphasia, apraxia, agnosia, or executive functioning disorders. At 60–70% of all cases of dementia in the elderly, Alzheimer's disease is the most common cause of the condition. When neurofibrillary tangles and senile plaques are found in the brains of dementia patients, Alzheimer's disease is strictly diagnosed as a neuropathological condition. Memory loss is often the first symptom of the disease, but eventually, a progressive global cognitive impairment sets in. The second most common cause of dementia in the elderly, after Alzheimer's disease, is vascular dementia. The loss of cognitive function brought on by ischemic, hypoperfusion, or hemorrhagic brain lesions as a result of cerebrovascular illness or cardiovascular pathology is known as vascular dementia. Vascular dementia diagnosis necessitates cognitive impairment, brain imaging evidence of vascular brain lesions, often primarily subcortical, a temporal correlation between dementia and stroke, and ruling out other dementia causes. Mixed dementia is likely the most prevalent kind of dementia because it is characterized by pathological changes in older people's brains that are most frequently caused by the combination of vascular dementia and Alzheimer's disease.

Although Alzheimer's disease was initially discovered over a century ago, only in the last 30 years has research into its signs, causes, risk factors, and treatments gathered steam. The exact physiologic alterations that precipitate the onset of Alzheimer's disease are still mostly unknown, even though research has provided a wealth of information about the disease. The only exceptions are a few uncommon, hereditary types of the illness that are known to result from genetic mutations. Although the symptoms of Alzheimer's disease vary from person to person, the most typical symptom pattern starts with a steadily declining memory for new information. This happens because the brain areas responsible for creating new memories are typically where disruptions in brain cell function start. People encounter additional challenges as the damage grows. Alzheimer's disease warning signs include memory loss that interferes with day-to-day functioning; difficulties organizing or solving problems; inability to finish familiar tasks at work, home, or leisure; confusion about time and place; difficulty understanding visual images and spatial relationships; new difficulties with words when speaking or writing; inability to remember where you put things or how to find them again; diminished or poor judgment; withdrawal from social or professional activities; and changes in mood and personality. The person's cognitive and functional abilities deteriorate as the illness worsens. People with advanced Alzheimer's disease require assistance with dressing, eating, taking a shower, and using the restroom, among other basic daily living tasks. As the illness progresses, a person loses their capacity for speech, becomes bedridden and dependent on 24-hour care, and is unable to identify loved ones. A person with Alzheimer's disease who has trouble moving is more susceptible to infections, such as pneumonia (lung infection).

4.1.3. Occurrence of Alzheimer's Disease

A disease's occurrence can be quantified as the number of new cases that arise within a given time frame in a population at risk of contracting the illness (incidence) or as the percentage of individuals in a defined population who are afflicted by the disease at a given time point (prevalence). Whereas the incidence represents the likelihood of contracting the disease, the prevalence represents the disease's impact on public health. Both the disease's incidence and duration determine its prevalence, which in some cases can be calculated as incidence × average disease duration.

4.1.4. Prevalence

Experts estimated that there are currently 24.3 million dementia sufferers, with 4.6 million new cases of dementia occurring annually (one new case every 7 seconds) based on the epidemiological data that is currently available. By 2040, there will be 81.11 million affected individuals, which doubles every 20 years. Prior reports have provided comparable estimates. Most dementia sufferers reside in developing nations. The number of people with dementia is highest in China and its western Pacific neighbors (6 million), followed by the United States (2.9 million), India (1.5 million), and the European Union (5.0 million). Globally, the rate of increase in dementia cases is not constant; between 2001 and 2040, numbers in developed nations are expected to rise by 100%, but in India, China, and other south Asian and western Pacific countries, they are expected to rise by more than 300%. Alzheimer's disease was identified as the cause of about 70% of these cases. Age-standardized prevalence in individuals 65 years of age and older was found to be 6 points 4 percent for dementia and 4 points 4 percent for Alzheimer's disease, according to pooled data from population-based studies conducted in Europe. Alzheimer's disease is 9 points 7 percent common in the US, according to a study done on a nationally representative sample of adults over the age of 70.

Globally, the estimated prevalence of dementia in individuals 60 years of age and older was 31.9%. Regionally, the prevalence was 11.6% in Africa, 4.0 percent in China and the Western Pacific, 4.6 percent in Latin America, 5.4 percent in Western Europe, and 6.4 percent in North America. A meta-analysis encompassing eighteen studies conducted in China between 1990 and 2010 revealed a 1.9% prevalence of Alzheimer's disease. Approximately 5 million new cases of dementia are diagnosed each year, affecting over 25 million people worldwide. The majority of these cases are caused by Alzheimer's disease. It is projected that the number of dementia cases will double every 20 years. The age-specific prevalence of AD has been found to be roughly similar across regions in several meta-analyzes and nationwide surveys, despite varying inclusion criteria (Figure 4.1). After 65 years of age, the age-specific prevalence of Alzheimer's disease nearly doubles every five years. In developed countries, one in 10 elderly individuals over 65 suffers from dementia to some extent, while over one-third of the very old (over 85) may exhibit dementia-related symptoms and indicators. The two most prevalent types of dementia, vascular dementia and Alzheimer's disease, account for 15% to 25% and 50% to 70% of all dementia cases, respectively. There is a similar pattern of dementia subtypes throughout the world.

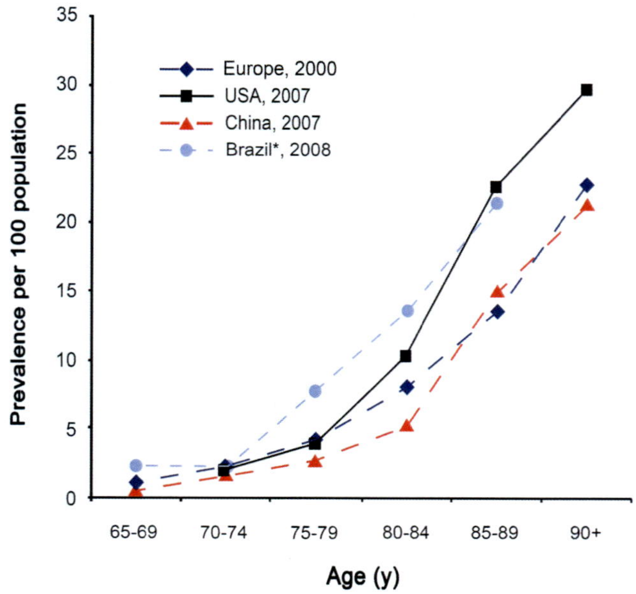

Figure 4.1. *Age-specific prevalence of Alzheimer's disease (per 100 population) across continents and countries.*

**prevalence of all types of dementia.*

Source: *Xu, W., Ferrari, C., & Wang, H. X. (2013). Epidemiology of Alzheimer's Disease. InTech. doi: 10.5772/54398.*

Recent years have seen a significant increase in interest in epidemiological studies of dementia and AD in low- and middle-income nations. According to a systematic review, 3 percent of people in developing nations were estimated to have Alzheimer's disease overall (95% confidence interval: 1 percent to 5 percent). In seven developing countries, the prevalence of dementia (according to the DSM-IV criteria) among individuals 65 years of age and older ranged greatly from less than 0.5 percent to more than 6 percent, which is significantly lower than in developed nations. In fact, dementia prevalence rates in rural Latin America and India were about 25% lower than those in European nations. However, the prevalence of AD among people 65 and older in Chinese cities was 3.5%, and it increased to 4.8% after post-hoc correction for negative screening errors. These figures are generally comparable with those from Western countries. Similar dementia prevalence rates have also been reported from Latin American urban populations, including 6 percent in Havana, Cuba, and 5 percent in São Paulo, Brazil (Harvey, Fox, & Rossor, 1999; Kalaria et al., 2008; Xu, Ferrari, & Wang, 2013).

4.1.5. Incidence

The yearly incidence of dementia worldwide is approximately 7.5 per 1,000 individuals. From about one case per 1,000 persons annually in those 60–64 years old to more than 70 cases per 1,000 persons annually in those 90 years and older, the incidence rate of dementia rises exponentially with age. When it comes to younger adults (less than 75 years old), dementia incidence rates vary less between regions, but they do more among older adults. In contrast to Europe and Asia, the USA has slightly lower rates, which may be the result of variations in study designs and case ascertainment techniques. In Europe, the aggregate incidence rate of Alzheimer's disease among those 65 and older was 19 per 1,000 person-year. The combined data from two extensive community-based studies conducted in the US, involving individuals over 65, in the Seattle and Baltimore areas, revealed an incidence rate of 15.0 (13.0 for men and 16.9 for women) per 1,000 person-year for Alzheimer's disease. Up until the age of 85, the incidence rate of Alzheimer's disease rises nearly exponentially with age (Figure 4.2).

Alzheimer's disease incidence that continuously increases exponentially with age implies that the disease is an inevitable part of aging, but a decline or convergence to a certain age may indicate that older individuals are less vulnerable, possibly due to environmental or genetic factors. The Cache County Study also discovered that, for both men and women, the incidence of AD rose with age, peaked, and then began to decline at very old ages. Nevertheless, a few meta-analyzes and extensive research conducted in Europe did not find any support for the hypothesis that the incidence of dementia and Alzheimer's disease may be declining among the oldest age groups. The apparent decline that some studies have suggested could be a result of the poor response rates and survival effects of these groups. Studies conducted in North America did not find a significant gender difference in the incidence of Alzheimer's disease, but several European studies found that women were more likely than men to have the disease, particularly in the oldest age groups.

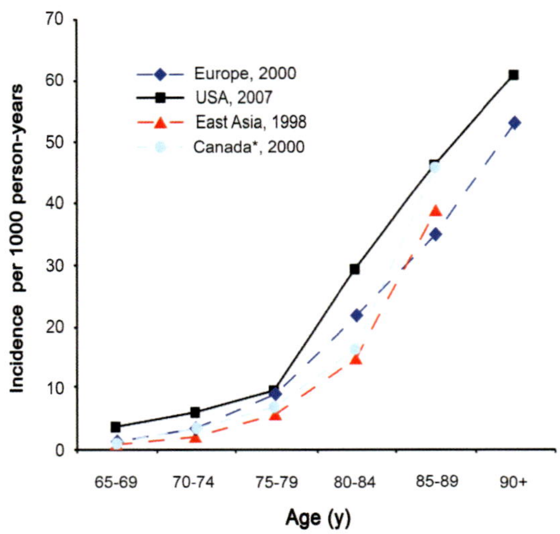

Figure 4.2. *Age-specific incidence of Alzheimer's disease (per 1,000 person years) across continents and countries.*

*Incidence of all types of dementia.

Source: *Xu, W., Ferrari, C., & Wang, H. X., (2013). Epidemiology of Alzheimer's Disease. InTech. doi: 10.5772/54398.*

There seem to be some regional differences in the prevalence of Alzheimer's. Eight European studies' combined data revealed a geographical dissociation across Europe, with higher incidence rates among the oldest old residents of northwest countries compared to those in southern countries. There have been reports that North America has somewhat lower incidence rates of Alzheimer's disease than Europe. Variations in approach, e.g., geographic variations may be partially explained by factors other than actual differences in the disease's regional distribution, such as variations in study design and case ascertainment procedures. There was no evidence of dementia incidence variation among the five areas in England and Wales according to a study conducted in the UK using the same methods. Research has shown that the incidence of AD is typically lower in developing nations than it is in North America and Europe. For instance, the incidence rate of AD in adults 65 years of age and older was 2.7 per 1,000 persons annually in Brazil and 3.2 per 1,000 persons annually in India.

4.1.6. Prognosis and Impact

One of the main causes of death for the elderly is dementia. However, even when several underlying causes of death are considered, death certificates grossly underreport the cause of death. The follow-up studies conducted in the community may yield trustworthy mortality data. The mortality rate from dementia was 2:04 per 100 person-year in the Swedish Kungsholmen Project, which included people 75 years of age or older. 70% of incident dementia cases passed away within five years of the diagnosis. Over half of the cases of dementia progressed to the severe stage within a three-year period. The percentage of severe dementia among prevalent cases in the Kungsholmen Project rose from 19% at baseline to 48% after three years and 78% after seven years. A decline in both cognition and function is the cause of this progression. Dementia has been found to be the primary predictor of developing dependence and functional decline over a three-year period, which explains its strong association with disability. The most common disorders among older adults residing in nursing homes or other institutions in industrialized countries are mental illness and cognitive impairment. Approximately half of those who developed functional dependence within three years can be attributed to dementia. However, the institutionalization of mentally ill patients varies according to age distribution, living in an urban or rural area, and other cultural factors. 70% of incident dementia cases in a population over 75 years old died within five years of the diagnosis, translating into a dementia-specific death rate of 2 points per 100 person-years. The chance of dying is tripled in dementia. At the societal level, the enormous and quickly expanding number of dementia patients' needs for healthcare and social services has a significant financial impact. According to estimates, the global direct costs of dementia in 2003 were estimated to be 156 billion USD, assuming a prevalence of 27.7 million dementia cases worldwide. It is clear that the dementing conditions will pose a significant challenge as a result of these costs and the anticipated rise in the number of elderly people in developing nations.

4.1.7. Risk and Protective Factors

Alzheimer's disease is a multifactorial disorder influenced by a person's genetic makeup, environment, and interactions with both. In the case of chronic multifactorial diseases like dementia, where the life-course approach should be taken into account, the primary epidemiological method for identifying influential factors is a population-based prospective study. Alzheimer's disease is primarily determined by age, with a small percentage of cases being caused by genetic mutations. The significant correlation between Alzheimer's disease and advancing age could be attributed in part to the cumulative impact of various protective and risk factors over an individual's lifetime, such as the intricate interplay between genetic predisposition, psychological variables, biological factors, and lifelong environmental exposures. While the etiologic roles of occupational exposures, inflammation, and dietary or nutritional factors, as well as vascular and psychosocial factors, are less well-established, epidemiological, neuroimaging, and neuropathological research all support the involvement of these factors in the development of Alzheimer's disease.

4.1.7.1. Genetic Factors

Presentilin-1, presenilin-2, and amyloid precursor protein mutations are the only causes of early-onset familial Alzheimer's disease, accounting for less than 5% of cases. Most AD cases occur randomly, and there is a great deal of variation in the neuropathological characteristics and risk profiles of these cases.

- **Apolipoprotein E ε4 (APOE ε4):** The only known susceptibility gene for both early- and late-onset Alzheimer's disease is the APOE ε4 allele. It is important to note that this gene is only susceptibility and is neither necessary nor sufficient for the onset of Alzheimer's disease. One of the three common forms of the APOE gene (ε2, ε3, and ε4), which codes for a protein that transports cholesterol in the bloodstream, is APOEε4. Each parent gives one copy of the APOE gene to each child. Individuals who receive a single APOE ε4 gene are more likely to experience Alzheimer's disease and to do so at a younger age compared to those who receive ε2 or ε3 forms of the gene. A higher risk is associated with two APOE-ε4 genes being inherited. It is not a guarantee that someone who inherits one or two copies of this form of the APOE gene will get Alzheimer's disease, unlike if they inherit a known genetic mutation for the disease. The APOE ε4 allele's risk effect diminishes with age; after age 75, the APOE genotype accounts for 15–20% of Alzheimer's cases. Numerous additional genes have been investigated as potential candidates, but the findings and reports are inconsistent. But not every (4-carrier) gets dementia. Research has indicated that having a high level of education, engaging in physically demanding hobbies, or maintaining good vascular health may lower the risk of dementia associated with APOE ε4. These ε4-carriers seem to have a dementia-free survival time that is comparable to that of non-ε4-carriers. Furthermore, there may be an interaction between the obese-related FTO gene and APOE ε4 that raises the risk of Alzheimer's disease.
- **Family History:** Compared to people without a first-degree relative with Alzheimer's, those who have a parent, brother, or sister with the illness are more likely to get it themselves. An even higher risk of Alzheimer's disease development is experienced by those who have multiple first-degree relatives affected by the illness. Heredity (genetics), shared environmental and/or lifestyle factors, or both, may be involved when diseases run in families.

4.1.7.2. Biological Risk Factors

One known risk factor for Alzheimer's disease is getting older. Every five years of age, the incidence of Alzheimer's disease nearly doubles. In particular, female sex is frequently linked to an elevated risk of AD in older adults. It appears that men are more likely than women to develop vascular dementia.

4.1.7.3. Vascular Disorders and Risk Factors

Alzheimer's disease has been associated with many vascular risk factors and disorders; however, the age at which an exposure is evaluated may affect the relationship between a given factor and the risk of Alzheimer's disease.

- **Blood Pressure:** High blood pressure in middle age has been linked to an increased risk of dementia and Alzheimer's disease, according to numerous studies. The brain's neurodegenerative markers have been linked to hypertension, indicating that chronically high blood pressure may either directly cause brain atrophy or contribute to the neurodegenerative process itself. Low blood pressure appears to be a predictor of dementia and Alzheimer's disease, while high blood pressure has less of an adverse effect in very old people. The longitudinal data from the Kungsholmen Project confirmed that low blood pressure in late life may be an indicator of impending illness due to the long latent period of dementia. This suggests that cerebral hypo-perfusion and low blood pressure in late life may play a role in the development of dementia and Alzheimer's disease. These results imply that there may be an age-dependent relationship between blood pressure and dementia.

The duration of treatment and the age at which people start taking the medications may have an impact on the preventive effect of antihypertensive therapy on dementia and AD, according to recent follow-up studies. Younger adults (i.e., <75 years) as well as individuals receiving ongoing care. The section on intervention trials towards primary prevention summarizes the evidence from clinical trials of dementia and antihypertensive therapy. Antihypertensive medication may delay the onset of atherosclerosis, lower the number of cerebrovascular lesions, and increase cerebral perfusion to prevent dementia and AD. Additionally, some antihypertensive medications (e.g., antagonists of the calcium channel) may provide neuroprotective benefits. Significantly fewer neuropathological alterations associated with Alzheimer's disease (i.e., neuritic plaque and neurofibrillary tangle densities) in the group receiving medication for hypertension compared to the non-hypertensive group, which may indicate a protective effect of antihypertensive therapy against neuropathology linked to Alzheimer's disease.

- **Cardiovascular Disease:** Maintaining a strong and healthy heart is essential for adequate blood flow to the brain. A study from the Cardiovascular Health Study found that individuals with cardiovascular disease, particularly those with peripheral arterial disease, were at a higher risk of developing Alzheimer's disease. This suggests that having extensive peripheral atherosclerosis can increase the likelihood of developing Alzheimer's. Other cardiovascular conditions, like heart failure and atrial fibrillation, have also been linked to a higher risk of dementia. In the Kungsholmen Project, individuals with heart failure were found to have more than an 80% increased risk of developing dementia and Alzheimer's disease.

- **Cerebrovascular Disease:** Dementia risk is increased by cerebral vascular abnormalities, including white matter changes, small and large ischemic cortical infarcts, hemorrhagic infarcts, and vasculopathies. An estimated two- to four-fold increased risk of incident dementia associated with clinical stroke (post-stroke dementia) is found by systematic reviews of population-based studies. Recurrent and strategic strokes, as well as multiple cerebral infarcts, are the primary risk factors for post-stroke dementia. White matter lesions found on neuroimaging and silent stroke are linked to an increased risk of dementia and cognitive decline. Brain emboli that occurred spontaneously were linked to VaD and AD. According to certain research, stroke and cognitive decline are related to Alzheimer's disease. When neurodegenerative damages are insufficient for an individual to exhibit dementia, cerebral vascular lesions may combine with neurodegenerative lesions to produce dementia syndrome. According to neuropathological research, cerebrovascular lesions, atherosclerosis, and neurodegenerative changes frequently coexist in the brain and may be related processes that combine to impair the aging brain further and enhance the clinical manifestation of dementia syndrome.
- **Diabetes Mellitus:** More than 80 years ago, a possible connection between diabetes and cognitive decline was first documented. It is now widely known that diabetes is linked to these cognitive alterations. A growing body of research indicates that type 2 diabetes is linked to cognitive impairment that affects executive function as well as memory. Numerous extensive, long-term studies conducted on a population-based sample have also demonstrated that older adults with type 2 diabetes experience an accelerated rate of cognitive decline. Several longitudinal studies have reported an increased risk of both vascular dementia and neurodegenerative type dementia in individuals with diabetes; a systematic review has confirmed this risk effect. Diabetes in middle age or diabetes for a longer period of time may be very important in dementia and Alzheimer's disease. Overall, diabetes increases the risk of dementia by 60% and causes a decline in cognitive function of 20–70%. Furthermore, a higher risk of dementia and Alzheimer's disease in the elderly is associated with borderline or prediabetes as well as impaired glucose tolerance.
- **Overweight and Obesity:** As with hypertension, obesity and dementia may be related for a person's lifetime, according to recent research. A higher middle-aged body mass index (BMI) was linked to a higher late-life risk of dementia. There was a higher BMI decline about 10 years before dementia symptoms appeared,

which is consistent with other research that links an earlier BMI decline to Alzheimer's disease. When measured less than 10 years before a clinical diagnosis of Alzheimer's disease, low BMI and weight loss can be interpreted as indicators of preclinical Alzheimer's disease. Low BMI and weight loss in later life may be associated with a higher risk of dementia and Alzheimer's disease. These results were supported by multiple follow-up studies of the elderly, which found a link between an accelerated BMI decline and the eventual onset of Alzheimer's disease. A 5- to 6-year period after a low BMI in late life was linked to an increased risk of Alzheimer's disease. Therefore, low body mass index and weight loss in later life may serve as indicators of preclinical Alzheimer's disease, especially if they are measured a few years before the disease is officially diagnosed.

- **Hyperlipidemia:** Certain studies have reported a correlation between middle-aged elevated cholesterol and a higher risk of Alzheimer's disease in later life. There have also been conflicting reports regarding the link between late-life cholesterol and the risk of dementia. Certain cohort studies discovered no correlation, or even the opposite, between total cholesterol and the risk of dementia. A decrease in total cholesterol was observed in a study at least 15 years before the onset of dementia. There has been recent evidence of a bidirectional relationship between cholesterol and cognition. Reduced cholesterol after midlife may indicate worsening cognitive status, but high cholesterol in midlife was linked to worse late-life cognition.
- **The Metabolic Syndrome:** Numerous studies have evaluated the association between the metabolic syndrome as a whole and the risk of Alzheimer's disease or cognitive decline, rather than examining the impact of its component parts. In recent years, there has been a growing focus on a group of interconnected metabolic risk factors, including diabetes, obesity, hypertension, and dyslipidemia. Individual metabolic syndrome components have been linked to cognitive outcomes. A prospective study discovered a link between cognitive decline and the metabolic syndrome. However, this result was not validated in an elderly population. In this age range, the metabolic syndrome concept might have less applicability. Ultimately, it was demonstrated by two studies that metabolic syndrome raised the risk of Alzheimer's disease.
- **Alcohol Consumption:** Overconsumption of alcohol can raise the risk of vascular dementia and cause alcoholic dementia. A higher chance of dementia in later life has been linked to middle-age alcohol consumption. On the other hand, a growing body of research indicates that moderate to light alcohol consumption may be linked to a lower risk of dementia and cognitive decline—an effect that

is also seen with cardiovascular disease. Light to moderate alcohol consumption was linked to a lower risk of dementia and Alzheimer's disease in a meta-analysis of 15 prospective studies on the impact of alcohol on dementia risk. The inverse association between moderate alcohol consumption and dementia may be the result of various factors such as information bias, the confounding of high socioeconomic status and healthy lifestyles, different methods used to assess alcohol consumption or outcome misclassification. Nevertheless, the significance of moderate alcohol consumption in dementia remains controversial.

- **Cigarette Smoking:** It's still unclear how smoking and cognitive decline are related. The majority of case-control research points to smoking as a risk factor for Alzheimer's disease. According to certain prospective studies, smoking is linked to a higher risk of Alzheimer's disease. The combined findings of 18 cross-sectional studies without industry affiliations revealed no association between smoking and Alzheimer's disease, according to a meta-analysis that looked at the relationship between smoking and the disease while taking tobacco industry affiliation into account. The risk of Alzheimer's disease was found to be significantly higher after 14 cohort studies that were not associated with the tobacco industry were analyzed. The Kungsholmen Project found that smoking had a greater impact on survival in individuals with Alzheimer's disease than in individuals without the disease. Additionally, smoking was no longer found to have a protective effect against Alzheimer's disease when incident cases of the disease were examined, indicating that the previously documented link between cigarette smoking and a low prevalence of dementia was likely the result of survival bias.
- **Diet and Nutrients:** Consumptions of seafood, fruits, and vegetables are rich in polyunsaturated fatty acids (PUFAs), which are antioxidants. High or additional vitamin C, E, B6, B12, and folate intake has been linked in certain observational studies to a lower risk of Alzheimer's disease. It has been discovered that there is a link between a higher risk of Alzheimer's disease and low levels of folate and B12. Research on how dietary PUFAs affect the likelihood of cognitive dysfunction was unable to conclude. Consuming PUFAs has been linked to a lower risk of dementia, Alzheimer's disease, and mild cognitive impairment, according to several studies. According to population-based studies, eating a moderate to high amount of unsaturated fats during midlife may be protective, while eating a moderate amount of saturated fats may raise the risk of dementia and Alzheimer's disease, particularly in those who carry the APOE ε4 gene. Through some pathways, including inflammation and atherosclerosis, fatty acids may influence dementia. Independent of vascular pathways,

adherence to the "Mediterranean diet," which calls for a higher intake of antioxidant-rich fruits, vegetables, and fish, has been linked to a lower risk of Alzheimer's disease.

4.1.7.4. Psychosocial Factors

Psychological factors include social economic status, education attainment in early life, and work complexity in adult-life and leisure activities. Evidence from epidemiological research has been accumulating that some psychosocial factors and a healthy lifestyle may postpone the onset of dementia, possibly by enhancing cognitive reserve.

- **Social Economic Status:** Social economic status, early educational attainment, adult work complexity, and leisure activities are examples of psychological factors. A growing body of epidemiological research data suggests that certain psychosocial variables and a healthy lifestyle may delay the onset of dementia, perhaps by improving cognitive reserve.
- **High Education:** Higher educational attainment in early life is consistently linked to a lower incidence of dementia, and specifically Alzheimer's disease, according to numerous longitudinal studies. Several surveys have found that highly educated people have a low prevalence of dementia. The risk of dementia may be lowered by lifetime mental activity linked to childhood education and educational attainment. According to the cognitive reserve hypothesis, education may improve neural and cognitive reserve, which could offer compensatory mechanisms to deal with degenerative pathological changes in the brain and postpone the onset of dementia syndrome. On the other hand, intelligence quotient, early life living conditions, and occupational toxic exposure experienced throughout adulthood may be substituted for or indicated by academic achievement (Harvey, Fox, Rossor, 1999; Kalaria et al., 2008; Xu, Ferrari, & Wang, 2013).
- **Physical Activity:** The idea that increased physical activity delays the onset of dementia is strongly supported by basic science and observational data on humans. Frequent exercise has been linked to a lower risk of dementia and cognitive decline, even low-intensity exercise like walking. In contrast to sports and any particular physical activity, the Kungsholmen Project found that physical activity that manifested itself in a variety of leisure activities was linked to a lower risk of dementia. Regular physical activity during middle age has been shown to have a strong protective effect against the development of dementia and Alzheimer's disease in later life, particularly in those who carry the APOE ε4 allele. While short bursts of exercise training may not have a significant impact on cognitive processes—since it can take years to reach high levels of physical fitness—they may nevertheless be noticeable in the subsets of cognitive domains that are more susceptible to age-related declines. In addition to supporting vascular

and overall health, physical activity also supports brain plasticity and may influence several neurotropic factors and gene transcripts that are crucial for the preservation of cognitive abilities. This theory is now being supported by a growing body of trial data regarding the advantages of exercise for cognitive function in both healthy older adults and those at risk for dementia. There aren't any RCTs that support the idea that dementia can be avoided with increased physical activity, though.

- **Mentally Stimulating Activity:** Numerous mentally taxing pursuits have been studied in connection with dementia and AD; these pursuits include knitting, gardening, dancing, playing musical instruments and board games, reading, participating in social and cultural events, and watching particular television shows, all of which have frequently been shown to have a protective effect. Due to individual and cultural differences in preference for particular activities, some researchers compiled mentally stimulating activities into a composite score. This composite score, which included participation in seven common activities with information processing as a central component, was linked to a lower risk of Alzheimer's disease (AD) even after adjusting for depressive symptoms, medical conditions, and the APOE ε4 allele. According to the Swedish Twin Study, working in more complex environments, especially when interacting with people, may lower the risk of Alzheimer's. High levels of complexity at work seemed to be linked to a lower risk of dementia, but mostly vascular dementia, according to the Canadian Study of Health and Aging. A high degree of complex mental activity throughout life was correlated with a lower rate of hippocampal atrophy, according to a recent neuroimaging study, which lends support to these findings.
- **Social Network and Social Engagement:** An increased risk of dementia has been linked to social disengagement or having a poor social network in later life. Longitudinal observational studies have provided evidence linking social disengagement or a weak social network to dementia and cognitive decline. Seniors who experience greater social isolation and fewer, unsatisfactory interactions with friends and family are also more vulnerable to dementia and AD. Moreover, a doubled risk of dementia and AD in later life was linked to low social engagement in late life and a decline in social engagement from middle age to late life. Better social support is implied by rich social networks and high levels of social engagement, which improves access to resources and material goods. Vast and rich social networks also offer intellectual and affective stimulation, which may have an impact on various health outcomes and cognitive function via behavioral, psychological, and physiological pathways. Last but not least, a recent study revealed that the personality trait linked to the lowest risk of dementia was low neuroticism combined with high extraversion; among socially isolated people, low neuroticism even appeared to reduce the risk of dementia.
- **Depression:** There is a strong correlation between depression and Alzheimer's disease, according to recent research. Major depression throughout one's lifetime has been linked to an increased risk of developing Alzheimer's disease in the future. The transition from mild cognitive impairment to Alzheimer's disease may

be impacted by the presence of depressive symptoms. The two main characteristics of an Alzheimer's disease brain, neuronal plaques and neurofibrillary tangles, are more prominent in the brains of patients with comorbid depression than in those without the illness. Conversely, patients with a history of depression have shown signs of neurodegenerative phenomena in various brain regions. Recent research indicates that the pathophysiology of Alzheimer's disease may be related to the molecular pathways and cascades that underpin the pathogenesis of major depression, such as hyper-activation of the hypothalamic-pituitary-adrenal (HPA) axis and chronic inflammation. According to a study, individuals with diabetes who experience depression have a higher risk of dementia (Harvey, Fox, Rossor, 1999; Kalaria et al., 2008; Xu, Ferrari, & Wang, 2013).

4.1.7.5. Other Factors

- **Inflammation:** It is well known that the atherosclerotic process involves inflammation. Serum inflammatory mediators may therefore be linked to dementia. There has been a correlation discovered in certain cohort studies, and the most promising marker for dementia risk prediction may be C-reactive protein. Furthermore, it has been proposed that long-term use of non-steroidal anti-inflammatory drugs is linked to a decreased risk of AD.
- **Hormone Replacement Therapy:** It has been widely reported that hormone replacement therapy in postmenopausal women is linked to a decreased risk of AD. Up until 2004, many observational studies had consistently shown a link between hormone replacement therapy and a lower risk of dementia and Alzheimer's disease in postmenopausal women. However, the Women's Health Study discovered a significantly higher risk of dementia associated with estrogenic therapy, rather than a protective effect.
- **Occupational Exposures:** There is a link between manual labor in the manufacturing of goods and a higher risk of AD and dementia. Employment and risks associated with it (e.g., heavy metals, and electromagnetic fields) could contribute to dementia and Alzheimer's disease. Data from the Kungsholmen Project demonstrated that manual labor in the production of goods was linked to a higher risk of dementia and Alzheimer's disease, with electromagnetic exposure being associated with a particular risk effect. Numerous follow-up studies have linked occupational exposure to extremely-low-frequency electromagnetic fields (ELF-EMF) to an increased risk of dementia and AD. According to a meta-analysis of epidemiological data, there may be a link between AD and occupational exposure to ELF-EMF.

- **Head Trauma and Traumatic Brain Injury:** Although head trauma has been thoroughly studied in numerous studies and has been proposed as a potential risk factor for Alzheimer's disease for a long time, there is ongoing debate regarding this connection. Compared to people who have never had a head injury, those who have moderate head injuries have a twofold increased risk of developing Alzheimer's disease, while those who have severe head injuries have a fivefold increased risk. A head injury is classified as moderate if it causes a loss of consciousness or post-traumatic amnesia that lasts longer than thirty minutes; if either condition persists for more than twenty-four hours, the injury is classified as severe. It has not been demonstrated that people with mild head injuries or those who suffer from a variety of common accidents, like bumping their head when getting out of a car, are at higher risk. Individuals who have sustained repeated head injuries, such as football players, boxers, and veterans of combat, may be more susceptible to dementia, late-life cognitive impairment, and autopsy evidence of tau tangles, a characteristic of Alzheimer's disease. To gain a deeper understanding of the correlation between brain injury and an elevated risk of Alzheimer's disease, more investigation is required (Harvey, Fox, Rossor, 1999; Kalaria et al., 2008; Xu, Ferrari, & Wang, 2013).

4.2. EPIDEMIOLOGY OF ALZHEIMER'S DISEASE MODIFIABLE RISK FACTORS AND PREVENTION

The most common type of dementia, Alzheimer's disease (AD), is characterized by a decline in cognition, function, and behavior. Usually, memory loss related to recent events is the first sign of AD. The two most important pathological characteristics found in the brain tissues of AD patients are elevated levels of hyperphosphorylated tau (p-tau), which aggregates intracellularly as neurofibrillary tangles (NFTs), and amyloid-β (Aβ), which forms extracellular senile plaques.

Around 50 million people worldwide suffer from dementia, and as the population ages, it is expected that this number will triple by 2050, increasing the risk of disability, the financial burden of illness, and the expense of medical care. Furthermore, there is no proven way to treat AD; existing treatments only manage symptoms. But because AD has a protracted prodromal phase, early prevention seems to be especially crucial to delaying the disease's progression. Therefore, to determine the risk and protective factors that have a significant impact on cognitive status, epidemiological studies are crucial.

It is actually true that underlying modifiable risk factors, which may alter a person's chance of developing AD, account for one-third of AD cases globally. To better understand the implications for AD prevention, we categorized these factors in this review into multiple categories, such as psychosocial factors, pre-existing diseases, lifestyle choices, and others. We also looked into any possible effects on cognition.

4.2.1. Descriptive Epidemiology of Alzheimer's Disease

The projected number of dementia patients worldwide is expected to reach 152 million by mid-century, with the greatest increase anticipated in low- and middle-income countries. In the United States, the number of Alzheimer's disease patients aged 65 and older is predicted to rise from 5.8 million to 13.8 million by 2050. Studies in Japan and China have shown a significant increase in Alzheimer's disease prevalence in recent decades, with women having a higher global prevalence and mortality rate compared to men. Additionally, deaths due to Alzheimer's disease in the United States increased by 146.2% from 2000 to 2018, making it the fifth leading cause of death among elderly Americans. Caregivers of Alzheimer's disease patients often experience mental stress and negative emotional effects. The burden of caring for these individuals is expected to be substantial and unsustainable. The focus of Alzheimer's disease care is on promoting well-being, as patients may experience a range of complex problems and symptoms across different domains. Epidemiological research suggests that behavioral and environmental factors play crucial roles in the development and progression of the disease. Individuals with cognitive dysfunction need to maintain physical health to protect their cognition. Many risk factors can contribute to the development of Alzheimer's disease, and some of these factors may also be symptoms of the disease. Accurate diagnosis is crucial for individuals experiencing cognitive decline. Despite the presence of Aβ and tau biomarkers in some individuals without symptoms, a pre-symptomatic diagnosis of Alzheimer's disease remains challenging. Future challenges in Alzheimer's disease research include the discovery of less invasive and more sensitive biomarkers for early screening and diagnosis. Exploring evidence-based strategies for prevention, particularly focusing on modifiable risk factors, will be a key area of future study.

4.2.2. Putative Modifiable Risk Factors and Prevention for Late-Onset Alzheimer's Disease

Evidence from observational studies has accumulated during the past few years and shown several potentially modifiable risk factors (Figure 4.3), concerning AD prevention some potential feasible suggestions are provided (Figure 4.4).

Pre-existing conditions, unhealthy lifestyles, and environmental exposures were the main risk factors; however, certain psychosocial conditions and healthy lifestyles may also provide protection against AD. Furthermore, certain factors—highlighted in bold—seemed to be both risk factors and AD symptoms, possibly as a result of reverse causality.

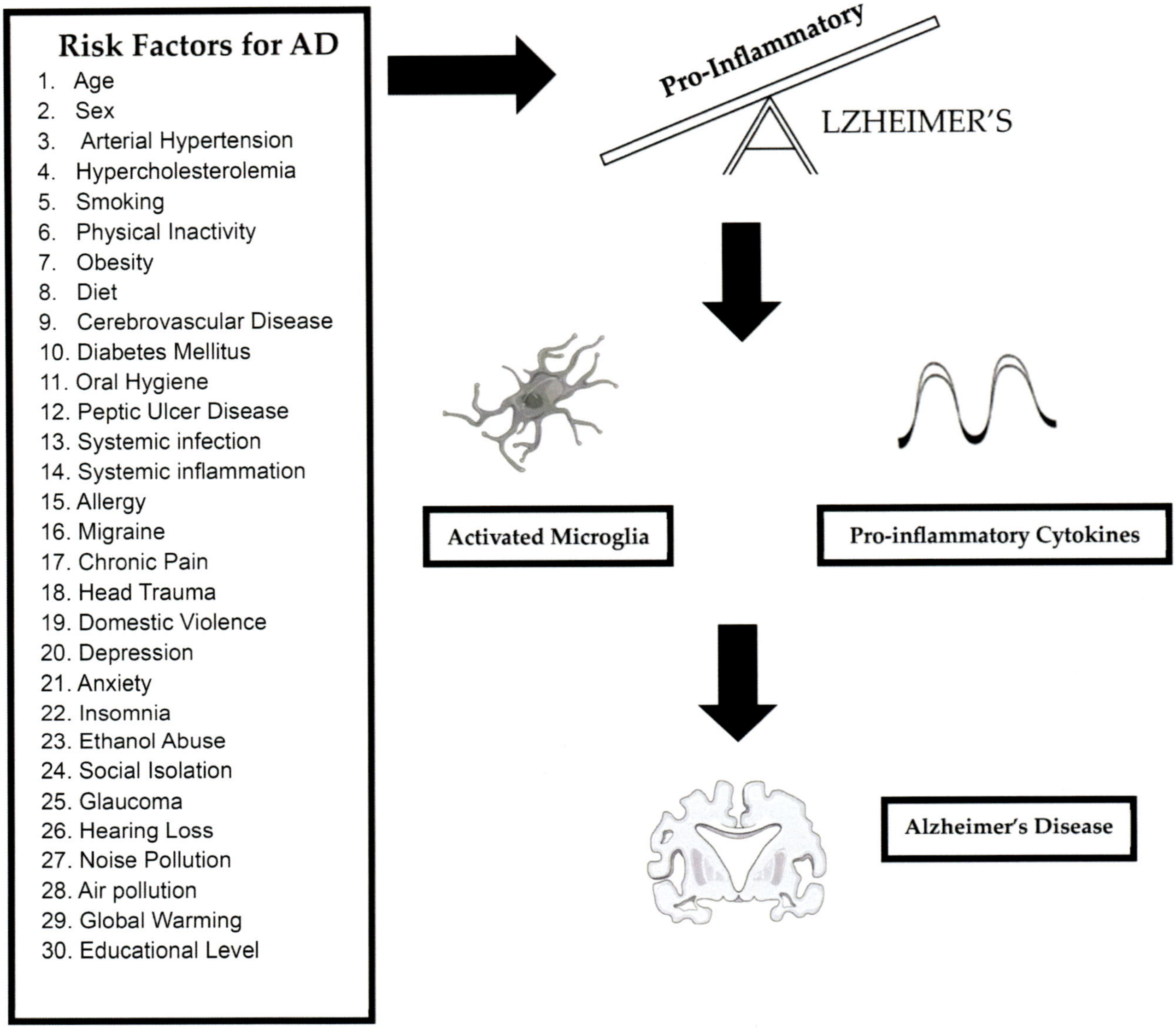

Figure 4.3. *Risk factors for Alzheimer's disease.*

Source: Weaver DF, (2024). Thirty risk factors for Alzheimer's disease unified by a common neuroimmune–neuroinflammation mechanism. Brain Sciences, 14(1), 41. https://doi.org/10.3390/brainsci14010041.

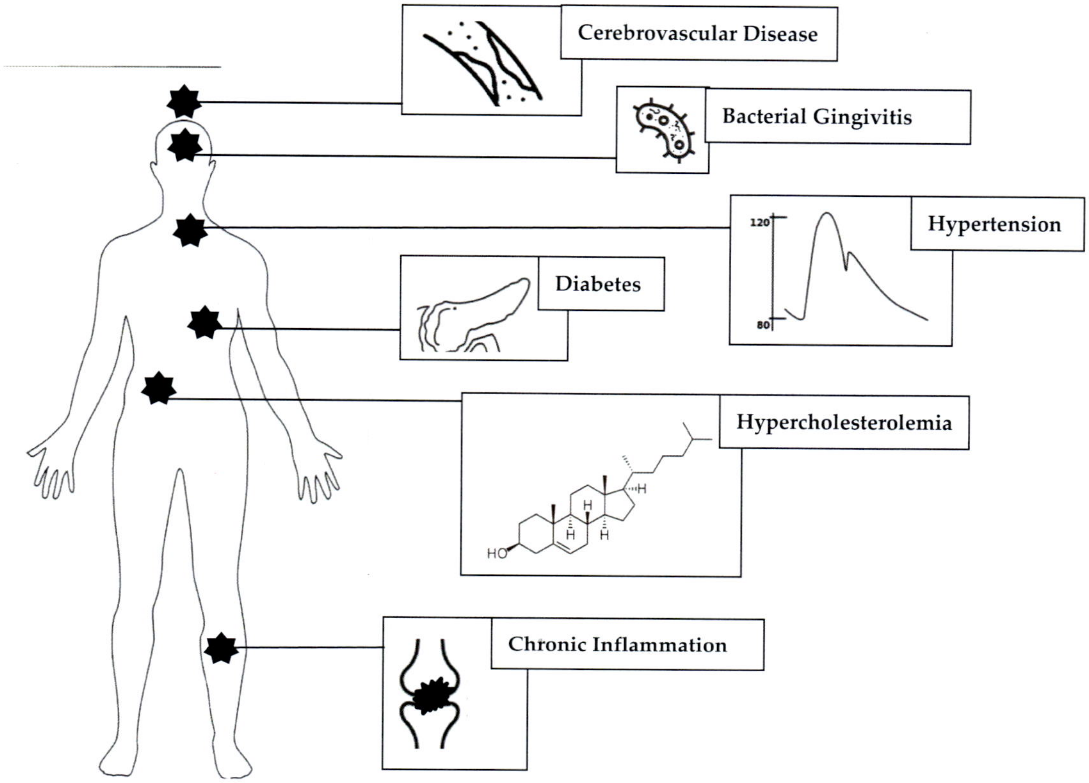

Figure 4.4. *Risk of Alzheimer's disease and slowing its progression.*

Source: *Weaver DF. (2024). Thirty risk factors for Alzheimer's disease unified by a common neuroimmune–neuroinflammation mechanism. Brain Sciences, 14(1), 41. https://doi.org/10.3390/brainsci14010041.*

4.2.2.1. Educational Attainment

Prolonged adult education may have positive effects on overall brain volume, including increased cortical surface area and thickness in the prodromal stage of AD. It may also improve language processing and intellectual abilities. Mendelian randomization research verified the causal relationships between education and both delayed AD onset [hazard ratio (HR) 0.76, 95% confidence intervals (CI) 0.67–0.85] and decreased AD risk [odds ratio (OR) 0.64, 95% confidence intervals (CI) 0.56–0.74]. Future research should thoroughly define these causal relationships.

- **Cognitive Activity and Bilingualism:** According to the Swedish study, engaging in cognitive activities actively was associated with a 46% lower risk of AD. Particularly, those who played more analog games showed a slower decline in memory and cognitive speed, which may have something to do with the strong connections between the superior frontal cortex and the hippocampal regions. As a component of cognitive reserve, bilingualism may improve neural efficiency through stronger functional connectivity in the default mode network for behavior control and the frontoparietal control network for executive control. Indeed, bilinguals outperformed monolinguals in both executive and visual-spatial functions. More specifically, lifelong bilinguals showed the first signs of AD significantly later than people who only spoke Cantonese or Mandarin. Gaining more education can increase brain volume and cognitive reserve, which can postpone the onset of AD. Likewise, bilingualism and cognitive exercise helped maintain normal cognitive functioning. To prevent AD, it is therefore necessary to broaden educational opportunities, particularly in language, and to encourage cognitive activities in general society.

- **Social Engagement:** Regularly interacting with friends was linked to a slightly lower risk of dementia because it helps build cognitive reserve early on through healthy social interaction. In particular, cultural activities within the community may also benefit the entire cognitive system. Healthy relationships between partners may have more of a protective effect on cognition, while widows—particularly those who carry the APOE ε4 gene—had a higher risk of AD (OR 7.67, 95% CI 1.6–40.0) than married individuals. In fact, widows had a higher chance of experiencing severe Aβ-related cognitive decline among older people who were still cognitively intact. Increased social interactions may improve language and memory skills, which could boost cognitive reserve even more. It is noteworthy that widowed or single people appeared to communicate with people less; therefore, it is advisable to build strong social networks and participate in more frequent social events (Harvey, Fox, & Rossor, 1999; Kalaria et al., 2008; Xu, Ferrari, & Wang, 2013).
- **Depression and Stress:** AD was significantly associated with depression (OR 1.65, 95% CI 1.42–1.92). According to an Australian study, the odds ratios for dementia related to mild, moderate, and severe depressive symptoms were 1.2, 1.7, and 2 points, respectively, with a 95% confidence interval between 1;2, and 1.4. Furthermore, citalopram treatment for longer than 4 years was highly associated with a 3-year delay in the development of AD from mild cognitive impairment (MCI). Citalopram has the noteworthy ability to decrease amyloid plaque in the cerebrospinal fluid (CSF) of both healthy volunteers and experimental transgenic AD mice, which has significant implications for clinical practice. Furthermore, depressed patients who were not taking medication had higher levels of microglial activation, a marker of neurodegenerative inflammation; as a result, effective treatment of depression may be important in preventing neurodegeneration. The prodromal stage of AD may share symptoms with depression, or the two conditions may have common causes like inflammation and neurodegeneration. As a result, depressive symptoms seem to be a prodromal marker of AD rather than

a causal risk factor. Furthermore, a mendelian randomization study did not support the causal association between depression and AD; as such, future research should delve deeper into this relationship. A higher incidence risk of AD (HR 1.36, 95% confidence interval 1.12–1.67) was observed in people with disorders related to stress. Another new risk factor for AD was long-term stress from one's job. Notably, stress may cause neuroinflammation and oxidative stress, which may accelerate the development of amyloid plaques. Controlling stress and regulating emotions would lessen the negative psychological effects on thinking.

4.2.3. Pre-Existing Diseases

4.2.3.1. Diabetes, Hypertension and Dyslipidemia

Based on 24 longitudinal studies, the evidence for the increased risk of AD in diabetics [relative risks (RR) 1.43, 95% confidence interval 1.25–1.62] was derived. Interestingly, the molecular link between diabetes and AD may be explained by the way Aβ interacts with islet amyloid polypeptide to exacerbate AD pathogenesis. The CSF p-tau level was higher in the untreated diabetics than in the antidiabetic or euglycemic adults, indicating that the antidiabetic medications may be able to lessen tau pathology. Furthermore, the use of metformin in conjunction with anti-diabetic medication may help to delay the onset of cognitive decline and lower the risk of dementia. The Framingham Offspring Study has also revealed a markedly elevated risk of AD (HR 1.73, 95% CI 1.02–2.94) in individuals with midlife and late-life high systolic pressure. However, a higher risk of AD was also associated with decreased systolic pressure from mid-to-late life (HR 2.12, 95% CI 1.12–4.00). People with high blood pressure variability had a risk of AD that was more than twice as high, suggesting that high blood pressure variation may contribute to the progression of AD. Thankfully, the use of antihypertensives reduced the risk of AD (RR 0.78, 95% CI 0.66–0.91); continued use of these medications may have markedly protective effects on cognition.

Blood lipids may be crucial in the development of AD. These include triglycerides (TG), total cholesterol (TC), low-density lipoprotein cholesterol (LDL-C), and high-density lipoprotein cholesterol (HDL-C). According to the Three-City Study, people with hypercholesterolemia had a significantly higher risk of AD; in particular, this association would be lessened after controlling for APOE ε4. Additionally, in the Adult Changes in Thought (ACT) Study, the cholesterol was separated into two subtypes: HDL-C and non-HDL-C. The results showed a U-shaped association between the non-HDL-C level and the risk of AD among individuals aged 60–69. When compared to 160 mg/dl of non-HDL-C, the HR was 1.29 (95% CI 1.04–1.61) at 120 mg/dl and 1.16 (95% CI 1.01–1.33) at 210 mg/dl. Notably, hypercholesterolemia may worsen the onset of AD by impairing the blood-brain barrier's integrity, increasing Aβ deposition, and causing neuroinflammation. Furthermore, elevated LDL-C levels were linked to an increased risk of AD, whereas HDL-C was probably protective against AD. There was no discernible correlation between TG level and AD risk. Positively, a meta-analysis showed that although the beneficial effects were not more pronounced in randomized controlled trials, the use of stain drugs was likely to reduce the risk of AD (RR 0.86, 95% CI 0.80–0.92) among individuals with hyperlipidemia in prospective studies. Young adults should adopt healthier lifestyles to prevent diabetes, hypertension, and hypercholesterolemia. Patients could use prescription drugs on a regular basis to manage these conditions. Regular use of antidiabetics was linked to a reduction in tau dysfunction, which slows the progression of AD. Antihypertensive medications and stain medications may be beneficial in reducing the incidence of AD in those patients (Harvey, Fox, Rossor, 1999; Kalaria et al., 2008; Xu, Ferrari, & Wang, 2013).

4.2.3.2. Obesity

Multiple studies suggest that middle-aged individuals with a higher BMI are at a greater risk of developing Alzheimer's disease (AD), whereas being overweight or obese later in life may have a protective effect on cognitive function. In particular, individuals with a high BMI in late life had a lower risk of AD, while those who experienced a significant decrease in BMI from midlife to late life had a higher risk. Additionally, obese elderly individuals tended to have lower levels of Aβ and larger hippocampus volume, possibly due to increased leptin production from adipocytes, which can promote neurogenesis in the hippocampus. It is important to consider age when evaluating the relationship between obesity and AD, with young adults advised to maintain a healthy weight and older individuals cautioned against significant weight loss.

4.2.3.3. Cardiovascular Diseases

The HR of AD after atrial fibrillation was 1.31 (95% confidence interval 1.20–1.43). Furthermore, over an extended period of 7.7 years, a significant increase in AD risk (HR 2.87, 95% CI 1.21–6.80) was also linked to mild reductions in cardiac index. The deterioration of cortical atrophy and neuropathological features may be explained by cerebral hypoperfusion, which is brought on by lower cardiac output in patients with atrial fibrillation. Positively, the risk of AD was decreased in patients with atrial fibrillation taking oral anticoagulants (HR 0.61, 95% CI 0.54–0.68). Interestingly, patients with atrial fibrillation treated with catheter ablation had a lower risk of AD compared to those receiving medical therapy (HR 0.77, 95% CI 0.61–0.97). A meta-analysis comprising six studies clearly demonstrated that stroke patients had an elevated risk of AD of approximately 59%. Therefore, useful techniques to lessen the severity of brain damage following a stroke may aid in delaying or stopping the onset of AD. The Rotterdam Study found a statistically significant increase in the risk of AD in people who had multiple cerebral microbleeds (HR 2.10, 95% CI 1.21–3.64). Additionally considered to be significant risk factors for AD were arteriolosclerosis (OR 1.20, 95% CI 1.04–1.40) and severe cerebral atherosclerosis (OR 1.33, 95% CI 1.11–1.58). Due to cerebrovascular diseases, neurovascular unit disorders may result in selective brain atrophies, disruptions of the blood-brain barrier, and decreased cerebral blood flow. These factors may cause direct damage to neurons and indirectly cause Aβ accumulation. Thus, with the right care, a deeper comprehension of these relationships may yield cognitive benefits. The primary goals for preventing AD should be early detection and treatment of vascular risks as well as maintaining optimal cardiovascular health. Patients with atrial fibrillation would have a much reduced risk of AD if they used pharmaceuticals such as oral anticoagulants and catheter ablation.

4.2.3.4. Traumatic Brain Injury

In both the Swedish study (OR 1.58, 95% CI 1.49–1.69) and the Danish study (HR 1.16, 95% CI 1.12–1.22), participants who had experienced traumatic brain injury (TBI) had a higher risk of developing AD. This finding may have been reinforced by specific findings about TBI, such as TBI involving the skull or spine, younger individuals with the injury, and multiple or severe TBI. According to their death certificates, athletes with a history of repeated head injuries were particularly vulnerable to AD-related mortality. Moreover, women with traumatic brain injuries had an increased chance of developing dementia among US military veterans. It's encouraging to know that stain medications, particularly rosuvastatin, may lower the risk of dementia in concussion sufferers due to their possible neuroprotective properties. To develop therapeutic strategies to reduce the risk and impact of AD, further research is necessary to concentrate on the likelihood that individuals with TBI will develop AD. Given the detrimental effects traumatic brain injury (TBI) has on cognitive function, it is imperative that individuals take precautions to protect their heads when participating in risky activities or employment.

4.2.3.5. Hyperhomocysteinemia

Blood homocysteine (Hcy) levels and AD risk have a linear dose-response relationship (HR 1.15, 95% CI 1.04–1.26, per 5 μmol/L increment), according to a meta-analysis that included 5 prospective studies. Nonetheless, certain results from long-term research indicate that this dose-dependent correlation was limited to high serum Hcy concentrations (approximately ≥10μmol/l). Large-scale prospective studies should be conducted to further evaluate these inconsistent exposure-response associations. Furthermore, in mouse models, elevated Hcy levels may influence tau hyperphosphorylation and Aβ deposition through the γ-secretase pathway and cdk5 kinase. Furthermore, supplementing with folic acid may help reduce hyperhomocysteinemia, suggesting that enhancing total homocysteine metabolism is a potential means of preventing AD.

4.2.3.6. Hearing Loss and Oral Diseases

Additionally, after hearing loss, the OR for AD was 1.39 (95% CI 1.05–1.84) in a case-control study. Due to poor listening conditions, people may find it difficult to understand speech, develop communication problems, or even become socially isolated. This reduces the amount of cognitive stimulation provided by the acoustic environment, which may worsen cognitive impairment caused by accelerated brain atrophy. In fact, there was a tendency for those with midlife hearing impairment to have significant temporal lobe volume loss. Positively, cochlear implants and hearing aids may be able to improve certain poorer listening conditions while also reducing the rate of cognitive decline. Early detection and treatment of hearing loss may also have a major impact on preventing AD. Tooth loss was a significant risk factor for AD, and oral diseases in general, especially chronic periodontitis and tooth loss, were major concerns for cognitive dysfunction. These conditions were likely mediated by local and systemic inflammatory responses. In particular, people with chronic periodontitis had a higher risk of AD (HR 1.707, 95% CI 1.152–2.528). Peripheral inflammation may be indirectly caused by proinflammatory cytokines or directly by periodontal pathogenic bacteria. To prevent AD, dental health should receive a lot of attention, particularly in developing nations (Harvey, Fox, Rossor, 1999; Kalaria et al., 2008; Xu, Ferrari, & Wang, 2013).

4.2.4. Lifestyles

- **Physical Activity:** A roughly half-decreased risk of AD was associated with higher daily physical activity participation. Furthermore, regular resistance exercise and choreographic intervention may have cognitive benefits that slow down the neurodegenerative process, particularly in areas linked to dementia conversion. Moreover, aerobic exercise improved oral fluency and executive function, two cognitive domains that may have benefited from its protective effects on hippocampal volume and neuronal health. A year of aerobic exercise training improved cardiorespiratory function, especially memory and cerebral perfusion. It is necessary to conduct additional research on the neurotrophic effects of active exercise, as its type, intensity, duration, and timing may have a greater impact on the prevention of AD. The association between active exercise and a lower risk of AD may be explained by reverse causality, as people in the preclinical stage of the disease tended to be less physically active than older, healthy individuals in the Whitehall II study, where physical activity was found to have no neuroprotective effects on cognitive functioning. Reverse causality's ability to account for the positive effects of physical activity on cognition is still up for debate.

- **Sleep Disturbances:** A higher accumulation of neurotoxic substances was observed in those with sleep disorders due to a decreased ability to clear metabolites, which was one of the risk factors for AD identified by insomnia and sleep disordered breathing. A 66% (95% confidence interval 1.03–2.68) higher risk of AD was observed in individuals with severe obstructive sleep apnea (≥30 vs. <5 apnea-hypopnea events/hour). Additionally, individuals with longer sleep length (> 9 hours) revealed a risk of AD that was more than twice as high; the RR of AD after a habitual sleep duration of less than 1 hour was 1.25 (95% CI 0.88–1.76). Furthermore, it showed a V-shaped relationship between daily sleep duration and cognitive decline and the ensuing risk for dementia. Both short duration (≤6 hours) and long duration (≥8 hours) had negative effects on cognitive function. Notably, individuals with inadequate or excessive nocturnal sleep duration tended to exhibit higher levels of amyloid deposition. Additionally, a mendelian randomization study found a causal link between increased cortical thickness and duration of sleep. Additionally, there might be a reciprocal relationship between the pathology of AD and sleep dysregulation; while sleep disorders may promote the build-up of tau and Aβ, the increased tau and Aβ aggregation may aggravate the development of sleep disturbances. To better investigate the possible function of sleep dysregulation as a biomarker of AD and the possible reciprocal relationship, more extensive longitudinal studies are required. Maintaining cognitive function greatly depends on getting enough sleep, so patients experiencing sleep issues should see a doctor and start therapy as soon as possible.
- **Coffee and Tea:** A J-shaped relationship between coffee consumption and AD was postulated; low consumption (1–2 cups/day) but not high consumption (>3 cups/day) was associated with an 18% reduction in the risk of

AD (RR 0.82, 95% CI 0.71–0.94, vs. <1 cup/day), with a greater tendency in women. This gender trait, however, differed from tea consumption. Green tea's cognitive-protective benefits were more pronounced in males. Drinking coffee or green tea may contain certain neuroprotective ingredients like caffeine and L-theanine. Green tea's anti-amyloid properties, which primarily inhibit Aβ aggregation and reduce Aβ-induced oxidative stress, may also protect against AD. The public should be encouraged to drink green tea and coffee in moderation. Those who regularly drank green tea had lower levels of CSF total-tau protein, most likely as a result of improved aberrant tau metabolism. On the other hand, neither black tea nor oolong tea demonstrated any cognitive advantages among the elderly Han participants in the study.

- **Diets:** The risk of AD was found to be inversely correlated with three dietary patterns: the Mediterranean diet (HR 0.46, 95% CI 0.26–0.79), the DASH diet (HR 0.61, 95% CI 0.38–0.97), and the MIND diet (HR 0.47, 95% CI 0.26–0.76). The protective effects of these dietary patterns on cognition may be attributed to anti-oxidant, anti-inflammatory, and anti-diabetic effects as well as adequate amounts of mono- and polyunsaturated fats. The Three-City study presented a novel diet pattern that includes a wider variety of foods like fresh fruits, vegetables, and seafood. It is worth noting that this diet pattern may have specific benefits for cognitive function. Ketogenic diets in particular may lower the risk of AD by changing the gut microbiota; in AD, the HR increased by 27% when a higher glycemic load was consumed. Furthermore, a meta-analysis comprising 21 cohort studies suggested that consuming more fish (RR 0.93, 95% CI 0.90–0.95) and dietary docosahexaenoic acid derived from marine sources (RR 0.63, 95% CI 0.51–0.76) could protect against the development of AD. Additionally, regular seafood consumption was linked to a decreased burden of AD brain pathology among APOE ε4 carriers, and this relationship held true even in the presence of elevated brain mercury levels.
- Others:
    - **Medications:** A 19% reduction in the risk of AD was linked to current or past use of nonsteroidal anti-inflammatory drugs (NSAIDs) (95% CI 0.70–0.94). In line with the meta-analysis, a randomized placebo-controlled trial found no convincing evidence to support the idea that aspirin could successfully reduce the risk of AD. Low-dose aspirin did not appear to enhance cognitive function in this meta-analysis. Thus, the question of whether NSAIDs would guard against AD is still up for debate. It was emphasized how anticholinergic drugs have a negative effect on thinking. Excessive anticholinergic use was linked to AD over

4 years (HR 1.63, 95% CI 1.24–2.14). It may be crucial to gradually reduce anticholinergic usage to protect cognitive function (Harvey, Fox, Rossor, 1999; Kalaria et al., 2008; Xu, Ferrari, & Wang, 2013).

- **Pollution:** We found some long-term cohorts investigating environmental factors linked to the chance of AD and cognitive decline. In children and young adults exposed to Mexico City's air pollution, the brainstem displayed abnormal aggregation and misfolding of p-tau and Aβ. Comparing the highest and lowest quartiles of NOx (≥26 vs. 2) in a Northern Swedish study, there was a 38% elevated risk for AD among those exposed to residential traffic-related air pollution (95% CI 0.87–2.19). <9 μg/m3). Particulate Matter2.5 (PM2.5), which is associated with gray matter atrophy, did, in fact, show that older women had a higher risk of AD (HR 1.24, 95% CI 1.14–1.34). Heart failure and ischemic heart disease are two cardiovascular disorders that may worsen the negative effects of air pollution on cognition. Most importantly, chronic air pollution may quicken the rate at which neurodegeneration develops through vascular illness, Aβ buildup, and neuroinflammation. As a result, it appears that lowering air pollution exposures is crucial for preventing AD. To better understand how environmental exposures affect AD and the possible mechanisms that underlie these relationships, more research is needed.

4.3. ANALYTIC EPIDEMIOLOGY OF ALZHEIMER'S DISEASE

Analytic epidemiology looks at relationships between exposures and outcomes within populations to gain a deeper understanding of the causes and determinants of diseases, such as Alzheimer's disease (AD). Analytical epidemiological studies in the context of AD seek to define risk factors, clarify disease mechanisms, and provide guidance for preventive measures. Cohort studies, case-control studies, and cross-sectional studies are examples of observational research, which is one of the main approaches in analytical epidemiology. Cohort studies track populations of people over time to look into how exposure to particular factors affects the prevalence of AD. Studies utilizing longitudinal cohorts offer significant insights into the temporal correlation between putative risk factors and the onset of AD. For instance, the Framingham Heart Study, a long-term cohort study, has advanced our knowledge of cardiovascular risk factors, including diabetes and hypertension, and how they relate to the likelihood of developing AD in later life. Cohort studies track the health and lifestyle characteristics of participants over many years, making it possible to identify modifiable risk factors that could be the focus of preventive interventions. Case-control studies evaluate differences in exposure to particular risk factors in the past by comparing people with AD (cases) to people without AD (controls). Studies using case-control methodology are especially helpful in the study of uncommon or slowly progressing illnesses such as AD. Case-control studies, for example, have shown links between AD and variables like dietary habits, degree of physical activity, and educational attainment. These results advance our knowledge of potential modifiable risk factors and intervention strategies.

Cross-sectional studies evaluate the prevalence of AD and how it is associated with different risk factors at one particular moment in time. Although they offer useful snapshots of the prevalence of risk factors and the disease burden, cross-sectional studies are unable to prove causality or establish time relationships. They may, however, give rise to theories that require more research.

The importance of addressing social determinants of health in AD prevention and management has been highlighted by cross-sectional studies that have found associations between AD and variables like socioeconomic status, social engagement, and cognitive reserve. Analytic epidemiology includes interventional research to assess the effectiveness of treatments or preventive measures for AD in addition to observational studies. The most reliable method for determining how effective an intervention is through randomized controlled trials or RCTs. Research on treatments aimed at delaying the onset or slowing the progression of AD includes pharmacotherapy, cognitive training, physical exercise, and dietary changes. To investigate heterogeneity in treatment effects and identify variables that may alter treatment response, analytical epidemiological techniques are used, such as subgroup analyzes and meta-analyzes.

4.3.1. Antecedent Risk Factors that Increase the Risk of Alzheimer's Disease

There are many factors linked to an increased risk of AD, but the most frequently reported are those related to cerebrovascular disease and its antecedents (Table 4.1). There is an increased risk if you have a history of diabetes, hypertension, smoking, obesity, or dyslipidemia. Curiously, cerebrovascular disease is a precondition for dementia in general. These conditions include cerebral hemorrhage, multiple small infarcts, large cortical infarcts, single strategically placed infarcts, cortical changes due to hypoperfusion, white matter changes, and vasculopathies.

Table 4.1. Factors that Modify the Risk of Alzheimer's Disease

Constitutive Factors	
1.	Age (neuroinflammation, proteopathy, vascular)
2.	Sex (neuroinflammation, proteopathy, vascular)
Personal Modifiable Factors	
3.	Arterial Hypertension (vascular, neuroinflammation, proteopathy)
4.	Hypercholesterolemia (vascular, neuroinflammation, proteopathy)
5.	Smoking (vascular, neuroinflammation, proteopathy)
6.	Physical Inactivity (vascular, neuroinflammation, proteopathy)
7.	Obesity (vascular, neuroinflammation, proteopathy)
8.	Diet (vascular, neuroinflammation, proteopathy)
9.	Diabetes Mellitus (vascular, neuroinflammation, proteopathy)
10.	Cerebrovascular Disease (vascular, neuroinflammation, proteopathy)
11.	Oral Hygiene (neuroinflammation, proteopathy)
12.	Peptic Ulcer Disease (neuroinflammation, proteopathy)
13.	Head Trauma (trauma, neuroinflammation, proteopathy)
14.	Depression (neuroinflammation, proteopathy)
15.	Anxiety (neuroinflammation, proteopathy)

16.	Insomnia (neuroinflammation, proteopathy)
17.	Ethanol Abuse (neuroinflammation, proteopathy)
18.	Social Isolation (neuroinflammation)
19.	Hearing Loss (neuroinflammation)
Societal Modifiable Factors	
20.	Domestic Violence (trauma, neuroinflammation, proteopathy)
21.	Noise Pollution (neuroinflammation)
22.	Air pollution (neuroinflammation)
23.	Global Warming (neuroinflammation)
24.	Educational Level (neuroinflammation, proteopathy)
Comorbidity or Concomitant Risk Factors	
25.	Systemic infection (neuroinflammation)
26.	Systemic inflammation (neuroinflammation)
27.	Chronic Pain (neuroinflammation)
28.	Chronic Migraine (neuroinflammation, proteopathy)
29.	Chronic Allergies (neuroinflammation)
30.	Glaucoma (neuroinflammation, proteopathy)

Source: Weaver DF, (2024). Thirty risk factors for Alzheimer's disease unified by a common neuroimmune–neuroinflammation mechanism. Brain Sciences, 14(1), 41. https://doi.org/10.3390/brainsci14010041.

- **Cerebrovascular Disease:** Purely vascular dementia is rare, although it is evident that cerebrovascular disease can manifest with dementia-like symptoms. More often than not, cerebrovascular illness and AD coexist, leaving evidence of both vascular illness and classic AD symptoms. It's interesting to note that the twofold increased risk of dementia following an incident stroke was unaffected by the degree or rate at which prestroke cognitive function changed. This suggests that prestroke cognitive function does not play a significant role in determining how much a stroke affects the risk of poststroke dementia. There are several theories as to how a stroke could cause cognitive impairment: it could cause atrophy and destroy brain parenchyma; it could cause damage in key areas that causes amnestic syndromes, like thalamic strokes; it could increase Aβ deposition; or it could combine vascular and Alzheimer-type pathology. A plausible explanation for the rise in Aβ could be the overexpression of p25 and cdk5, which leads to hypoperfusion-induced ischemia and hypoxia. This, in turn, raises BACE1 levels and accelerates the processing of amyloid precursor protein (APP). Patients with dementia frequently have white matter hyperintensities detected by MRI, but it is unknown how these changes in white matter contribute to cognitive decline. Furthermore, no clear mechanism exists to explain the impact on cognition or their involvement in Alzheimer's disease because hypertension, diabetes, and microvascular disease are all linked to these alterations. Cognitive tasks involving the frontal and temporal lobes, such as memory retrieval and storage, can be more difficult to perform when thalamic vascular disease is present (Harvey, Fox, Rossor, 1999; Kalaria et al., 2008; Xu, Ferrari, & Wang, 2013).

- **Hypertension:** Studies, both longitudinal and cross-sectional, suggest that blood pressure may play a role in dementia in later life. It appears that middle-aged hypertension raises the risk of dementia in later life. This is supported by observational studies that link middle-aged hypertension to late-life cognitive impairment. The relationship between hypertension and dementia in later life is not entirely clear-cut, as dementia is linked to both abnormally high and low blood pressure. Blood pressure starts to drop with the onset and progression of Alzheimer's disease; this is likely due to changes in the autonomic regulation of blood flow, weight loss, and vessel stiffening. Although hypertension is a medical condition that can be treated, clinical trials involving antihypertensive drugs have been attempted in AD patients, with varying degrees of success.
- **Type II Diabetes:** Having type II diabetes increases the risk of developing AD by approximately twofold. Diabetes may contribute to the accumulation of Aβ in the brain by causing hyperinsulinemia, which interferes with Aβ clearance. Receptors for advanced glycation end-products, implicated in diabetes pathogenesis, have been found in cells associated with AD pathology. Excess adipose tissue can also lead to diabetes, as adipokines and cytokines produced by adipose tissue correlate with insulin resistance and hyperinsulinemia, potentially impacting AD risk. Meta-analysis of longitudinal studies revealed a pooled effect size of 1.54 for diabetes in increasing AD risk.
- **Body Weight;** Several cross-sectional and case–control studies found that low body mass index and being underweight were apparent risk factors for dementia and age-related brain changes such as atrophy. In contrast, several prospective studies linked both low and high body weight, weight loss and weight gain to risk of AD. The strongest effect was in a meta-analysis associating obesity (assessed by high body mass index) and the risk of AD (odds ratio, OR, 1.59 95% CI 1.02–2.5; $z = 2.0$; $p = 0.42$). The mechanisms by which body weight alters disease risk are unknown, but may include effects such as insulin resistance or the co-incidence of type II diabetes.
- **Smoking:** Initially, case-control studies suggested that smoking reduced the risk of Alzheimer's disease; however, later prospective studies found no association or an increased risk. Smoking may raise the risk of dementia by upregulating cholinergic nicotinic receptors in the brain, which increases cholinergic metabolism. AD brains are always associated with cholinergic deficits, which are defined by

decreased levels of acetylcholine, choline acetyl transferase, and/or nicotinic acetylcholine receptors. On the other hand, nicotine itself enhances information processing and attention by increasing acetylcholine release and nicotinic receptor density. Elevated oxidative stress brought on by smoking may work against these actions. Oxidative stress has been linked to AD through the production of free radicals and disruption of inflammatory-immune systems, which can then trigger phagocytes that produce more oxidative damage.

- **Traumatic Brain Injury:** People who have experienced traumatic brain injury are more likely to develop dementia than people without a history of trauma, especially if they have the APOE-ε4 allele. According to a meta-analysis, men with a history of traumatic brain injury are more likely to develop dementia than women. There is evidence to support a connection between human brain injury and increased Aβ deposition and intraneuronal tau pathology, even in younger patients, according to both postmortem and experimental studies. Additionally, there is an overproduction of APP and elevated CSF Aβ levels (Harvey, Fox, Rossor, 1999; Kalaria et al., 2008; Xu, Ferrari, & Wang, 2013).

4.3.2. Protective Factors that Reduce Risk of Alzheimer's Disease

4.3.2.1. Cognitive Reserve

People who lead intellectually stimulating lives—that is, who achieve high levels of education and/or employment—are less likely to exhibit clinical signs of AD pathology. While some studies found no correlation between educational attainment and AD risk, numerous other studies conducted worldwide have found that subjects with higher education had a lower overall dementia risk. Studies on "normal aging" have shown that people with higher levels of education experience slower cognitive and functional decline. This suggests that education may play a role in age-related cognitive decline. According to these studies, the same education-related variables that postpone the onset of dementia of the AD type also help people deal with the cognitive changes that come with normal aging. A more literate population in New York City was also linked to a slower decline in memory, executive function, and language skills in an ethnically diverse cohort of older adults without dementia.

A plethora of research has also investigated the connection between recreational pursuits and incident dementia. In China, gardening and communal activities were also protective against incident dementia. Participating in intellectual, social, and other constructive activities was linked to a lower risk of incident dementia, and having a large social network protected against dementia development. Engaging in a range of recreational pursuits classified as cerebral (e.g., reading, engaging in gaming, attending classes) or social activities (e.g., visiting friends or family) was evaluated in a different population study of senior citizens in New York who were not suffering from dementia. Subjects who engaged in a lot of leisure activities had a 38% lower risk of dementia during follow-up. Another prospective study examined the frequency of engagement in typical cognitive tasks (i.e., reading a book, magazine, or newspaper) for 801 elderly Catholic nuns, priests, and brothers who were not suffering from dementia at baseline. Lastly, leisure activities such as reading, playing board games or musical instruments, dancing, and playing music were linked to a lower risk of incident dementia in another prospective cohort from New York. In this study, lower rates of memory decline were also linked to higher engagement in cognitive activities. A meta-analysis looked at cohort studies that looked at how premorbid IQ, mental activities, education, and occupation affected the risk of dementia. Based on an integrated total of 29,279 individuals from 22 studies, a summary analysis was conducted. The follow-up period was 7 1 years on average. When comparing people with high brain reserve to those with low brain reserve, the summary odds ratio for incident dementia was 0.54 (95% confidence interval [CI] 0.49–0.59, $p < 0.0001$), indicating a 46% lower risk. Of the 33 data sets, 25 showed a significant protective effect and 8 showed no significant effect.

Several studies of AD patients revealed that those with higher cognitive reserve have worse outcomes, in contrast to the above studies where higher reserve was linked to better outcomes (Table 4.1). Patients with higher levels of education or occupational attainment died earlier than those with lower levels in prospective studies involving AD subjects matched for clinical severity at baseline. Similarly, in patients with diagnosed AD, a faster rate of cognitive decline has been linked to higher levels of education or occupational attainment, increased leisure activity, and greater lifetime cognitive activity. These results seem counterintuitive at first, but they are in line with the cognitive reserve theory. According to the hypothesis, patients with a higher cognitive reserve will have more advanced underlying pathology of Alzheimer's disease at any given level of clinical severity assessment. Incidence studies reviewed above suggest that when pathology was more advanced, the clinical disease would emerge. This variation in pathological severity would also exist at later clinical stages of the illness. The higher level of pathology in the high-reserve patients would eventually cause them to pass away more quickly. Alzheimer's disease patient cognitive decline has also been linked to higher educational attainment, increased leisure time engagement, and lifetime cognitive activities.

4.3.2.2. Diet

Dietary fats have the potential to raise cholesterol levels, which may raise the risk of cerebral vascular disease. The likelihood of AD may also rise with this sequence. A doubling of the risk of incident Alzheimer's disease was linked to dietary fat intake in the fifth (highest) quintile when compared to the first quintile. The highest intake of n-6 polyunsaturated fats and monounsaturated fat decreased the risk of AD, while trans-unsaturated fats were linked to a three-fold increased risk of the disease. Higher intakes of total and saturated fat have also been linked to an increased risk of AD; however, there is no evidence of a correlation with polyunsaturated fat. Dietary components rich in omega-3 fatty acids are crucial for the development of the developing brain. Consuming fish or omega-3 fatty acids has been linked in numerous studies to a lower risk of AD. For instance, a French study discovered that regular consumption of omega-3 rich oils was linked to an increased risk of all forms of dementia, while weekly consumption of fish was associated with a lower risk of AD. Higher dietary vitamin D intake was linked to a lower risk of Alzheimer's disease in two studies. This association was not seen in a third study, possibly because the subjects had lower levels of vitamin D intake.

Additionally, there has been conflicting evidence linking total homocysteine to AD. Certain B vitamins play a major role in determining homocysteine concentrations. Two studies provided preliminary evidence that low folate levels are linked to an increased risk of AD based on serum folate levels. Conflicting results were reported by some studies that used self-reported information to estimate dietary intake of folate and B vitamins. While one study found a link between higher folate intake and a lower risk of AD, another did not find a statistically significant reduction in AD risk linked to folate intake. There was no correlation between the risk of AD and vitamins B6 or B12. The lack of consideration for potential additive and interactive (antagonistic or synergistic) effects among nutritional components may account for discrepancies in the literature currently available regarding some of the dietary elements mentioned above and the risk of AD. These effects might be better captured in a composite dietary pattern like the Mediterranean diet. High consumption of fruits, vegetables, legumes, and cereals; high consumption of unsaturated fatty acids (mostly from olive oil); low consumption of saturated fatty acids; moderately high consumption of fish; low to moderate consumption of dairy products (mostly from cheese or yogurt); low consumption of meat and poultry; and regular but moderate consumption of ethanol, mostly from wine and usually during meals, are the characteristics of the latter. Higher Mediterranean diet adherence was linked to a lower risk of AD (hazard ratio, 0.91; 95% CI, 0.83–0.98; p = 0.015) in one study. Subjects in the middle tertile had an AD hazard ratio of 0.85 (95% CI, 0.63–1.16) compared with those in the lowest Mediterranean diet tertile, and those in the highest tertile had a hazard ratio of 0.60 (95% CI, 0.42–0.87) (p for trend = 0.007). A follow-up analysis revealed that the Mediterranean diet was also linked to a lower risk of mild cognitive impairment and the development of AD from mild cognitive impairment (Harvey, Fox, Rossor, 1999; Kalaria et al., 2008; Xu, Ferrari, & Wang, 2013).

4.3.2.3. Physical Activity

Exercise can promote brain vascularization, stimulate neurogenesis, activate brain plasticity mechanisms, remodel neuronal circuitry in the brain, and improve learning in both young and old animals. Additionally, it might boost brain-derived neurotrophic factor levels, improve neuronal survival and resistance to brain insults, activate gene expression profiles that are thought to support brain plasticity, and lower inflammatory markers like interleukin-6 and C-reactive protein. According to a Cochrane review, aerobic exercise interventions were linked to improvements in cognitive function in eight out of eleven randomized controlled trials of exercise in older adults without known cognitive impairment. While some research has not found a link between physical activity and dementia, other studies have found that physical activity has positive effects. A combined investigation into the relationship between diet and physical activity and the risk of Alzheimer's disease was conducted on 1880 community-dwelling elders in New York City who were free of dementia. The risk of AD was found to be significantly lower when a strict Mediterranean-style diet and regular physical activity were combined, as opposed to no or very little physical activity.

4.3.2.4. Cognitive Enhancement

Specifically, the effects of cognitive engagement on the risk of AD have been the subject of several studies. The frequency of participation in particular activities that may have a cognitive component was self-reported in the studies. Analysis was done on 5698 individuals 65 years of age and older who were dementia-free in the

Three-City cohort study. Recreational activities that stimulate the mind were substantially linked to a lower risk of AD (hazard ratio (HR) = 0.39). This finding held true even after controlling for vascular risk factors, depressive symptoms, and physical functioning. It was also independent of other proxies of cognitive reserve (Harvey, Fox, Rossor, 1999; Kalaria et al., 2008; Xu, Ferrari, & Wang, 2013).

4.3.3. Genetic Epidemiology

4.3.3.1. Rare Variants

Familial early-onset disease has been strongly linked to rare mutations in three genes: APP, PSEN1, and PSEN2 (Table 4.2). These mutations result in enhanced relative levels of the $A\beta_{42}$ peptide, its aggregation, and an early onset of disease, usually starting in the fourth or fifth decade of life. They are highly penetrant and mostly inherited in an autosomal dominant pattern. An even smaller percentage (less than 1% of all AD patients) have APP mutations. Occasionally, families of patients with familial Alzheimer's disease with later onset will see rare variants like these. Since all APP missense mutations are located in or close to the Aβ-coding exons (16 and 17) of APP, they have an impact on the proteolytic processing and/or aggregation of APP. Microduplication at the APP locus on Ch 21 is another feature of the mutation spectrum. As of this writing, 401 families had 182 distinct AD-related mutations found in PSEN1, while only 23 families had 14 mutations found in PSEN2. Small deletions and insertions have also been reported, but single-nucleotide substitutions account for the majority of PSEN mutations. PSEN mutations modify the proteolytic cleavage of APP by γ-secretase, leading to an elevated $A\beta_{42}/A\beta_{40}$ ratio through an increase in $A\beta_{42}$ and/or a decrease in $A\beta_{40}$. This suggests a mechanism of partial loss-of-function in PSEN instead of a gain-of-function. While mutations in these three genes are uncommon causes of AD, their identification provides strong evidence that Aβ plays a critical role in the etiology of AD. This amyloid hypothesis, also known as the Aβ hypothesis, postulates that imbalances between Aβ production and Aβ clearance lead to neurodegenerative processes and raise the possibility that additional genes involved in these pathways could also be risk factors.

Table 4.2. Common Susceptibility Genes and Their Related SNPs in AD and IS

Mapped Gene	Region	SNP	Position Relative to Gene	Risk Allele	*p* Value	Risk to	References
ALDH1A2	15q21.3	rs4775044	intron variant	N.A	4.0×10^{-6}	AD	Schwartzentruber et al. (2021)
		rs4471613	intron variant	A	5.0×10^{-7}	IS	Carty et al. (2015)
ANKRD22	10q23.31	rs147285445	intron variant	T	4.0×10^{-6}	AD	Mez et al. (2017)
		rs11202867	intron variant	N.A	1.0×10^{-5}	IS	Kumar et al. (2021)

ANTXR1	2p13.3	rs7561207	intron variant	N.A	4.0×10^{-6}	AD	Nazarian et al. (2019)
		rs149587156	intergenic variant	N.A	5.0×10^{-6}	IS	Kumar et al. (2021)
DIO2-AS1	14q31.1	rs7155666	intron variant	A	8.0×10^{-10}	AD	Chung et al. (2022)
		rs11846182	intron variant	T	9.0×10^{-6}	IS	Lee et al. (2017)
HDAC9	7p21.1	rs117756856	intron variant	A	9.0×10^{-6}	AD	Mez et al. (2017)
		rs11984041	intron variant	T	5.0×10^{-9}	IS	Network NSG. (2016)
		rs2023938	3'prime UTR variant	G	8.0×10^{-7}	IS	Malik et al. (2017)
		rs71524263	intron variant	N.A	2.0×10^{-12}	IS	Traylor et al. (2017)
		rs2107595	regulatory region variant	N.A	4.0×10^{-15}	IS	Malik et al. (2018)
JPH3	16q24.2	rs117760708	non coding transcript exon variant	T	3.0×10^{-6}	AD	Mez et al. (2017)
		rs12445022	intergenic variant	A	9.0×10^{-8}	IS	Traylor et al. (2021)
KCNN3	1q21.3	rs16830122	intron variant	A	2.0×10^{-6}	AD	Jun et al. (2016)
		rs114812453	intergenic variant	N.A	3.0×10^{-7}	IS	Kumar et al. (2021)
LNC-LBCS	6p22.3	rs62402815	intron variant	N.A	2.0×10^{-6}	AD	Nazarian et al. (2019)
		rs9348394	intron variant	N.A	5.0×10^{-6}	IS	Kumar et al. (2021)
MMP12	11q22.2	rs12808148	intergenic variant	N.A	1.0×10^{-6}	AD	Kamboh et al. (2012)
		rs72983521	intergenic variant	N.A	3.0×10^{-8}	IS	Malik et al. (2018)
MMP3	11q22.2	rs12808148	intergenic variant	N.A	1.0×10^{-6}	AD	Kamboh et al. (2012)
		rs72983521	intergenic variant	N.A	5.0×10^{-8}	IS	Malik et al. (2018)

PCSK6	15q26.3	rs146322114	intron variant	A	2.0×10^{-6}	AD	Mez et al. (2017)
		rs528002287	intron variant	N.A	6.0×10^{-6}	IS	Kumar et al. (2021)
RBMS3	3p24.1	rs17022021	intron variant	T	8.0×10^{-6}	AD	Mez et al. (2017)
		rs115182009	intron variant	N.A	9.0×10^{-7}	IS	Kumar et al. (2021)
RNU6-909P	5p14.1	rs150631144	intron variant	T	1.0×10^{-7}	AD	Mez et al. (2017)
		rs13354619	intron variant	N.A	2.0×10^{-6}	IS	Kumar et al. (2021)

Abbreviation: AD: Alzheimer's disease; IS: ischemic stroke; N.A: not available; SNP: single nucleotide polymorphisms. ×

Source: Dong W, & Huang Y, (2023). Common genetic factors and pathways in Alzheimer's disease and ischemic stroke: Evidences from GWAS. Genes, 14(2), 353. https://doi.org/10.3390/genes14020353.

4.3.3.2. Common Variants

Apolipoprotein E (APOE), a three-allele polymorphism (ε2, ε3, and ε4), is the strongest common genetic variant for typical late-onset AD starting after age 65, ε3 is thought to be a neutral allele, ε4 to be a high-risk allele, and ε2 to be a protective allele (Table 4.2). The ε4 allele has a dose-dependent effect on age at onset. Nonetheless, over 50% of patients with late-onset illness lack the high-risk ε4 allele. A 20% population-attributable risk has been estimated for APOE-ε4. As potential susceptibility loci, variations in CLU, PICALM, CR1, and BIN1 have been found by genome-wide association (GWA) studies. Other Hispanic and non-Hispanic populations have confirmed the presence of these genetic variants. The odds ratios for these genes range from 1.16 to 1.20 for CR1, CLU, and PICALM, and are significantly lower than those for APOE (OR = are 3.2 and 14.9 for ε3/ε4 and ε4/ε4, respectively) (Harvey, Fox, Rossor, 1999; Kalaria et al., 2008; Xu, Ferrari, & Wang, 2013).

4.3.3.3. Familial Late-Onset Alzheimer's Disease

Strong correlations between LOAD and a locus on chromosome 14q31 have been found; however, the underlying locus's identity is unknown and it might be a modifier of onset age. Single-nucleotide polymorphisms on chromosome 10p14 in CUGBP2 with genome-wide significance were found in individuals with one APOE ε4 allele, according to the results of GWA studies in the NIA-LOAD Family Study, which involved 900+ families stratified by APOE genotype. These findings were confirmed in a separate Caribbean-Hispanic cohort. The variants in BIN1 were also replicated by the NIA-LOAD Family Study, which also offered some modest confirmation for CLU but not for CR1 or PICALM following APOE adjustment. It is unknown how these genes contribute to the pathophysiology of Alzheimer's disease, but it is evident that the detection of these potential gene variants has been made possible by large sample sizes. Lastly, late-onset AD is linked to variations in SORL1, which codes for a protein involved in APP trafficking. The SORL1 connections have small effect sizes, but they are consistent with other recently discovered genetic connections for AD. Variants in SORCS1, the SORL1 homolog, have a weak correlation with AD as well. In cultured cells, overexpression of either gene causes Aβ levels to drop, whereas RNAi-induced inhibition causes Aβ levels to rise. Thus, both genes might be involved in the pathophysiology of AD. While the published GWA study results are instructive, functional validation of the genetic associations is still necessary. Although GWA studies are a means of screening the genome, their capacity to identify genuine associations is limited. If the true effect is less than what was seen in the initial study, the findings of such studies may be challenging to repeat. Furthermore, associations with single rare variants (minor allele frequency <5%) or multiple rare variants at a single site (better identified by linkage studies) may not be detected by GWA studies. Lastly, these types of investigations are insufficient to establish the biological significance of a detected genetic association or to demonstrate causation (Harvey, Fox, & Rossor, 1999; Kalaria et al., 2008; Xu, Ferrari, & Wang, 2013).

A Closer Look

Familial Patterns in Alzheimer's Epidemiology

Familial patterns in Alzheimer's disease epidemiology highlight the significant role of genetics in the development and progression of this neurodegenerative disorder. Alzheimer's disease (AD) is characterized by the accumulation of beta-amyloid plaques and tau protein tangles in the brain, leading to cognitive decline and memory loss. While sporadic cases of AD are prevalent, familial forms of the disease underscore the influence of genetic factors in its etiology. Within families affected by Alzheimer's, there is often a clustering of cases, suggesting a hereditary component. Understanding familial patterns is essential for elucidating the genetic mechanisms underlying AD and informing strategies for early detection and intervention.

A key aspect of familial patterns in Alzheimer's epidemiology is the identification of genetic mutations associated with an increased risk of developing the disease. Mutations in genes such as amyloid precursor protein (APP), presenilin 1 (PSEN1), and presenilin 2 (PSEN2) have been implicated in familial forms of early-onset Alzheimer's disease. These mutations disrupt the processing of amyloid precursor protein, leading to the overproduction and accumulation of beta-amyloid plaques in the brain. Similarly, mutations in the apolipoprotein E (APOE) gene, particularly the ε4 allele, are associated with an increased risk of late-onset Alzheimer's disease, the most common form of the disorder. Familial studies have provided valuable insights into the genetic architecture of Alzheimer's and have facilitated the identification of novel therapeutic targets.

Furthermore, familial aggregation studies have demonstrated that individuals with a family history of Alzheimer's are at a higher risk of developing the disease themselves compared to those with no family history. This familial clustering suggests a shared genetic predisposition among affected individuals within families. However, it is essential to recognize that genetic susceptibility alone does not determine the onset of Alzheimer's disease. Environmental factors and lifestyle choices also play a significant role in modifying disease risk, even among individuals with a familial predisposition.

The study of familial patterns in Alzheimer's epidemiology has also shed light on the concept of genetic penetrance—the likelihood that a specific genetic mutation will result in the clinical manifestation of the disease. While some mutations, such as those in the PSEN1 gene, exhibit high penetrance and almost invariably lead to Alzheimer's, others, like the APOE ε4 allele, demonstrate variable penetrance and may interact with other genetic and environmental factors to influence disease risk. Understanding the factors that modulate penetrance is crucial for predicting individual susceptibility to Alzheimer's and developing personalized prevention and treatment strategies.

Summary

- Alzheimer's disease, a progressive neurodegenerative disorder, presents a significant public health challenge worldwide due to its prevalence, impact on individuals and families, and healthcare burden.
- The aging of populations has become a worldwide phenomenon. In 1990, 26 nations had more than 2 million elderly citizens aged 65 years and older, and the projections indicate that an additional 34 countries will join the list by 2030.
- Dementia is defined as a clinical syndrome, and is characterized by the development of multiple cognitive deficits that are severe enough to interfere with daily functioning, including social and professional functioning.
- Dementia is one of the leading causes of death in older people. However, death certificates grossly underreport its cause, even when multiple underlying causes of death are taken into account. The community-based follow-up studies could provide reliable data on mortality.
- Alzheimer's disease is a multifactorial disorder that is determined by genetic and environmental factors as well as their interactions. A population-based prospective study is the major epidemiological approach to identifying influential factors for chronic multifactorial diseases such as dementia, in which the life-course approach should be taken into consideration.
- A healthy heart helps ensure that enough blood is pumped through blood vessels to the brain.
- Cerebrovascular changes such as hemorrhagic infarcts, small and large ischemic cortical infarcts, vasculopathies, and white matter changes all increase the risk of dementia. Systematic reviews of population-based studies reveal an approximately two- to four-fold increased risk of incident dementia associated with clinical stroke (post-stroke dementia).
- Excessive alcohol intake can cause alcoholic dementia and may increase the risk of vascular dementia. Heavier alcohol intake in middle age was associated with an increased risk of late-life dementia.

References

1. American Psychiatric Association. (1987). *Diagnostic and Statistical Manual of Mental Disorders (3rd ed., revised)*. Washington, DC: Author.
2. American Psychiatric Association. (1994). *Diagnostic and Statistical Manual of Mental Disorders (4th ed.)*. Washington, DC: Author.
3. Bennett, D. A. (2007). Editorial comment on 'Prevalence of dementia in the United States: The aging, demographics, and memory study' by Plassman et al. *Neuroepidemiology, 29*(1–2), 133–135. https://doi.org/10.1159/000109825.
4. Centers for Disease Control and Prevention. (2003). Public health and aging: Trends in aging—United States and worldwide. *JAMA, 289*(11), 1371–1373. https://doi.org/10.1001/jama.289.11.1371.

5. Corrada, M. M., Brookmeyer, R., Berlau, D., Paganini-Hill, A., & Kawas, C. H. (2008). Prevalence of dementia after age 90: Results from the 90+ study. *Neurology, 71*(5), 337–343. https://doi.org/10.1212/01.wnl.0000310773.65918.cd.

6. Ferri, C. P., Prince, M., Brayne, C., Brodaty, H., Fratiglioni, L., Ganguli, M., et al. (2005). Global prevalence of dementia: A Delphi consensus study. *The Lancet, 366*(9503), 2112–2117. https://doi.org/10.1016/S0140-6736(05)67889-0.

7. Fratiglioni, L., Winblad, B., & von Strauss, E. (2007). Prevention of Alzheimer's disease and dementia: Major findings from the Kungsholmen Project. *Physiology & Behavior, 92*(1–2), 98–104. https://doi.org/10.1016/j.physbeh.2007.05.059.

8. Harvey, R., Fox, N., & Rossor, M. (1999). *Dementia Handbook.* London: Martin Dunitz.

9. Kalaria, R. N., Maestre, G. E., Arizaga, R., Friedland, R. P., Galasko, D., Hall, K., et al. (2008). Alzheimer's disease and vascular dementia in developing countries: Prevalence, management, and risk factors. *The Lancet Neurology, 7*(9), 812–826. https://doi.org/10.1016/S1474-4422(08)70169-8.

10. Kinsella, K., & Velkoff, V. A. (2002). The demographics of aging. *Aging Clinical and Experimental Research, 14*(3), 159–169. https://doi.org/10.1007/BF03324427.

11. Korczyn, A. D., & Vakhapova, V. (2007). The prevention of the dementia epidemic. *Journal of the Neurological Sciences, 257*(1–2), 2–4. https://doi.org/10.1016/j.jns.2007.02.006.

12. Llibre Rodriguez, J. J., Ferri, C. P., Acosta, D., Guerra, M., Huang, Y., Jacob, K. S., et al. (2008). Prevalence of dementia in Latin America, India, and China: A population-based cross-sectional survey. *The Lancet, 372*(9637), 464–474. https://doi.org/10.1016/S0140-6736(08)61002-8.

13. Lobo, A., Launer, L. J., Fratiglioni, L., Andersen, K., Di Carlo, A., Breteler, M. M., et al. (2000). Prevalence of dementia and major subtypes in Europe: A collaborative study of population-based cohorts. *Neurology, 54*(11 Suppl 5), S4–S9.

14. Lunenfeld, B. (2008). An aging world—Demographics and challenges. *Gynecological Endocrinology, 24*(1), 1–3. https://doi.org/10.1080/09513590801921526.

15. Plassman, B. L., Langa, K. M., Fisher, G. G., Heeringa, S. G., Weir, D. R., Ofstedal, M. B., et al. (2007). Prevalence of dementia in the United States: The aging, demographics, and memory study. *Neuroepidemiology, 29*(1–2), 125–132. https://doi.org/10.1159/000109998.

16. Qiu, C., Kivipelto, M., & von Strauss, E. (2009). Epidemiology of Alzheimer's disease: Occurrence, determinants, and strategies toward intervention. *Dialogues in Clinical Neuroscience, 11*(2), 111–128. https://doi.org/10.31887/DCNS.2009.11.2/cqiu.

17. Reitz, C., Brayne, C., & Mayeux, R. (2011). Epidemiology of Alzheimer's disease. *Nature Reviews Neurology, 7*(3), 137–152. https://doi.org/10.1038/nrneurol.2011.2.

18. Roman, G. C. (2003). Vascular dementia: Distinguishing characteristics, treatment, and prevention. *Journal of the American Geriatrics Society, 51*(5 Suppl Dementia), S296–S304. https://doi.org/10.1046/j.1532-5415.51.5s.1.x.

19. von Strauss, E., Viitanen, M., De Ronchi, D., Winblad, B., & Fratiglioni, L. (1999). Aging and the occurrence of dementia: Findings from a population-based cohort with a large sample of nonagenarians. *Archives of Neurology, 56*(5), 587–592. https://doi.org/10.1001/archneur.56.5.587.

20. Wimo, A., Winblad, B., Aguero-Torres, H., & von Strauss, E. (2003). The magnitude of dementia occurrence in the world. *Alzheimer's Disease and Associated Disorders, 17*(2), 63–67. https://doi.org/10.1097/00002093-200304000-00002.

21. Xu, W., Ferrari, C., & Wang, H.-X. (2013). Epidemiology of Alzheimer's disease. Intech. https://doi.org/10.5772/54398.

22. Zhang, Y., Xu, Y., Nie, H., Lei, T., Wu, Y., Zhang, L., et al. (2012). Prevalence of dementia and major dementia subtypes in the Chinese populations: A meta-analysis of dementia prevalence surveys, 1980–2010. *Journal of Clinical Neuroscience, 19*(10), 1333–1337. https://doi.org/10.1016/j.jocn.2012.02.021.

23. Zhang, Z. X., Zahner, G. E., Roman, G. C., Liu, J., Hong, Z., Qu, Q. M., et al. (2005). Dementia subtypes in China: Prevalence in Beijing, Xian, Shanghai, and Chengdu. *Archives of Neurology, 62*(3), 447–453. https://doi.org/10.1001/archneur.62.3.447.

Chapter 5

DIAGNOSIS OF ALZHEIMER'S DISEASE

Contents

Introduction 150
5.1. Importance of the Diagnosis of Alzheimer's Disease 152
5.2. Alzheimer's Disease Biomarkers 156
5.3. Diagnosis and Management of Alzheimer's Disease 170
Summary 187
References 187

INTRODUCTION

Alzheimer's disease diagnosis requires a comprehensive evaluation that may include neuroimaging, clinical assessment, and cognitive testing. To start the right treatments and support, an early diagnosis is essential. However, because Alzheimer's has a gradual onset and shares symptoms with other types of dementia or normal aging, diagnosing the disease can be difficult.

A thorough medical history is usually the first step in the diagnostic process in order to detect any cognitive issues, behavioral abnormalities, or functional decline. It is very helpful to get details about the person's symptoms and how they change over time from family members or caregivers. Subtle indicators of cognitive impairment, such as issues with memory, language, or executive function, may be discovered during a neurological examination. A key component of the diagnostic assessment of Alzheimer's disease is cognitive testing. Standardized assessments, like the Montreal Cognitive Assessment (MoCA) and the Mini-Mental State Examination (MMSE), evaluate a range of cognitive domains, including language, memory, attention, and visuospatial skills. These assessments aid in the diagnosis and tracking of disease progression by measuring the degree of cognitive impairment and tracking changes over time.

Neuroimaging methods like positron emission tomography (PET) and magnetic resonance imaging (MRI) shed light on the structure and function of the brain. A brain's structural alterations, such as hippocampal atrophy, which is frequently linked to Alzheimer's disease, can be found with an MRI scan. Alzheimer's pathology can be detected in the brain through PET imaging using radiotracers that target tau or amyloid protein deposition, supporting the diagnosis. Cerebrospinal fluid (CSF) biomarkers have become a useful diagnostic tool for Alzheimer's disease in recent years. Examination of CSF biomarkers, including tau and amyloid-beta proteins, can reveal information about the underlying pathology of Alzheimer's disease. Nevertheless, obtaining CSF samples is usually limited to specialized diagnostic centers as it involves an invasive procedure. It is noteworthy that the diagnosis of Alzheimer's disease is achieved by ruling out other possible causes of cognitive impairment, such as depression, thyroid dysfunction, or vitamin deficiencies. Furthermore, it can be difficult to differentiate Alzheimer's from other types of dementia, such as vascular dementia or Lewy body dementia, but doing so is crucial for directing care and treatment.

A thorough assessment that integrates clinical assessment, cognitive testing, and neuroimaging findings is necessary for the diagnosis of Alzheimer's disease. Early detection improves outcomes for people and their families by enabling prompt intervention and support. Even though there are still difficulties, research is continuing to improve diagnostic standards and broaden our knowledge of this intricate neurodegenerative condition.

Orientation and Directional Terms

Terms	Definition	Illustration
Disease	A disease is a particular abnormal condition that adversely affects the structure or function of all or part of an organism and is not immediately due to any external injury.	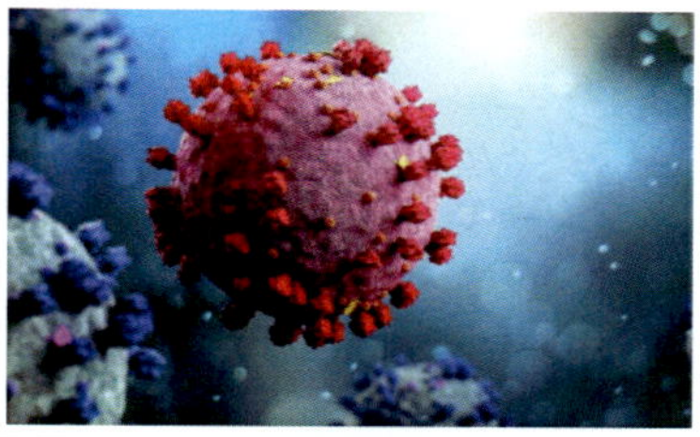
Magnetic Resonance Imaging	Magnetic resonance imaging is a noninvasive medical imaging test that produces detailed images of almost every internal structure in the human body, including the organs, bones, muscles and blood vessels.	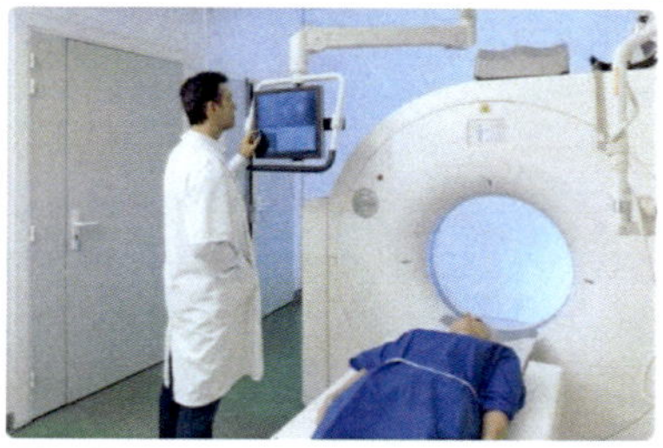
Positron Emission Tomography	Positron emission tomography (PET) is a type of nuclear medicine procedure that measures the metabolic activity of the cells of body tissues.	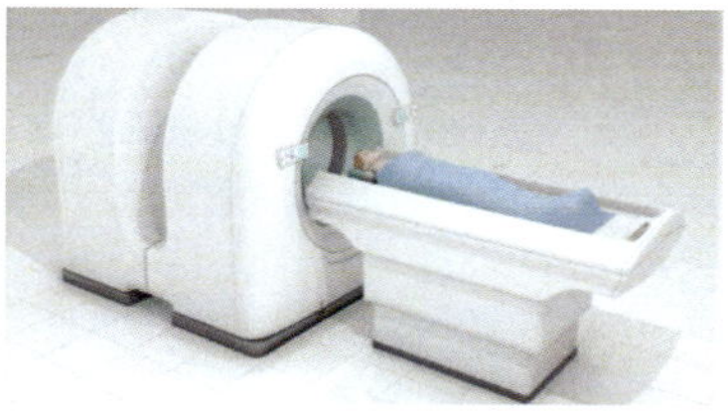
Pathology	Pathology is a branch of medical science that is focused on the study and diagnosis of disease.	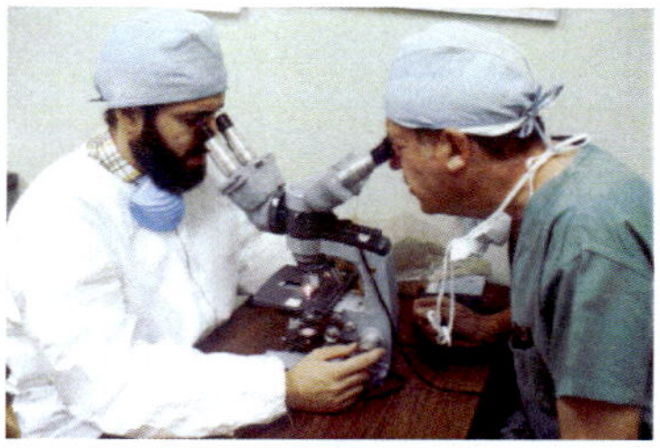
Hypometabolism	Hypometabolism, characterized by decreased brain glucose consumption, is a common feature of many neurodegenerative diseases.	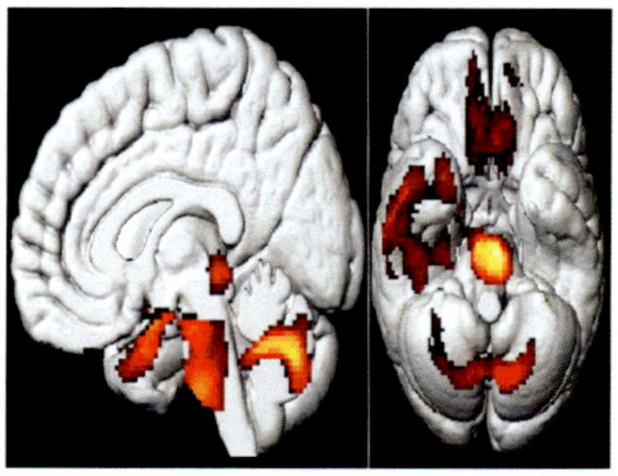

5.1. IMPORTANCE OF THE DIAGNOSIS OF ALZHEIMER'S DISEASE

The ability to explain symptoms is a key component in Alzheimer's disease diagnosis. It is helpful to get feedback on your symptoms and how they affect your day-to-day activities from a close friend or family member. Cognitive and memory tests are useful in the diagnosis of Alzheimer's disease.

Tests for blood and imaging can rule out other possible reasons for the symptoms. Alternately, they might make it easier for your doctor to determine which illness is causing your dementia symptoms. Alzheimer's disease was previously only identified with certainty after a person passed away and a microscope examination showed plaques and tangles in the brain. Researchers and medical professionals can now more accurately diagnose Alzheimer's disease in its early stages of life. Plaques and tangles are detectable through biomarkers. Certain kinds of PET scans and assays that quantify tau and amyloid proteins in blood and cerebral spinal fluid are examples of biomarker tests.

5.1.1. How Is Alzheimer's Disease Diagnosed?

To help determine whether a patient experiencing thinking or memory issues has Alzheimer's disease, doctors employ a variety of techniques and instruments.

To diagnose Alzheimer's, doctors may:

- Ask the person experiencing symptoms, as well as a family member or friend, questions about overall health, use of prescription and over-the-counter medicines, diet, past medical problems, ability to carry out daily activities, and changes in behavior and personality.
- Conduct tests of memory, problem solving, attention, counting, and language.
- Order blood, urine, and other standard medical tests that can help identify other possible causes of the problem.
- Administer a psychiatric evaluation to determine if depression or another mental health condition is causing or contributing to a person's symptoms.
- Collect cerebrospinal fluid (CSF) via a spinal tap and measure the levels of proteins associated with Alzheimer's and related dementias.
- Perform brain scans, such as computed tomography (CT), magnetic resonance imaging (MRI), or positron emission tomography (PET), to support an Alzheimer's diagnosis or rule out other possible causes for symptoms.

To get the most accurate picture of how a patient's memory and other cognitive abilities are changing over time, doctors might wish to repeat these tests. The tests can also aid in the diagnosis of other conditions that may be causing memory issues, including an infection, Parkinson's disease, stroke, tumors, sleep disorders, adverse drug reactions, or other kinds of dementia. A few of these ailments might be curable and even reversible. Individuals experiencing memory issues ought to visit their physician every six to twelve months.

Before the early 2000s, an autopsy—a process carried out after death—was the only reliable method of determining whether a person had Alzheimer's disease. Lab and imaging tests are now available to help a doctor or researcher see biological signs of the disease, or biomarkers, in a living person thanks to research advancements. For instance, many doctors can now do so, subject to state-specific availability. According to Food and Drug Administration guidelines, a blood test should be ordered to determine the levels of beta-amyloid, a protein that abnormally accumulates in the brains of Alzheimer's patients. There are many more blood tests being developed. Currently, blood test results should be considered in conjunction with other tests rather than being used in isolation to diagnose dementia. Nonetheless, these diagnostic tests are still not widely available. Research teams funded by the NIA are still exploring possibilities for less invasive, less costly, and quicker methods of diagnosing Alzheimer's (Balasa et al., 2011; Altomare et al., 2019; Villain & Dubois, 2019; Werry, 2019; Dubois et al., 2021).

5.1.1.1. What Happens if a Doctor Thinks It's Alzheimer's Disease?

If a primary care doctor suspects Alzheimer's, he or she may refer the patient to a specialist who can provide a detailed diagnosis or further assessment. Specialists include:

- **Geriatricians**: who manage health care in older adults and know how the body changes as it ages and whether symptoms indicate a serious problem.
- **Geriatric Psychiatrists**: who specialize in the mental and emotional problems of older adults and can assess memory and thinking problems.
- **Neurologists**: who specialize in abnormalities of the brain and central nervous system and can conduct and review brain scans.
- **Neuropsychologists**: who can conduct tests of memory and thinking.

Memory clinics and Alzheimer's disease Research Centers are equipped with teams of specialists collaborating to diagnose cognitive issues. Furthermore, these specialized facilities have the necessary equipment for advanced brain scans and diagnostic tests.

5.1.1.2. What Are the Potential 0Benefits of an Early Alzheimer's Diagnosis?

Over time, Alzheimer's disease gradually gets worse. Individuals with this disease progress at varying rates; mild Alzheimer's occurs when a person first notices symptoms, while severe Alzheimer's occurs when a person becomes totally dependent on others for everyday care, like feeding themselves.

For several reasons, some people may benefit from an early and accurate diagnosis. Despite the lack of a cure, medications are being developed to slow the disease's progression. In addition to coping mechanisms to handle behavioral problems, medications are also available to treat certain Alzheimer's symptoms. People who are in the early or middle stages of the disease respond best to the majority of currently available medications. Study up on Alzheimer's disease therapies.

In addition, having an early diagnosis helps people with Alzheimer's and their families:

- Plan for the future
- 5Take care of financial and legal matters
- Address potential safety issues
- Learn about living arrangements
- Develop support networks

5.1.2. Specialists for Diagnosis

The possibility of being referred to a specialist for diagnosing Alzheimer's disease is determined by various factors, such as the proficiency of your primary care provider, the severity of your symptoms, and the presence of specialized resources in your location. In some instances, primary care physicians can start the diagnostic procedure and handle early-stage Alzheimer's disease with assistance from neurologists, geriatricians, or psychiatrists as necessary.

On the other hand, your primary care physician might refer you to a specialist for additional assessment and treatment if they suspect Alzheimer's disease or have trouble diagnosing it. Neurologists with experience in cognitive disorders or memory clinics that specialize in dementia assessment and care are frequently consulted for the diagnosis of Alzheimer's disease. These experts might have access to cutting-edge diagnostic resources that can help confirm the diagnosis and direct treatment choices, such as advanced neuroimaging techniques, specialized neuropsychological testing, or cerebrospinal fluid biomarker analysis.

Additionally, comprehensive diagnostic evaluations involving a team of specialists, including neurologists, neuropsychologists, geriatricians, social workers, and other healthcare professionals, may be provided by multidisciplinary memory clinics or Alzheimer's disease centers. These clinics enable a comprehensive approach to diagnosis and treatment by offering individualized care and support catered to the specific requirements of patients and their families. Ultimately, the clinical judgment of your healthcare provider and the resources available in your healthcare system will determine whether or not to refer you to a specialist for an Alzheimer's disease diagnosis. It's critical to be open and honest with your healthcare provider about any memory or cognitive changes you may be experiencing to ensure prompt evaluation and appropriate management (Balasa et al., 2011; Altomare et al., 2019; Villain & Dubois, 2019; Werry, 2019; Dubois et al., 2021).

5.1.3. What Other Health Problems Can Cause Memory Trouble?

Memory trouble can be attributed to various health problems beyond Alzheimer's disease. Some common medical conditions and factors that can affect memory include:

- **Vascular Dementia**: This type of dementia occurs when there is damage to the brain's blood vessels, leading to impaired blood flow and oxygen delivery to brain cells. Symptoms may include memory loss, confusion, and difficulties with executive function.
- **Stroke**: A stroke occurs when there is a sudden interruption of blood flow to the brain, depriving brain cells of oxygen and nutrients. Depending on the location and severity of the stroke, memory problems can arise along with other neurological deficits.
- **Traumatic Brain Injury (TBI)**: Head injuries resulting from accidents, falls, or sports-related incidents can cause cognitive impairments, including memory difficulties. The extent of memory problems can vary depending on the severity and location of the injury.

- **Parkinson's Disease**: While Parkinson's disease primarily affects movement, it can also lead to cognitive changes, including memory impairment. The accumulation of alpha-synuclein protein in the brain contributes to cognitive decline in Parkinson's disease.
- **Depression and Anxiety**: Mental health conditions like depression and anxiety can impact cognitive function, including memory. Persistent feelings of sadness, worry, or stress can interfere with attention, concentration, and memory encoding and retrieval processes.
- **Thyroid Disorders**: Both hypothyroidism (underactive thyroid) and hyperthyroidism (overactive thyroid) can affect cognitive function, including memory. Thyroid hormones play a crucial role in brain development and function, and imbalances can lead to cognitive symptoms.
- **Nutritional Deficiencies**: Inadequate intake of essential nutrients, such as vitamin B12, thiamine (vitamin B1), and folate, can impair cognitive function and memory. These nutrients are vital for maintaining healthy brain function and nerve transmission.
- **Medication Side Effects**: Certain medications, including sedatives, anticholinergics, antihistamines, and benzodiazepines, can cause memory problems as a side effect. It's essential to review medication lists with healthcare providers to identify any potential cognitive effects.
- **Sleep Disorders**: Chronic sleep disturbances, such as insomnia, sleep apnea, or restless leg syndrome, can interfere with memory consolidation and cognitive function. Adequate sleep is crucial for memory formation and overall brain health.
- **Chronic Medical Conditions**: Chronic illnesses like diabetes, hypertension, and heart disease can impact vascular health and increase the risk of cognitive impairment and memory problems over time.

If you or a loved one is experiencing memory problems, it's crucial to speak with a healthcare professional to identify the underlying cause and the best course of action. Reversible causes can be addressed, cognitive function and quality of life can be enhanced, and early detection and intervention can help.

5.1.4. Brain Scan Needed to Diagnose Alzheimer's Disease

The diagnosis of Alzheimer's disease frequently combines neuroimaging, cognitive testing, and clinical assessment. Although cognitive testing and clinical assessment offer important insights into cognitive impairment, neuroimaging methods are essential for confirming the diagnosis and comprehending the underlying brain abnormalities linked to Alzheimer's disease. The diagnosis and differential diagnosis of Alzheimer's disease are aided by structural and functional brain scans, two types of neuroimaging modalities that offer important information about the structure, function, and pathology of the brain.

The structural anatomy of the brain can be seen in great detail thanks to structural neuroimaging methods like magnetic resonance imaging (MRI). When diagnosing Alzheimer's disease, MRI scans can reveal changes in brain volume, cortical thickness, and the presence of structural abnormalities. Hippocampal atrophy, which is characterized by shrinkage of the hippocampus, a region essential for memory formation, is one of the distinguishing characteristics of Alzheimer's disease on MRI. Hippocampal atrophy is a sensitive biomarker for Alzheimer's disease that correlates with cognitive decline and the advancement of the disease, according to studies. Furthermore, MRI can identify additional structural abnormalities linked to Alzheimer's disease, including white matter hyper-intensities, ventricular enlargement, and cortical thinning. These abnormalities may help differentiate Alzheimer's from other types of dementia or cognitive impairment.

Functional brain imaging techniques, such as positron emission tomography (PET) and functional magnetic resonance imaging (fMRI), offer valuable insights into brain function and connectivity. PET imaging using radiotracers that target amyloid-beta and tau proteins enables the visualization and quantification of these pathological features, which are characteristic of Alzheimer's disease. Detection of elevated levels of amyloid and tau in specific brain regions is indicative of Alzheimer's pathology and supports the diagnosis of the disease. Additionally, PET imaging can evaluate cerebral glucose metabolism, which is often impaired in Alzheimer's disease, indicating neuronal dysfunction and synaptic loss in affected brain areas. On the other hand, fMRI can measure changes in blood flow and oxygenation levels in the brain, providing information on brain activity and functional connections. Studies have demonstrated disruptions in functional connectivity networks in Alzheimer's disease, underscoring the disease's impact on brain networks and cognitive function.

Although neuroimaging methods offer important insights into the pathology of Alzheimer's disease, they are not used alone for diagnosis; rather, they are used in conjunction with clinical assessment and cognitive testing. To establish a comprehensive diagnosis of Alzheimer's disease, neuroimaging findings should be interpreted in conjunction with clinical symptoms, cognitive assessment results, and other diagnostic tests. Furthermore, by differentiating Alzheimer's disease from other neurodegenerative diseases, vascular dementia, or other causes of cognitive impairment, neuroimaging can help with differential diagnosis. Furthermore, neuroimaging methods can be used to measure the course of a disease over time, track how well a treatment is working, and assess the effectiveness of disease-modifying medications in clinical trials.

Neuroimaging is essential for the diagnosis and treatment of Alzheimer's disease because it offers important insights into the pathology, structure, and function of the brain. The underlying brain abnormalities linked to Alzheimer's disease can be better understood by using structural and functional brain scans, such as MRI, PET, and fMRI. These scans can help with diagnosis, differential diagnosis, and tracking the course of the disease. To create a thorough diagnosis and direct treatment choices for people with Alzheimer's disease, neuroimaging results should be interpreted in concert with clinical evaluation and cognitive testing (Balasa et al., 2011; Altomare et al., 2019; Villain & Dubois, 2019; Werry, 2019; Dubois et al., 2021).

5.2. ALZHEIMER'S DISEASE BIOMARKERS

The word "biomarker," which is short for "biological marker," refers to a medical indicator or trait seen in living organisms in general. Measurable biological changes known as biomarkers can indicate the presence of an illness or a person's susceptibility to one. By identifying and measuring biomarkers, scientists and medical professionals can screen for specific diseases. A few techniques are getting samples of bodily fluids such as blood, saliva, urine, and cerebrospinal fluid (a clear, colorless liquid that surrounds the brain and spinal cord) and performing imaging scans. One common biomarker of diabetes is a high blood glucose (sugar) level, which is used to make the diagnosis.

5.2.1. Biomarkers in Alzheimer's Disease: Role in Early and Differential Diagnosis and Recognition of Atypical Variants

The most prevalent type of dementia, accounting for roughly two-thirds of cases worldwide, is Alzheimer's disease (AD). Roughly 25% of dementia cases are clinically identified globally, leaving an estimated 41 million people living with dementia who are still undiagnosed. AD is a neurodegenerative disease characterized by neuropathologic alterations such as amyloid-beta (Aβ) plaques made of aggregated Aβ and neurofibrillary tangles made of aggregated tau proteins. It has different pathobiological subtypes and clinical presentations. These neuropathologic alterations are linked to reactive astrogliosis, neuroinflammation, transmitter deficits, synapse and neuronal loss, and ultimately cognitive impairment.

Although dementia with a subtle onset, slow progression, and prominent amnestic impairment is the classic clinical phenotype of AD, accounting for about 85% of cases, a significant minority of patients with AD pathology also exhibit non-amnestic cognitive impairment. AD is difficult to diagnose because of its varied pathobiological characteristics (e.g., composition, location, and severity), hereditary variables, brain resiliency, and the consequent unique clinical presentation (e.g., frontal AD, corticobasal syndrome (CBS), posterior cortical atrophy (PCA), logopenic variant of primary progressive aphasia (lvPPA), etc. Particularly in the aging brain, AD pathology can often co-occur with other neurodegenerative and vascular diseases. For this reason, prompt differential diagnosis is essential to providing the right care, support, and customized treatment regimens.

AD patients may have advanced into later stages of the disease at the time of diagnosis, with an average interval of 2 and a half years between the onset of symptoms and diagnosis. Patients with AD experience varying degrees of cognitive impairment, which correspond to distinct stages in the disease's progression. These stages include preclinical disease, which is characterized by the presence of biomarkers of AD pathology but lacks or has subtle cognitive impairment, prodromal AD, which is characterized by mild cognitive impairment due to AD, mild dementia, and moderate-to-severe dementia due to AD.

In order to fully benefit from symptomatic medications that have been shown to reduce symptoms and postpone the clinical decline of AD, early diagnosis is crucial. Furthermore, new disease-modifying therapies (DMTs) for AD are currently being developed or approved. Early diagnosis of AD is even more important because these are thought to be most effective in the early stages of the disease, and clinical trials have concentrated on participants with early AD (mild cognitive impairment due to AD or early AD dementia). As an illustration, the US Food and Drug Administration recently approved aducanumab, a monoclonal antibody that targets aggregated Aβ, for the treatment of early Alzheimer's disease. Furthermore, a number of additional treatments for AD are presently being developed and may eventually be put to clinical use.

The development of in vivo biomarkers has allowed for a shift in diagnosing Alzheimer's Disease (AD) from later dementia stages to earlier stages, enabling the possibility of pre-symptomatic diagnosis. The recent recommendations of the International Working Group suggest that diagnosis of AD in clinical settings is limited to individuals with specific AD phenotypes and biomarker findings. Those who are unimpaired cognitively but test positive for biomarkers should be considered at risk for developing AD dementia. Clinical diagnosis is primarily based on phenotype, but biomarkers are increasingly used to differentiate between disorders and AD subtypes, particularly in early stages, and to identify individuals at risk for presenting with symptoms of AD.

5.2.2. The Clinical Phenotypes of 0AD

Amnestic syndrome is the most common phenotype of AD, accounting for about 85% of cases. Less frequently occurring AD phenotypes are lvPPA and PCA. Additional abnormalities encompass CBS, behavioral or dysexecutive variations of frontal AD, and additional variations (e.g., split into two categories: semantic variant primary progressive aphasia (svPPA) and non-fluent primary progressive aphasia (nfPPA). The composition of one published clinical sample, illustrating the prevalence of typical and atypical clinical phenotypes of AD, is shown (Figure 5.1).

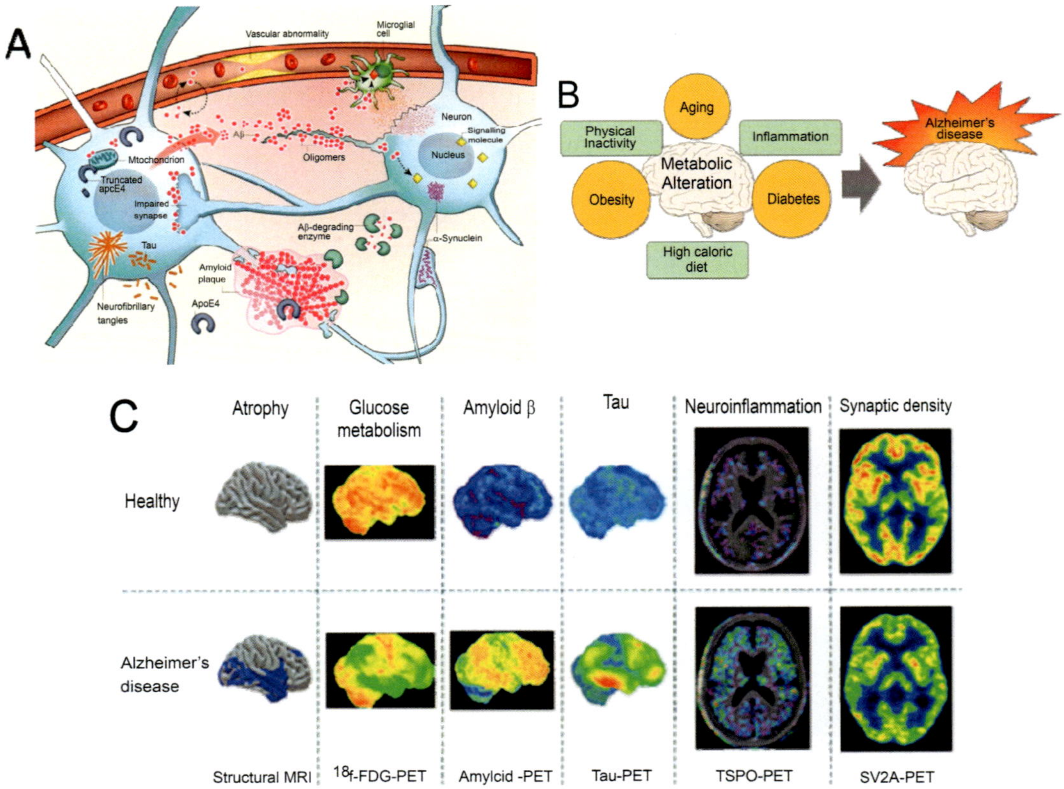

Figure 5.1. *Clinical analysis.*

Source: Passeri E, Elkhoury K, Morsink M, Broersen K, Linder M, Tamayol A, Malaplate C, & Yen FT, (2022). Arab-tehrany e. Alzheimer's disease: Treatment strategies and their limitations. International Journal of Molecular Sciences, 23(22), 13954. https://doi.org/10.3390/ijms232213954.

The clinical sample included 523 patients with AD who were subsequently referred to a specialized dementia clinic; 42 patients had motor cognitive impairment (MCI) and are not shown in the pie chart. Although it's possible, patients with language presentation most likely had lvPPA rather than nfPPA. Alzheimer's disease (AD); corticobasal syndrome (CBS); non-fluent primary progressive aphasia (nfPPA); mild cognitive impairment (MCI); posterior cortical atrophy (PCA); and semantic variant primary progressive aphasia (svPPA).

Semantic cueing is used to assess amnestic syndrome, which is typically characterized by deficits in learning and recall of recently acquired information (e.g., for efficient information encoding and retrieval, such as the Free and Cued Selective Reminding Test, which uses controlled learning. Individuals suffering from amnestic syndrome exhibit reduced overall recall and poor free recall (e.g., inadequate cueing effectiveness or poor recognition), suggesting that information is not retained and that retrieval is not made easier.

Single-word retrieval, sentence repetition, and motor speech abilities (including phonemic paraphasia) are impaired in patients with lvPPA. The function of the bilateral occipital and parietal cortices, as well as the dorsal and ventral visual streams, is impaired in PCA, resulting in a decline in visuospatial and visuoperceptual abilities (accompanied by visual inattention or Balint's syndrome) and poor reading and math skills.

Alien limb phenomena, myoclonus, eye and limb apraxia, parkinsonian rigidity, and cortical sensory deficits are characteristics of CBS. Frontal AD is characterized by a progressive clinical syndrome that may include disproportionate executive dysfunction or prominent frontal behavioral features. Initially, cognitive difficulties are more common in patients with behavioral and dysexecutive variants of frontal AD than behavioral changes (25% or less). A smaller percentage of cases initially present with motor symptoms, or a combination of behavioral, cognitive, and/or motor symptoms. Apathy, disinhibition, loss of empathy, perseverative or compulsive behavior, hyperorality, and dietary changes are among the behavioral symptoms; on the other hand, the dysexecutive variant is characterized by a decline in core executive cognitive function, including working memory and cognitive flexibility. There are other primary progressive aphasia phenotypes that are less likely to be associated with AD pathology. These include svPPA, which is known for difficulties understanding word meanings, and nfPPA, which is characterized by poor grammar in both spoken and written form along with impaired syntactic comprehension and bucco-facial apraxia. Compared to 20% of nfPPA cases and 16% of svPPA cases, 86% of all lvPPA cases are caused by AD (Balasa et al., 2011; Altomare et al., 2019; Villain & Dubois, 2019; Werry, 2019; Dubois et al., 2021).

The clinical symptoms associated with the different phenotypes of AD are summarized in Table 5.1.

Table 5.1. Clinical Features of the Different Phenotypes of AD

A. Insidious onset. Symptoms have a gradual onset over months to years, not sudden over hours or days B. Clear-cut history of worsening of cognition by report or observation; and C. The initial and most prominent cognitive deficit are evident on history and examination in one of the following categories a. Amnestic presentation is the most common syndromic presentation of AD dementia. The deficits should include impairment in learning and recall of recently learned information. There should also be evidence of cognitive dysfunction in at least one other cognitive domain b. Nonamnestic presentations: • Language presentation: The most prominent deficits are in word-finding, but deficits in other cognitive domains should be present • Visuospatial presentation: The most prominent deficits are in spatial cognition, including object agnosia, impaired face recognition, simultagnosia, and alexia. Deficits in other cognitive domains should be present • Executive dysfunction: The most prominent deficits are impaired reasoning, judgment, and problem solving. Deficits in other cognitive domains should be present	
Possible AD	Atypical course A. Atypical course meets the core clinical criteria in terms of the cognitive deficits for AD dementia, but either has a sudden onset of cognitive impairment or demonstrates insufficient historical detail or objective cognitive documentation of progressive decline or Etiologically mixed presentation B. Etiologically mixed presentation meets all core clinical criteria for AD dementia but has evidence as the following: a. Concomitant cerebrovascular disease, defined by a history of stroke temporally related to the onset or worsening of cognitive impairment; or the presence of multiple or extensive infarcts or severe white matter hyperintensity burden; or b. Features of Dementia with Lewy bodies other than the dementia itself; or c. Evidence for another neurological diseases or a non-neurological medical comorbidity or medication use that could have a substantial effect on cognition

Probable AD with Three Levels of Evidence of AD Pathophysiology	Intermediate Aβ unavailable or indeterminate Neuronal injury positive Intermediate Aβ positive Neuronal injury unavailable or indeterminate High Aβ positive Neuronal injury positive
Possible AD (Atypical Presentation) with Evidence of AD Pathophysiology	High but does not rule out second etiology Aβ positive Neuronal injury positive
Dementia-Unlikely Due to AD	1. Does not meet clinical criteria for AD dementia. 2. a. Regardless of meeting clinical criteria for probable or possible AD dementia, there is sufficient evidence for an alternative diagnosis such as HIV dementia, dementia of Huntington's disease, or others that rarely, if ever, overlap with AD. b. Regardless of meeting clinical criteria for possible AD dementia, both Aβ and neuronal injury biomarkers are negative

Source: Xu, W., Marseglia, A., Ferrari, C., & Wang, H.-X. (2013). Alzheimer's Disease: A Clinical Perspective. InTech. doi: 10.5772/54539.

Co-pathologies such as α-synuclein accumulation, vascular pathology, TAR DNA-binding protein 43 pathology, and non-AD tauopathies can impact the clinical presentation of AD, especially in the aging population, since co-pathologies tend to get worse with age. The existence of co-pathologies typically causes symptoms to manifest more subtly or with differences in effect. The majority of non-AD neurodegenerative diseases lack biomarkers for their underlying pathology, so post-mortem analysis or the discovery of a biomarker-supported phenotype are the only ways to distinguish AD from these diseases. The canonical biomarkers of AD are present in both atypical and typical phenotypes; in vivo confirmation of AD pathology can be achieved through fluid biomarkers and molecular neuroimaging.

5.2.3. Biomarker Profiles for Typical and Atypical Phenotypes of AD

Most AD biomarkers fall into one of two categories: topographic biomarkers or pathophysiologic biomarkers. Both types of biomarkers can aid in the identification, distinction, and diagnosis of AD phenotypes by clinicians. Amyloid positron emission tomography (PET), amyloid and tau protein concentrations in cerebrospinal fluid (CSF), and plasma concentrations of these and other protein biomarkers are examples of pathophysiologic biomarkers associated with AD lesions. Topographic biomarkers, such as regional hypometabolism on fluorodeoxyglucose (FDG)-PET, tau PET, and regional/local atrophy on structural magnetic resonance imaging (MRI), are associated with the regional effects of AD pathology. Although no fluid biomarker has been definitively connected to a specific clinical phenotype of AD to date, there are corresponding molecular, metabolic, and degenerative imaging biomarkers for the various phenotypes of AD based on differences in their regional distribution (Figure 5.2). The existing literature is predominantly focused on biomarkers of AD pathology, where the main clinical value of their uses is to discriminate between phenotypes that are associated with AD vs. non-AD pathologies, as well as to gauge biological advancements like phosphorylated tau (pTau) levels in plasma and CSF. The necessity of clinical evaluation is emphasized by the fact that there is currently no single biomarker or biomarker algorithm that can distinguish between AD phenotypes with definitive diagnostic accuracy.

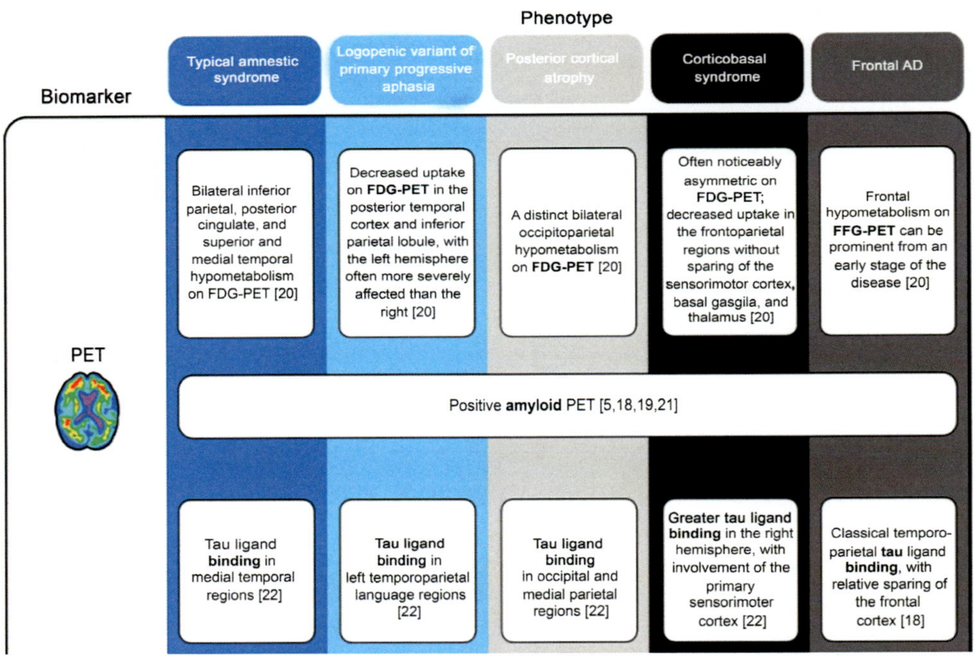

	Specificity	Sensitivity
Biomarkers of Aβ Deposition		
CSF Aβ [83]	90%	86%
PET amyloid imaging [78]	56.2%	93.5%
Biomarkers of Neuronal Injury		
CSF tau [83]	90%	81%
Medial temporal lobe atrophy on MRI [75]	88%	85%
FDG-PET imaging [78]	74%	78.7%

Figure 5.2. *Summary of anticipated biomarker results for the different clinical phenotypes of AD.*

Source: Xu, W., Marseglia, A., Ferrari, C., & Wang, H.-X. (2013). Alzheimer's Disease: A Clinical Perspective. InTech. doi: 10.5772/54539.

5.2.4. PET Markers

Using a range of ligands for PET imaging, physicians can differentiate between other neurodegenerative diseases and determine the underlying pathology of both typical and atypical phenotypes of AD. of PET imaging across the clinical phenotypes of AD are shown (Figure 5.3).

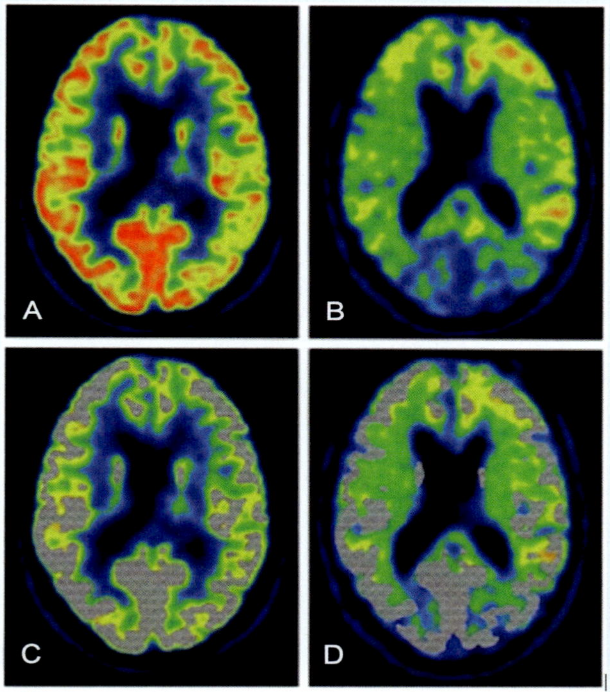

Figure 5.3. *FDG-PET for the clinical phenotypes of AD.*

Source: Høilund-Carlsen PF, Revheim M-E, Costa T, Kepp KP, Castellani RJ, Perry G, Alavi A, & Barrio JR, (2023). FDG-PET versus amyloid-PET imaging for diagnosis and response evaluation in Alzheimer's disease: Benefits and pitfalls. Diagnostics, 13(13), 2254. https://doi.org/10.3390/diagnostics13132254.

A topographic biomarker called FDG-PET can be used to distinguish between typical and atypical AD. Regional hypometabolism patterns in AD variants reflect clinical deficits. Bilateral hypometabolism in the parietal and medial temporal regions, including the precuneus, is a common feature in AD patients. In order to facilitate differential diagnosis, this imaging technique can also identify patterns of hypometabolism typical of dementias other than AD, such as frontotemporal dementia (FTD) and dementia with Lewy bodies. Although FDG-PET is less common than MRI, it offers more diagnostic information.

Amyloid PET is primarily utilized in the research context and is capable of visualizing brain fibrillar or insoluble Aβ plaques, but not other Aβ peptide forms. The most thoroughly tested biomarker for identifying amyloid plaques is amyloid PET, which has shown excellent accuracy in imaging-to-autopsy studies (specificity: 100%; sensitivity: 92%). In contrast to other imaging modalities, patients with typical and atypical AD have similar amyloid distribution as seen by PET.

Tau PET is the only autopsy-validated (sensitivity, 92–100%; specificity, 52–92%) direct marker of neurofibrillary tangles; fluid markers have not shown comparable accuracy. Tau PET is primarily used in the research setting. As tau PET is associated with short-term progression (3–5 years) in cognitively unimpaired individuals, it has been demonstrated to predict cognitive decline in comparison to amyloid PET. This makes tau PET highly relevant for clinical settings. Tau PET is a topographic technique, and its deposition patterns are more indicative of the clinical phenotype than those of amyloid PET. Greater levels of Tau PET ligand binding have been observed in patients with the amnestic form of AD, left frontal regions in logopenic aphasia, and occipital regions in posterior cortical atrophy. Typical (amnestic form) and atypical AD have different tau PET patterns, which may help to characterize the biology underlying the respective phenotypes. Currently being studied as additional PET biomarkers to assist in the diagnosis of AD are translocator protein PET for neuroinflammation and synaptic vesicle glycoprotein 2A PET for synaptic density. Notably, rather than being used for differential diagnosis, these biomarkers would be used for disease staging and prognostication. Furthermore, there is very little use of these PET tracers in clinical settings (Balasa et al., 2011; Altomare et al., 2019; Villain & Dubois, 2019; Werry, 2019; Dubois et al., 2021).

5.2.5. MRI Markers

Topographic biomarkers of AD include changes in MRI, and structural MRI in AD patients reveals gray matter atrophy and volume loss, which point to neurodegeneration. Since serial structural MRI imaging has less variance than single structural MRI, it is frequently used to track the progression of disease. Given that clinical trials could be conducted with smaller sample sizes than would be feasible with traditional clinical assessments, some data suggest that serial structural MRI may have the potential to assess therapeutic efficacy in clinical practice. T2-weighted or susceptibility-weighted MRI is used to measure vascular activity and identify cerebral amyloid angiopathy. Diffusion tensor imaging MRI is used to evaluate white matter damage. Resting state functional MRI is used to evaluate changes in functional brain connectivity that are thought to precede structural brain changes. Although these methods are not currently employed in most clinical trials or standard clinical practice, they might become more crucial in the management of amyloid-related imaging abnormalities (ARIA) when anti-amyloid medications are used.

While in atypical AD, atrophy is typically most prominent in regions corresponding to clinical symptoms and is frequently hippocampal-sparing in early-stage disease, in the typical form of AD, atrophy starts in the medial-temporal lobe and progresses to involve the lateral-temporal and parietal cortices on structural MRI. While MRI changes mirror those observed in FDG-PET, they typically manifest later in the course of the illness. It has been demonstrated that hippocampal volume measured by structural magnetic resonance imaging in patients with AD correlates with memory scores on the Free and Cued Selective Reminding Test in patients with amnestic syndrome.

5.2.6. CSF Biomarkers

0Both tau and Aβ peptides can be identified using CSF biomarkers, and in the majority of patients, changes in these biomarkers can be identified before changes in neuroimaging biomarkers. While an increase in pTau is more specific to AD pathology in both typical and atypical presentations, CSF tau indicates neuronal death and can therefore be elevated in atypical phenotypes as well as non-AD dementias. Aβ (1–42) (Aβ42), Aβ (1–40) (Aβ40), pTau 181 (pTau181), pTau 217 (pTau217), and total tau (tTau) are examples of CSF biomarkers. Even in the pre-symptomatic and prodromal stages of the disease progression, these markers have been proven to reliably identify biologic changes associated with AD, and some have even shown promise in predicting cognitive decline.

The degree of Aβ plaque deposition is inversely correlated with CSF Aβ42 concentration and Aβ42/40 ratio, while the degree of neurodegeneration and neurofibrillary tangles is correlated with tTau and pTau concentrations, respectively. Even in individuals with atypical clinical features or irregular CSF findings for other analytes, the presence of a decreased CSF Aβ42/40 ratio usually indicates AD pathology. Regarding a "FTD-phenotype," the pTau181/Aβ42 ratio is helpful in distinguishing frontal AD patients from frontotemporal dementia patients as well as in identifying the behavioral and semantic variants of the disease. Another pTau epitope that has shown promise for early AD diagnosis and detection of AD pathology incipient is CSF pTau 231 (pTau231). This epitope is not limited to the clinical phenotype.

Because of its high sensitivity, neurofilament light chain (NfL) has taken the place of tau as a biofluid indicator of neurodegeneration in certain clinics. Other CSF biomarkers that are being studied to help diagnose AD include neurogranin and other synaptic biomarkers, glial fibrillary acidic protein (GFAP), and chitinase 3-like 1 (also known as YKL-40). Notably, rather than being used for differential diagnosis, these biomarkers would be used for disease staging and prognostication (Balasa et al., 2011; Altomare et al., 2019; Villain & Dubois, 2019; Werry, 2019; Dubois et al., 2021).

5.2.7. Blood-Based Biomarkers (BBBMs)

BBBMs are becoming valuable instruments to help identify the pathology linked to AD; blood levels of pTau and Aβ peptides have shown correlations with both PET positivity and the corresponding levels in CSF. Commercially available in the US, assays measuring the plasma Aβ42/40 ratio have demonstrated potential in detecting Aβ positivity across the entire AD spectrum. Additional validation of these assays is necessary because of possible robustness issues, specifically to determine whether the plasma Aβ42/40 ratio would be sufficiently scalable to support clinical diagnosis in a timely manner. Plasma pTau181, pTau217, and pTau231 have demonstrated potential in identifying tau-related AD pathology that is progressing. Furthermore, blood GFAP has shown promise in both differentiating FTD from AD and predicting cognitive decline to AD dementia in patients with mild cognitive impairment.

A recent study found that NfL levels are higher in patients with primary progressive aphasia compared to controls, and can help differentiate between different subtypes of the disease with 81% sensitivity and 67% specificity. While Aβ peptides and pTau levels in plasma may be better at distinguishing Alzheimer's disease from other conditions, NfL shows promise in aiding the diagnosis of Alzheimer's-related primary progressive aphasia, especially in one particular subtype. In the future, Blood-Brain Barrier Markers (BBBMs) are expected to be a valuable tool for detecting Alzheimer's disease, ensuring that patients receive necessary assessments and tests promptly. While biomarker profiles cannot replace clinical evaluation entirely, BBBMs are likely to be used in conjunction with clinical information and imaging to support clinical decision-making.

One blood-based genetic biomarker for AD is apolipoprotein E (APOE), and having the APOE ε4 genotype increases the risk of the disease. APOE ε4 gene carrier status is one of the factors that can increase the risk of progression to symptomatic AD; APOE ε4 homozygotes have an extremely high risk of developing clinical AD. Thus, the likelihood of amyloid pathology is supported by the presence of APOE ε4 in a person exhibiting symptoms similar to AD. The most effective method for identifying people who are more likely to develop dementia may involve combining APOE status with polygenic risk scores that do not include the APOE region in order to assess the contribution of non-APOE genes. In terms of clinical phenotypes, the APOE ε4 allele promotes the typical amnestic phenotype, while the atypical non-memory phenotypes frequently arise when the APOE ε4 allele is absent (Balasa et al., 2011; Altomare et al., 2019; Villain & Dubois, 2019; Werry, 2019; Dubois et al., 2021).

5.2.8. Biomarkers Should be Complementary to Clinical Assessment for AD Diagnosis

In the past, the diagnosis of AD was exclusively determined by clinical criteria. Nevertheless, contemporary guidelines for AD diagnosis also take biologic marker presence into account. The National Institute on Aging and Alzheimer's Association (NIA-AA)-based "ATN" research framework can be used for the neuropathologic diagnosis of AD using biomarkers. This framework suggests defining AD independent of clinical phenotypes and even in the absence of cognitive symptoms, based on amyloid abnormalities ('A'), tau protein changes ('T'), and evidence of neurodegeneration ('N'). According to the ATN research framework guidelines, neuropathologists are qualified to attest to the existence of AD pathology in the brain, but they are not qualified to diagnose the clinicopathologic syndrome that is identified as AD.

There is discussion regarding the application of the NIA-AA "ATN" research framework in clinical practice because its intended use is for research. In order to support or validate the clinical diagnosis of AD, biomarkers should be used in addition to clinical assessment, as they are not adequate on their own. While tau PET has demonstrated the ability to predict cognitive decline in individuals without cognitive impairment, biomarker-only diagnosis of AD typically has a modest predictive accuracy in cognitively unimpaired individuals because these subjects may have amyloid positivity without ever exhibiting clinical symptoms. According to current estimates, 44–74% of cognitively unimpaired individuals with amyloidosis have a lifetime dementia risk. It is significant to remember that there is no direct biological or clinical progression comparison between tau PET and CSF tau measurements. As previously mentioned, tau alterations are typically indicative of a more rapid progression. Moreover, a diagnosis of AD based solely on biomarkers may be detrimental to a patient in the absence of clinical assessment or clinical symptoms. It is important for patients to understand the varied nature and progression of AD, as well as the possibility that symptoms may not appear during their lifetime in the case of a positive biomarker result. Individuals with AD diagnosed clinically might not exhibit biomarker positivity. The AD phenotype is not always a reliable indicator of AD pathology in the brain, as up to 35% of patients with a clinical diagnosis of AD have amyloid PET negativity.

The significant variation in the course of the disease among those who are biomarker-positive is another significant drawback of the biomarker-only AD diagnosis approach. The likelihood of advancement is contingent upon various factors and may be linked to various mechanisms, including brain resistance (i.e., demonstrated minimal or nonexistent pathology in spite of significant AD risk factors), resilience (i.e., maintaining a normal cognitive function in spite of severe AD pathology), and reserve (i.e., pre-morbid physiologic capacity). A significant percentage of individuals maintain cognitive normalcy throughout their lives, only exhibiting signs of Alzheimer's disease (AD) pathology, such as amyloidosis, upon autopsy or in vivo imaging (~30%).

The etiology of many dementias is mixed, and because most non-AD pathologic changes lack biomarkers, it can be difficult to distinguish non-AD dementias. Phenotype or post-mortem examination plays a major role in differential diagnosis. The diagnostic accuracy for a clinical diagnosis of AD is only approximately 75–80%, even among specialists. However, based on a comprehensive clinical work-up that includes neuroimaging, CSF biomarkers (Aβ42, pTau181, and tTau) alone can distinguish between AD and non-AD dementias (such as dementia with Lewy bodies, FTD, vascular dementia, and Parkinson's disease dementia) with a diagnostic accuracy of 82.7%, which is comparable to the clinical diagnostic accuracy of 81.6%. Furthermore, it has been shown that tau PET and amyloid PET can distinguish between frontotemporal lobar degeneration and AD. In AD, amyloid and tau PET are positive; in non-AD disorders, they are negative.

Table 5.2. Summary for Diagnosing Alzheimer's Disease

Test Name	Type	Description
Physical and neurological exam	Physical	A medical professional will conduct a physical examination. The neurological examination may encompass the evaluation of reflexes as an assessment component. The current topic of discussion pertains to the physiological aspects of muscle tone and strength. The capacity to rise from a seated position and ambulate to a different location within a given space. The faculties of vision and audition, coordination, and balance.
Lab test	Blood	The utilization of blood tests can aid in excluding alternative etiologies of cognitive impairment and amnesia, such as hypothyroidism or inadequate vitamin concentrations. Beta-amyloid protein and tau protein levels can also be quantified through blood tests. However, the accessibility of these tests is limited, and coverage may be restricted.
Magnetic resonance imaging (MRI)	Brain Imaging	Magnetic resonance imaging (MRI) employs a combination of radio waves and a potent magnetic field to generate comprehensive visual representations of the brain. However, exhibiting atrophy in specific brain regions linked to Alzheimer's, MRI scans also eliminate alternative ailments. In the assessment of dementia, an MRI is typically favored over a CT scan.
Computerized tomography (CT)	Brain Imaging	The computed tomography (CT) scan, a specialized form of X-ray imaging, can generate cross-sectional visual representations of the human brain. Typically, it excludes the presence of neoplasms, cerebrovascular accidents, and cranial traumas. Magnetic resonance imaging (MRI) employs radiofrequency waves and a potent magnetic field to generate intricate visual representations of the human brain. However, exhibiting atrophy in specific brain regions linked to Alzheimer's, MRI scans also eliminate alternative ailments. In the assessment of dementia, an MRI is typically favored over a CT scan.
Positron emission tomography (PET)	Brain Imaging	Positron emission tomography (PET) can acquire visual representations of the pathological progression. In the process of conducting a PET scan, a radiopharmaceutical tracer of low intensity is administered intravenously to enable the identification of a specific cerebral characteristic.
Genetic test	Genetic	The utilization of genetic testing is not advised for the majority of individuals undergoing evaluation for Alzheimer's disease. Individuals with a familial background of early-onset Alzheimer's disease may contemplate the matter.

Source: *Dara OA, Lopez-Guede JM, Raheem HI, Rahebi J, Zulueta E, & Fernandez-Gamiz U, (2023). Alzheimer's disease diagnosis using machine learning: A survey. Applied Sciences, 13(14), 8298. https://doi.org/10.3390/app13148298.*

It is significant to remember that the "ATN" research framework is a constrained set of biomarkers that should be taken into account when diagnosing AD. Inflammatory biomarkers, beta-synuclein (synaptic degeneration), NfL (neurodegeneration), and GFAP (astrogliosis) are additional biomarkers that should be taken into account for incorporation into the framework (Balasa et al., 2011; Altomare et al., 2019; Villain & Dubois, 2019; Werry, 2019; Dubois et al., 2021)

5.2.9. Biomarkers to Support Clinical Decision Making

Confirmatory roles for AD biomarkers are crucial in clinical decision making, especially with the development of anti-Aβ DMTs (Figure 5.4). Early intervention in the course of the disease is desirable because these DMTs are intended to postpone the onset or slow the progression of cognitive changes. Biomarkers can help in the early diagnosis of AD and may even be able to identify patients at risk of the disease before they manifest clinically, depending on the underlying pathology. Clinically validated AD biomarkers include tau PET, FDG-PET, MRI, CSF measurements of tau and amyloid, and plasma biomarkers, which are almost ready for approval.

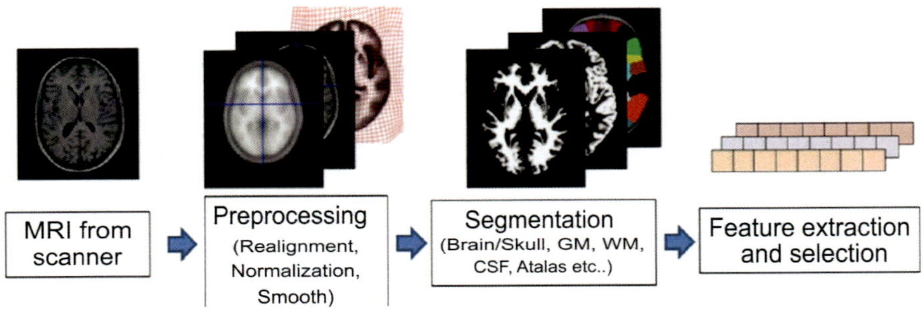

Figure 5.4. *The role of AD biomarkers in the clinical setting.*

Source: Dara OA, Lopez-Guede JM, Raheem HI, Rahebi J, Zulueta E, & Fernandez-Gamiz U, (2023). Alzheimer's disease diagnosis using machine learning: A survey. Applied Sciences, 13(14), 8298. https://doi.org/10.3390/app13148298.

Utilizing biomarkers in clinical practice shows promise in aiding drug development for individuals with or at risk of AD. For instance, APOE ε4 homozygotes are a high-risk group for preclinical AD research and trials. While APOE ε4 status may not play a key role in diagnosing AD, it could be significant in the era of anti-Aβ DMTs due to APOE ε4 carriers having a higher risk of ARIA. Amyloid PET quantifies amyloid plaque burden and assists in AD diagnosis, though its cost and availability may limit its use in clinical settings. Plasma biomarkers like pTau181 and pTau217 show promise in predicting AD progression in individuals without cognitive impairment and may aid in participant selection and monitoring in clinical trials. FDG-PET, on the other hand, could be a more accessible tool for predicting AD progression in those with mild cognitive impairment and estimating disease-free time.

Improved *in vivo* detection of amnestic and non-amnestic AD phenotypes is made possible by biomarkers. Compared to patients presenting with typical AD, patients with atypical AD clinical syndromes frequently receive a later diagnosis. According to one study, patients with young-onset AD who presented atypically were more likely to receive the wrong diagnosis (53%) than those who presented typically (4%). These patients can now be more confidently identified and diagnosed earlier in the course of the disease thanks to the availability of AD biomarkers and the inclusion of atypical AD phenotypes in diagnostic algorithms. As a result, they can receive customized information, appropriate care and support, and the creation of unique treatment plans. Giving patients and their families information about their prognosis can help them cope with the news and make plans and decisions based on the information at hand. These developments will facilitate more patient access to DMT clinical trials, which frequently turn away individuals with unusual phenotypes (Balasa et al., 2011; Altomare et al., 2019; Villain & Dubois, 2019; Werry, 2019; Dubois et al., 2021).

5.2.10. Who Should Attend Alzheimer's Disease Testing and Diagnosis?

Several medical specialists often collaborate to diagnose and treat Alzheimer's patients to provide comprehensive care. Depending on the healthcare system, the resources at hand, and the case's complexity, different people may be involved.

Some key professionals who may be involved in Alzheimer's disease testing and diagnosis:

- **Primary Care Physician (PCP)**: The primary care physician often serves as the initial point of contact for individuals with cognitive concerns. They conduct an initial evaluation, gather medical history, perform cognitive screening tests, and may initiate further diagnostic workup. PCPs play a crucial role in coordinating care and referring patients to specialists as needed.
- **Neurologist**: Neurologists specialize in the diagnosis and treatment of neurological disorders, including Alzheimer's disease and other forms of dementia. They may conduct a more in-depth neurological evaluation, interpret neuroimaging results, and provide specialized expertise in diagnosing and managing cognitive disorders.
- **Geriatrician**: Geriatricians specialize in the care of older adults and may play a significant role in Alzheimer's disease diagnosis, particularly in elderly populations. They have expertise in managing age-related health conditions, cognitive impairment, and complex medical issues often associated with Alzheimer's disease.
- **Neuropsychologist**: Neuropsychologists are trained in assessing cognitive function and identifying patterns of cognitive impairment. They conduct comprehensive neuropsychological evaluations, including standardized testing of memory, language, attention, and executive function, which can aid in diagnosing Alzheimer's disease and differentiating it from other cognitive disorders.
- **Radiologist**: Radiologists interpret neuroimaging studies, such as MRI and PET scans, to identify structural and functional abnormalities in the brain. They provide valuable insights into brain changes associated with Alzheimer's disease, supporting the diagnostic process and treatment planning.
- **Clinical Psychologist or Psychiatrist**: Clinical psychologists and psychiatrists may be involved in the assessment and management of mood and behavioral symptoms associated with Alzheimer's disease. They provide support for individuals with Alzheimer's and their families, addressing psychological and emotional needs

throughout the diagnostic process and beyond.

- **Caregivers and Family Members**: Caregivers and family members play a crucial role in Alzheimer's disease testing and diagnosis by providing essential information about symptoms, medical history, and functional status. They may accompany the individual to appointments, assist with cognitive testing, and provide ongoing support throughout the diagnostic process and beyond.
- **Social Worker or Case Manager**: Social workers or case managers help coordinate care, provide resources, and support individuals and families coping with Alzheimer's disease. They offer assistance with accessing community services, long-term care planning, and navigating the healthcare system.

A multidisciplinary team of medical experts, including primary care doctors, neurologists, geriatricians, neuropsychologists, radiologists, psychologists, social workers, and caregivers, are frequently involved in the testing and diagnosis of Alzheimer's disease. A thorough assessment, prompt diagnosis, and a customized treatment plan catered to the needs and circumstances of the individual are guaranteed by collaborative care (Balasa et al., 2011; Altomare et al., 2019; Villain & Dubois, 2019; Werry, 2019; Dubois et al., 2021).

5.3. DIAGNOSIS AND MANAGEMENT OF ALZHEIMER'S DISEASE

The progressive neurological condition known as Alzheimer's disease poses particular difficulties for both diagnosis and treatment. Although it can be difficult to detect early because of its gradual onset and progression, early detection is vital. Together with a neurological examination and medical history, the diagnosis usually entails a thorough evaluation of cognitive function, including memory, language, executive function, and visuospatial abilities. The diagnosis can be confirmed with the help of sophisticated neuroimaging methods like MRI and PET scans, which can spot distinctive brain abnormalities like amyloid buildup and atrophy. Alzheimer's disease management becomes complex after a diagnosis, with a focus on both pharmacological and non-pharmacological interventions. The goal of pharmacotherapy is to reduce symptoms and possibly halt the course of the illness. Medications that block cholinergic neurotransmission, like galantamine, rivastigmine, and donepezil, are frequently prescribed to treat cognitive decline and functional impairment. Moreover, memantine, an NMDA receptor antagonist, might be recommended to control symptoms and modulate glutamatergic activity.

However, medication by itself is unable to fully address the intricacies of Alzheimer's disease. Therefore, non-pharmacological interventions are essential for improving the general quality of life of both Alzheimer's patients and their carers. In order to support cognitive reserve and functional independence, these interventions include cognitive stimulation programs that involve participants in a variety of mentally stimulating activities. Moreover, exercise has become a very promising intervention due to its potential neuroprotective effects, mood-enhancing properties, and cognitive benefits. Two equally important aspects of managing Alzheimer's disease are social support and caregiver education. Because of the significant financial, emotional, and physical demands they frequently bear, caregivers require specialized interventions to meet their needs. Caregivers can benefit greatly from support groups, respite care services, and caregiver education programs, which can help them manage the demands of caregiving more skillfully while still preserving their own wellbeing.

Furthermore, treating related comorbidities and enhancing general health are essential components of a holistic approach to managing Alzheimer's disease. Controlling cardiovascular risk factors, such as diabetes, hyperlipidemia, and hypertension, may lessen the impact of blood vessels on cognitive decline. Furthermore, encouraging a brain-healthy lifestyle through social interaction, regular exercise, a balanced diet, and enough sleep may improve general wellbeing and cognitive function. Alzheimer's disease diagnosis and treatment require a thorough, multidisciplinary approach. Timely intervention is facilitated by early detection, and the disease's complex nature is addressed through a combination of pharmaceutical and non-pharmacological approaches. To further improve the quality of life for both Alzheimer's patients and their carers, Alzheimer's disease management strategies also include assisting caregivers and maximizing general health.

Diagnosing Alzheimer's disease (AD) involves a two-stage process. In the first stage, the dementia syndrome is identified based on neuropsychological and neuropsychiatric components, as well as deficits in daily activities. This stage aims to differentiate AD from other conditions such as delirium, physical illness, drug side effects, and normal memory loss. The second stage involves determining the cause of dementia, with AD being the most common diagnosis followed by vascular dementia, Lewy body dementia, frontal lobe dementia, and other secondary causes.

A mixed Alzheimer's/vascular dementia presentation is common, with AD typically showing a gradual onset of cognitive deficits while vascular dementia may have abrupt onset, fluctuating symptoms, hypertension, and neurological signs. In Lewy body dementia, memory loss may not be an early symptom, with marked fluctuations and distressing psychotic symptoms and behavioral disturbances.

Diagnostic tests should be minimally invasive and cost-effective, including routine blood tests, chest x-rays, and electrocardiograms when necessary. Referral to a cardiologist or neurologist may be needed in the presence of cerebrovascular signs, and computed tomography may be used if an intracranial lesion is suspected. An accurate diagnosis allows healthcare providers to communicate the disease course to the family and discuss any genetic implications (Balasa et al., 2011; Altomare et al., 2019; Villain & Dubois, 2019; Werry, 2019; Dubois et al., 2021).

5.3.1. Clinical Assessment of Dementia

AD diagnosis is basically a two-step procedure. The first step in diagnosing dementia is to rule out other conditions. These include delirium, depression, concurrent physical illness, drug treatment, learning disabilities, the effects of living in a severely impoverished environment, and normal aging-related memory loss. The second step in treating dementia is figuring out what causes the clinical syndrome. After vascular dementia, Lewy-body dementia, and frontal lobe dementia, AD is the most common cause. Dementia has numerous "secondary causes," some of which are curable. There are three main ways that dementia manifests as a clinical syndrome. First, there is a neuropsychological component that includes amnesia (loss of memory); aphasia (either expressive or receptive; the latter is more noticeable in conversation; nominal aphasia tested by directly questioning the naming of objects); apraxia (the inability to perform tasks despite intact sensory and motor nervous systems, manifest in dementia most usually by an inability to dress, often described as putting on a shirt or coat back to front, or the inability to use a knife and fork correctly); and agnosia (the inability to recognize objects, such as one's own mirror reflection or a family member; note that this is different from forgetting someone's name).

Secondly, a significant number of patients exhibit symptoms associated with neuropsychiatry, including behavioral disorders and psychiatric disturbances. Noncognitive features, neuropsychiatric features, and, more recently, behavioral and psychological symptoms of dementia (BPSD) have all been used to characterize these symptoms. The most prevalent are (approximate frequencies in brackets): hallucinations (15%, most commonly auditory; suspect an intercurrent delirium or Lewy-body dementia if persistent visual hallucinations are present); depression (up to 66% at some point during their dementia); paranoid ideation (30%); misidentifications (20%, usually based on agnosia, often manifest as a failure to recognize others, sometimes coupled with the delusional belief that people or objects have been duplicated); aggressiveness (20%); and wandering (20%). Third, deficiencies in day-to-day living activities. As dementia progresses, it can cause noticeable difficulties with dressing, eating, and using the restroom—basic daily activities. Early signs of them include not washing or dressing to one's usual standard. For single people, self-neglecting one's diet can result in weight loss, while ignoring household chores can lead to remarks about how clean the home is (instrumental activities of daily living).

5.3.1.1. Features of Dementia

- **Neuropsychologic:** Amnesia, aphasia, apraxia, agnosia
- **Neuropsychiatric:** Psychiatric disorders (e.g., delusions, depression, hallucinations) behavioral disturbances (e.g., aggression, agitation)
- Activities of daily living (basic and instrumental)

All forms of dementia share this trio of symptoms, with the clinical presentation, the existence of additional features, and additional elements of the history and examination serving as the basis for differentiation. Dementia's clinical manifestation.

5.3.1.2. Clinical Presentation of Dementia

Individuals suffering from dementia typically seek the assistance of specialized services only when their symptoms become unbearable and interfere with their daily activities. By then, the patient frequently cannot recall a precise past and might even contest the existence of an issue. An informant's history is crucial. A spouse passing away, moving from a familiar neighborhood, or taking a vacation abroad can all seem to be sudden triggers for the onset of dementia; however, these events may only have served to draw attention to the condition or hastened its decline due to an abrupt change in surroundings. Support from a spouse or other professional can help reduce issues that don't surface until after a death in the family. An in-depth history provided by an informant typically reveals the truth. Adherence to strict routines, which are disrupted when the sufferer moves away from familiar surroundings, can minimize failing cognitive function.

- Presentation of Dementia
  - Often noticed by others
  - Often precipitated by another event, e.g., a holiday or house move
  - Death of a spouse may reveal previously unnoticed problems
  - Informant history essential

5.3.1.3. Symptoms of Alzheimer's Disease

Memory loss and spatial disorientation are likely the most prevalent of AD's early symptoms, which are typically cognitive in nature. Particularly affected is short-term memory, and families and other people (including professionals) may not fully understand the significance of this change and may dismiss it as a typical age-related decline. In retrospect, personality changes can be considered among the first indications of dementia and are frequently reported in the advanced stages. The personality changes that make up the consensus criteria for Alzheimer's disease diagnosis are listed below. These criteria have been published and extensively verified.

- **Personality Changes in Dementia**
  - Increased rigidity
  - Increased egocentricity
  - Impairment of regard for the feelings of others
  - Coarsening of affect
  - Impairment of emotional control
  - Hilarity in inappropriate situations
  - Diminished emotional responsiveness
  - Sexual misdemeanor
  - Hobbies relinquished
  - Diminished initiative or growing apathy
  - Purposeless hyperactivity

5.3.1.4. Symptoms of Vascular Dementia

Because AD and vascular dementia frequently coexist, differentiating between the two conditions can be challenging. Vascular dementia typically develops suddenly, though it occasionally happens after an identifiable cerebrovascular accident. The course is typically characterized as a progressive one that includes periods of confusion and varying degrees of cognitive impairment.

- **Diagnostic Criteria for Dementia of the Alzheimer's Type**
  - Development of multiple cognitive deficits with both:
  - Memory impairment
  - One or more of amnesia, apraxia, agnosia,
  - Gradual onset of symptoms
  - Symptoms interfere with work and social activities
  - Absence of any other illness (systemic or cerebral) causing the dementia

Compared to AD, there is more mood instability and a higher propensity for anxiety and depression. Rarely, mild lacunar infarcts may be linked to progressive mental decline in the absence of focal symptoms. It is believed that the two forms of dementia can be distinguished by the patchy nature of the psychological deficits as opposed to the overall impairment of AD, with vascular dementia showing comparatively more personality and insight preservation.

- **Features Suggestive of Vascular Dementia**
  - Abrupt onset
  - Stepwise deterioration
  - Fluctuating course
  - Nocturnal confusion
  - Preserved personality
  - Depression
  - Somatic complaints
  - Emotional incontinence
  - Hypertension
  - History of strokes

- Associated atherosclerosis
- Focal neurological signs
- Focal neurological symptoms

- **Diagnostic Criteria for Vascular Dementia**
  - Presence of dementia
  - Focal neurological signs and symptoms or neuroimaging evidence of cerebrovascular disease judged to be etiologically related to the dementia
  - Symptoms not occurring in the course of delirium

Compared to patients seen in most elderly psychiatry services, the initial study group's patients were younger and had milder illness effects. A bimodal distribution of scores was discovered, indicating that patients with a score of 4 or higher had vascular dementia and those with a score of less than 4 had Alzheimer-type dementia. Individuals with a score of four to seven were considered to have a mixed picture. Table 5.3 lists the essential characteristics of vascular dementia. More recently, there has been debate regarding the usefulness of the Ilachinski score in distinguishing vascular dementias from other kinds of dementias. Some have criticized Ilachinski's score for not being sensitive enough. Furthermore, the Ilachinski checklist does not consider the findings of neuroradiological tests, and higher scores on the test do not necessarily indicate a diagnosis of vascular dementia. A mixed picture is common because older adults, including those with AD, frequently experience infarctions. The characteristics that have been found to be most accurate in separating Alzheimer-type dementia from vascular dementia include abrupt onset, history of strokes, hypertension, and neurological signs and symptoms.

Table 5.3. Blood Biomarkers and VCID

Author, Year [Reference]	**Population**	**Biomakers**	**Outcome**	**Results**
Murr J et al. (2014)	670 cognitively normal subjects	Plasma oxidized low-density lipoprotein (OxLDL) levels	Risk Factor follow-up: 4.8 years (2.2–10.3)	No association between OxLDL and risk of all-cause dementia, AD, and vascular dementia or subtypes was found.
Dong H et al. (2015)	127 AD patients, 30 MCI and 30 VaD patients.	Serum circulating miRNAs	Differential diagnosis	The panel of miR-31, miR-93 and miR-146a can be used to discriminate AD from VaD.
Duits FH et al. (2015)	52 AD patients, 24 VaD patients, 26 cognitively normal subjects.	Plasma and CSF levels of MMP2, MMP9, MMP10, TIMP1 and TIMP2. CSF levels of amyloid-β(1–42) (Aβ42), tau, and tau phosphorylated at threonine-181 (p-tau).	Differential diagnosis	AD patients showed higher plasma MMP2 levels compared to VaD patients ($p < 0.05$).

Hatanaka H et al. (2015)	72 AD, 27 VaD, 24 Mixed Dementia (MD) patients and 53 cognitively normal subjects.	Plasma levels of diacron reactive oxygen metabolite (dROM) and biological anti-oxidant potential (BAP).	Differential diagnosis	The dROM levels were significantly higher in the AD and MD groups than in the control group. The BAP levels were significantly lower in the MD group than in the control, AD and VaD groups.
Hilal S et al. (2015)	41 cognitive impairment with no dementia (CIND) subjects and 46 demented subjects with burden of cerebrovascular diseases (CeVD); 37 CIND and 34 cases with dementia without CeVD; 35 cognitively normal subjects.	Plasma NTpro-BNP and high sensitivity cardiac troponin T (hs-cTnT) levels.	Differential diagnosis	Plasma concentrations of hs-cTnT were associated significantly with CeVD in both CIND and dementia. NTpro-BNP was associated with dementia with CeVD
Teunissen CE et al. (2015)	295 subjects including healthy controls (*n* = 65), patients with subjective memory complaints (*n* = 99), patients with AD (*n* = 100), and patients with vascular dementia (*n* = 31).	Serum leptin levels	Differential diagnosis	Serum leptin levels are not altered in AD or vascular dementia patients compared to healthy controls and were not related to cognitive decline.
Wang C et al. (2015)	10 cognitively healthy subjects and 10 age-matched VaD subjects.	Differentially expressed proteins (DEPs)	Differential diagnosis	High-degree proteins were detected in the protein-protein (PPI) interaction network, such as ATP5B (ATP synthase subunit β) in VaD.
Castellazzi M et al. (2016)	232 MCI, 65 VaD, 175 AD, 88 MD, 104 Multiple Sclerosis (MS) patients, 165 cognitively healthy controls.	Serum High-density lipoprotein (HDL)-bound paraoxonase-1 (PON-1) levels	Differential diagnosis	Serum arylesterase, but not paraoxonase, levels were significantly lower in patients affected by MCI, VaD, AD, MD as well as those with MS as compared to healthy controls.

Chen Z et al. (2016)	52 subcortical ischemic vascular disease patients with no dementia (SIVDND), 55 patients with mild cognitive impairment (SVMCI), 54 patients with vascular dementia (VaD), 54 cognitively healthy controls.	Serum thyroid-stimulating hormone (TSH), total triiodothyronine (TT3), free triiodothyronine (FT3), total thyroxine (TT4) and free thyroxine (FT4), thyroglobulin antibody (TGA), and antithyroid peroxidase antibody (TPO-Abs).	Correlation with cognitive status	Serum TT3 and FT3 levels decreased, whereas serum TSH level increased, with the decline in cognitive functions in SIVD.
Dukic L et al. (2016)	235 participants, divided in 4 groups: AD (*N* = 70), VaD (*N* = 67), MCI (*N* = 48) and Cognitively Healthy Participants (*N* = 50).	Serum kallikrein 6 (KLK6), clusterin (CLU), adiponectin (ADPN) and interleukin-6 (IL-6)	Differential diagnosis	Serum concentrations of KLK6, CLU and ADPN did not differ between AD, VaD, MCI and cognitively healthy control group of participants, whereas IL-6 was significantly higher in VaD patients than in AD, MCI and healthy individuals.
Horvath I et al. (2016)	40 nondemented controls, 11 stable mild cognitive impairment (SMCI), 6 MCI due to AD (MCI-AD), 40 AD and 7 VaD. patients.	CSF concentration of Aβ1–42, S100A8, S100A9 and Tau.	Differential diagnosis	The S100A9 and Aβ1–42 levels correlated with each other: their CSF content decreased already at the SMCI stage and declined further under MCIAD, AD, and VaD conditions.
Kitagawa K et al. (2016)	466 cognitively healthy subjects	serum high-molecular-weight (HMW) adiponectin level	Risk factor (median follow-up period: 6.9 years)	Risks of dementia in patients with high versus low HMW adiponectin levels were almost identical. No association was found between adiponectin levels and Alzheimer's disease dementia or vascular dementia in the whole group or amongst men and women separately.
Levada OA et al. (2016)	21 patients with AD; 22 patients with subcortical vascular dementia; 16 cognitively healthy subjects.	Plasma levels of brain-derived neurotrophic factor (BDNF)	Differential diagnosis	At baseline there was lower BDNF levels in both AD and VaD groups, which was significant only in subjects with AD.

Mirza SS et al. (2016)	357 AD patients; 32 VaD patients.	Serum N-terminal pro B-type natriuretic peptide (NT-proBNP) levels	Risk factor	Higher NT-proBNP was associated with a higher risk of dementia, with a particularly strong association with vascular dementia.
Nilsson ED et al. (2016)	374 incident dementia cases: 120 AD patients, 84 VaD and 102 MD patients.	Plasma level of copeptin	Risk factor (median follow-up period: 4.2 years)	Baseline level of copeptin predicted incident VaD.
Pan X et al. (2016)	Exploration phase: 338 control subjects and 43 AD patients; Validation phase: 861 control subjects, 81 AD patients, 70 vascular dementia patients and 13 frontotemporal dementia patients.	Blood Thiamine diphosphate (TDP), thiamine monophosphate, and thiamine levels	Differential diagnosis	TDP exhibited significant and consistent values for AD diagnosis in both exploration and validation phases. TDP can effectively distinguish AD from vascular dementia.
Bednarska-Makaruk M et al. (2017)	205 patients with dementia (89 with AD, 47 with VaD, 69 with mixed dementia (MD)), 113 persons with MCI and 107 controls.	Serum adiponectin, leptin and resistin levels, IL-6, CRP, chitotriosidase, 25-OH vitamin D, HDL-cholesterol and paraoxonase 1, glucose, insulin and HOMA-IR.	Differential diagnosis	Vascular and mixed dementia are characterized by an increase of resistin. Positive correlation of resistin with inflammation indicators may suggest the potential pro-inflammatory role of resistin in the development of dementia, especially in dementia of vascular mechanism.
Busse M et al. (2017)	60 AD patients, 20 VaD patients, 12 frontotemporal dementia patients and 24 cognitively healthy persons.	Innate and adaptive cell populations in whole blood.	Differential diagnosis	Monocytes and NK cells were diminished in VaD, but not in AD and FTD. B cell and T cell numbers were decreased in all investigated forms of dementia. Changes in the contribution of naïve/memory T cells were only present in AD.

Holm H et al. (2017)	120 AD patients, 83 VaD, 102 MD and 68 other etiology.	Plasma N-terminal prosomatostatin (NT-proSST)	Risk factor (follow-up period of 4.6 ± 1.3 years)	Higher levels of circulating NTproSST are associated with increased incidence of vascular dementia.
Holm H et al. (2017)	A population-based cohort of 5347 individuals without prevalent dementia	Plasma midregional pro-atrial natriuretic peptide (MR-proANP), C-terminal endothelin-1 (CT-proET-1) and midregional proadrenomedullin (MR-proADM).	Risk factor (follow-up period of 4.6 ± 1.3 years)	Elevated plasma concentration of MR-proANP is an independent predictor of all-cause and vascular dementia. Pronounced increase in CT-proET-1 indicates higher risk of vascular dementia.
Hsu PF et al. (2017)	1436 individuals from a national representative sample in Taiwan.	CRP levels were determined.	Risk Factor (11.04 years (median) of follow-up)	260 individuals (18.11%) were diagnosed with dementia. Those with high CRP had a 55% higher risk of dementia compared with those with normal CRP. After adjusting for possible confounding cardiovascular risk factors, high CRP was independently associated with VaD, but not AD.
Moretti R et al. (2017)	543 patients: 456 patients suffering from subcortical vascular dementia (sVAD), 87 AD and healthy age-matched controls	Clinical laboratory measurements, including serum total cholesterol, triglycerides, and high-density lipoprotein (HDL) cholesterol, have been determined enzymatically and low-density lipoprotein (LDL) cholesterol was calculated using Friedewald's formula. Serum levels of 25(OH)D, the level of calcium and PTH were measured. The level of folate, vitamin B12 levels and Homocysteine were also tested.	Correlation	Vitamin D deficiency was present in demented cases, as well as low levels of folate and high levels of homocysteine, more pronounced in sVAD cases.
Prabhakar P et al. (2017)	204 patients with small vessel VaD; 200 cognitively normal subjects.	Plasma miRNA profiling.	Differential diagnosis	plasma miR-409–3p, miR-502–3p, miR-486–5p and miR-451a could be used to differentiate small vessel VaD patients from healthy controls.

Quinlan P et al. (2017)	342 patients with subjective or objective mild cognitive impairment	Serum IGF-I concentrations at baseline	Risk factor (mean follow-up: 3.6 years)	In a memory clinic population, low serum IGF-I was a risk marker for subsequent VaD whereas low IGF-I did not associate with the risk of AD. High serum IGF-I was not related to the risk of conversion to dementia.
Suridjan I et al. (2017)	29 possible vascular mild cognitive impairment patients and 89 controls)	Serum lipid peroxidation markers levels. Ratios of early- (lipid hydroperoxides, LPH) to late-stage (8-isoprostane, 8-ISO; 4-hydroxy-2-nonenal, 4-HNE) lipid peroxidation products were calculated.	Correlation with cognitive status	A global effect of group on lipid peroxidation markers was observed, adjusting for sex, years of education, and cardiopulmonary fitness. Lower lipid peroxidation at baseline, as determined by lower 8-ISO concentration, was associated with greater improvement in verbal memory (F (1, 64) = 4.738, p = 0.03) and executive function (F(1, 64) = 5.219, p = 0.026) performance. Higher ratios of 8-ISO/LPH and 8-ISO+4-HNE to LPH, were associated with less improvement in executive function performance over a 24-week exercise intervention.
Tang SC et al. (2017)	172 Ischemic Stroke (IS) patients, including 73 with CDR = 0, 63 with CDR = 0.5, and 36 with CDR ≥ 1 (VaD patients).	Plasma concentration of receptor for advanced glycation end products (soluble RAGE (sRAGE); endogenous soluble form of RAGE (esRAGE))	Correlation with cognitive status	Plasma sRAGE and esRAGE were elevated in patients with dementia compared with those without dementia among IS patients.
Vishnu VY et al. (2017)	118 subjects, 68 with dementia (MCI-AD and AD: 52; MCI VaSC and VaD:16).	Plasma IL-6; C-Reactive Protein (CRP); plasma fibrinogen; plasma D-dimer.	Differential diagnosis	Plasma Fibrinogen and D dimer: were higher in Vascular group; no difference in IL-6 and CRP.

Wang R et al. (2017)	88 patients with dementia (43 AD patients, 45 VaD patients) and 45 healthy age-matched controls	Plasma Cystatin C (Cys C) and HDL levels	Differential diagnosis	Plasma Cys C levels were higher in patients with AD/VaD than in healthy subjects. Plasma HDL levels were lower in patients with AD/VaD than in healthy subjects.
Yang R et al. (2017)	51 healthy subjects and 41 elderly patients (with 6 participants affected by vascular mild cognitive impairment (Va-MCI)), 9 with VaD, 8 with MCI due to AD and 18 with AD	Plasma GDF-11 and β2-MG levels	Differential diagnosis	No differences in circulating GDF-11 levels amongst the healthy advanced age and four cognitive impairment groups. β2-MG levels increased with age, but there was no significant difference between healthy elderly males and advanced age males. Increased levels of β2-MG were observed in the dementia group compared with the healthy advanced age group.
Brombo G et al. (2018)	320 elderly individuals (≥65 years old): 60 patients with normal cognition; 60 patients with VaD; 100 patients with AD; 100 patients with MCI.	Plasma Klotho levels	Differential diagnosis	Lower levels of plasma Klotho (1st tertile) were associated with higher prevalence of VaD, but not AD.
Latourte A et al. (2018)	1598 people.	Serum Uric Acid (SUA)	Risk Factor (median follow-up duration: 10.1 years)	Association for development of dementia was stronger with vascular or mixed dementia (HR = 3.66 (95% CI 1.29 to 10.41), p = 0.015) than Alzheimer's disease (HR = 1.55 (95% CI 0.92 to 2.61), p = 0.10).
Lauriola M et al. (2018)	116 patients: 32 healthy controls, 39 with diagnosis of VaD, 14 MCI and 31 AD.	Erythrocyte associated Aβ (iAβ40 and iAβ42) levels	Differential diagnosis	AD showed different iAβ42 levels as compared to VaD. Conversely, no differences were found for iAβ40.

Shang J et al. (2018)	266 patients with AD, 44 MCI, 33 VaD and 200 ischemic stroke (IS) in comparison to 130 healthy controls.	Plasma fatty acids [eicosapentaenoic acid (EPA) and docosahexaenoic acid (DHA)], adiponectin, reptin, plasma markers of inflammation [high-sensitivity C-reactive protein (hsCRP) and serum amyloid A (serum AA)], and plasma lipids [high-density lipoprotein and low-density lipoprotein (LDL)]	Differential diagnosis	Lower EPA and DHA levels and higher reptin and LDL levels were associated with AD and IS. The reptin/ adiponectin ratio was strongly associated with IS. The hsCRP level was more strongly associated with VaD and IS, and the serum AA level was associated with all three cognitive diseases and IS.
Staszewski J et al. (2018)	123 patients (age, mean ± SD: 72.2 ± 8 years, 49% females), with lacunar stroke (*n* = 49), vascular dementia (*n* = 48), and vascular parkinsonism (*n* = 26).	Soluble intercellular cell adhesion molecule-1 (sICAM-1), soluble platelet selectin (sP-selectin), CD40 ligand (sCD40 L), platelet factor-4 (PF-4) and homocysteine; combined high-sensitivity C-reactive protein (hsCRP), interleukin-1α and -6 (IL-1α and IL-6, respectively) and tumor necrosis factor-α (TNF-α).	Correlation with radiological status	Lacunes are associated with different inflammatory markers.
Yang TT et al. (2018)	101 MCI, 107 AD, 30 Parkinson's disease with dementia (PDD), 20 VaD patients	Serum levels of exosomal miR-135a, -193b, and -384	Differential diagnosis	Both serum exosome miR-135a and miR-384 were up-regulated while miR-193b was down-regulated in AD patients compared with normal controls and non-AD dementias.
Staszewski et al. (2019)	130 patients with marked MRI features of SVD and recent lacunar stroke (*n* = 52,LS), vascular Parkinsonism (*n* = 28,VaP) or dementia (*n* = 50,VaD).	IL-1α, IL-6, hs-CRP, sICAM-1, sP-selectin, TNF-α, homocysteine, fibrinogen, D-dimer, serum total cholesterol (TC), high density lipoprotein cholesterol (HDL-C), low-density lipoprotein cholesterol (LDL-C), triglycerides (TG), eGFR, serum FG, HbA1c, albumin and uric acid (UA).	Risk Factor (mean follow-up time: 22.3 ± 4.3 months)	IL-1α, IL-6, homocysteine, d-dimer were significantly associated with the event of death or stroke, even after adjusting for age, sex and SVD radiological markers.

Source: Cipollini V, Troili F, & Giubilei F, (2019). Emerging biomarkers in vascular cognitive impairment and dementia: From pathophysiological pathways to clinical application. International Journal of Molecular Sciences, 20(11):2812. https://doi.org/10.3390/ijms20112812.

5.3.1.5. Symptoms of Lewy-Body Dementia

The clinical features of Lewy-body dementia include a variable course, marked behavioral disturbance, distressing psychotic symptoms, and periods of lucidity during which the degree of cognitive impairment appears to be relatively mild compared to the severity of the behavioral disturbance.

- **Clinical Features of Lewy-Body Dementia**
  - Progressive cognitive decline interfering with social or occupational functioning; memory loss may not be an early feature
  - One or two features of:
  - Fluctuating cognition with pronounced variation in attention and alertness
  - Recurrent visual hallucinations
  - Spontaneous motor features of parkinsonism (Balasa et al., 2011; Altomare et al., 2019; Villain & Dubois, 2019; Werry, 2019; Dubois et al., 2021).

5.3.2. Assessment of Dementia

Establishing a diagnosis and looking for coexisting disorders are the goals of investigations. A precise diagnosis facilitates a suitable dialog regarding treatment and prognosis with the patient and their relatives. Families will become concerned about the genetic ramifications upon receiving an AD diagnosis. By distinguishing between Alzheimer's disease and vascular dementia, the physician can provide the family with details regarding the illness's progression. The most crucial part of the investigation is getting the patient to provide a complete history, along with additional information from relevant sources like family members. The family doctor is a crucial source of information about the patient's medical and personal history, premorbid personality, social circumstances, and family dynamics.

It is easy to determine the beginning and length of the presenting problem by having a conversation with a trustworthy informant. All people experience memory problems and personality changes. The first thing that may stand out as a change is difficulties with hobbies, like playing bridge or following an intricate knitting pattern. It's critical to understand how the disease progresses in order to differentiate AD from vascular dementia. Family members may provide proof of psychotic symptoms like delusions or hallucinations.

A mental health examination will reveal any signs of self-neglect, physical illness that may be obvious, disinhibited or inappropriate behavior, as well as signs of agitation or retardation that may indicate depression. Hostile or guarded behavior could be a sign of underlying paranoid thoughts. A noticeable sign of clouding of consciousness, such as a poor attention span, can help distinguish dementia from delirium. Aphasia or dysarthria will be evident in the patient's speech. Advanced dementia is associated with abnormal speech patterns such as perseverance (the patient answering new questions with the same response to the previous one), palilalia (repeating a question's last word more frequently), logoclonia (repeating the last syllable), and logorrhea (words flowing out of one's mouth without meaning). The patient may exhibit echolalia, or speech or movement imitating the examiner, or echopraxia. Although the patient's thinking is frequently poor in dementia, probing will show whether delusions or depressive ideas are present, and the patient may go into detail about psychotic experiences. Agitation, anxiety, and irritability are indicative of affective symptoms, which are frequently observed in conjunction with dementia and may be the presenting feature. Perception disorders are common in dementia patients, and the history may reveal characteristics suggestive of visual or auditory hallucinations. It is not unusual to witness a patient experiencing hallucinations while the examiner is present. Asking the right questions will expose psychotic symptoms like misidentifications or paranoid thoughts.

- **Main Features of Mental State Examination**
  - Observe for agitation, retardation, self-neglect
  - Enquire about symptoms of depression
  - Enquire about psychotic symptoms
  - Observe any obvious manifestations of physical illness
  - Carry out cognitive function tests

A standard test like the Mini-Mental State Examination (MMSE) greatly aids in the assessment of cognitive function. The MMSE is worth thirty points, 10 of which are awarded for location and time orientation, and the remaining points are awarded for attention, registration, recall, language, information manipulation, and praxis tests. A cutoff score of 23 or 24 on the MMSE has been proposed as a good way to distinguish between cognitive dysfunction and normalcy. An effective screening tool for clinical evaluation is the MMSE. When a patient is referred with possible dementia, the MMSE is a helpful screening tool. It takes little time to complete, is sensitive to changes over time, and in patients with AD, is predicted to decline by about 3 points annually.

It is important to perform a physical examination paying particular attention to the central nervous system. Vascular disease is indicated by high blood pressure and focal neurological symptoms. Evaluation of eyesight and hearing is crucial since deficiencies can exacerbate cognitive dysfunction. Certain investigations are considered necessary by the majority of doctors, while others are based primarily on the individual's experience and, to some extent, what is available locally. The question of which screening tests are required is up for debate. Some contend that these tests are unnecessary because there are few curable causes of dementia. The most beneficial investigations are reasonably priced and require little physical intervention. A typical screening would comprise a complete blood count, erythrocyte sedimentation rate, serum B12 and folate, urea and electrolytes, thyroid function tests, liver function tests, and serological tests for syphilis if there are any unusual or atypical features.

- **Useful Information from an Informant Regarding Dementia**
  - Onset of illness: gradual or sudden
  - First symptoms
  - Amount of social support
  - Presence of psychotic symptoms
- • **Assessment Instruments Useful in Dementia**
  - Cognitive function
  - Mini-Mental State Examination (MMSE)
  - Clock Drawing Test

- Global assessment
  - Clinical Dementia Rating
  - Global Deterioration Scale
- Psychiatric symptoms
- Cornell Scale for Depression in Dementia
- Neuropsychiatrie Inventory
- Activities of daily living
  - Bristol Activities of Daily Living scale
  - Disability Assessment of Dementia

5.3.3. Assessment Instruments for Dementia

A number of different instruments have been developed to assess various aspects of dementia. A selection is summarized below:

- **Cognitive Function**
  - **Mini-Mental State Examination (MMSE):** This is the most widely used test of cognitive function. It is scored out of 30, and tests the domains of orientation, language, writing, memory, and praxis.
  - **Standardized Mini-Mental State Examination (SMMSE):** This is a standardized version of the Mini-Mental State Examination, which comes with complete rating instructions leading to slightly improved validity.

Abbreviated Mental Test Score (AMTS) this is a much briefer screening tool, scored out of 10, which tests only orientation and memory.

  - **Alzheimer's Disease Assessment Scale (ADAS):** This is now a standard cognitive scale used in drug trials. It assesses a number of cognitive functions including memory, language, and practice, and also has a section devoted to non-cognitive features.
  - **Clock Drawing Test (CDT):** This is a relatively new development, is very easy to administer, and is very popular in primary care because of its simplicity.
- **Global Measures**
  - **Clinical Dementia Rating (CDR):** This is probably the most widely used global scale to give an overall severity rating in dementia, ranging from 0 (none), 0.5 (questionable dementia), through mild and moderate to severe dementia. Each is rated in 6 domains: memory, orientation, judgment and problem solving, community affairs, home and hobbies, and personal care.
  - **Global Deterioration Scale (CDS):** This consists of the description of 7 stages of dementia from 1 (normal) to 7, where all verbal ability is lost. The scale has been used extensively and validated with postmortem findings.
- Psychopathology
  - **Cornell Scale for Depression in Dementia (CSDD):** This is a 19-item scale, which specifically assesses depression in people with dementia in 5 main domains: mood related

signs, behavioral disturbance, physical signs, cyclic functions, and ideation disturbance. A mixture of informant-rated and observational ratings makes it ideal for the assessment in patients with cognitive impairment where information from the patient might not always be available. A score of 8 or above suggests significant depressive symptoms.

- **BEHAV-AD:** this is a 25-item scale, which measures many of the psychiatric symptoms and behavioral disturbances associated with dementia. They are rated on a 3 -point scale, and a second part of the scale is a global rating of the severity of the symptoms, the BEHAV-AD is particularly useful in the assessment of patients in drug trials.
- **Neuropsychiatrie Inventory (NPI):** 12 behavioral areas are assessed in the NPI (delusions, hallucinations, agitation, depression, anxiety, euphoria, apathy, disinhibition, irritability, aberrant motor behavior, nighttime behaviors, and appetite/eating disorders), each of which is rated on a 4-point scale of frequency and 3-point scale of severity. Distress in carers is also measured.
- **MOUSEPAD:** This is based on the longer Present Behavioral Examination and measures a number of behavior and psychiatric symptoms, with particular reference to their development over the life of the dementia syndrome.

- **Functional Ability**
  - **Bristol Activities of Daily Living Scale (DADLS):** This is a 20-item scale rated on a 5-point severity looking at basic activities of daily living (e.g., feeding, eating, and toileting) and instrumental activities of daily living (which refer to the performance of more complex tasks such as shopping, traveling, answering the telephone, and handling finances).
  - **Interview for Deterioration in Daily Living Activities in Dementia (IDDD):** This contains 33 self-care items rated on a 4-point scale and has been used extensively to assess the effects of drugs.
  - **Disability Assessment for Dementia (DAD):** A rating of activities of daily living in dementia separating them into the different areas of initiation, planning and organization, and affective performance; basic activities and instrumental of activities daily living are assessed.
  - **Alzheimer's Disease Functional Assessment and Change Scale (ADFACS):** This is an 18-item scale looking at a wide range of basic activities and instrumental activities of daily living (Balasa et al., 2011; Altomare et al., 2019; Villain & Dubois, 2019; Werry, 2019; Dubois et al., 2021).

A Closer Look

Heart Disease Risk

Heart disease prediction has never been a precise science. Some factors can help predict future risk, including smoking, diabetes, high blood pressure, and high cholesterol (especially LDL or bad cholesterol). However, it's not always simple to identify atherosclerosis, the condition that causes the majority of heart attacks. A coronary artery calcium (CAC) scan could be useful in this situation. It gauges the calcium content of the heart's arteries, elevated calcium levels being linked to heart disease.

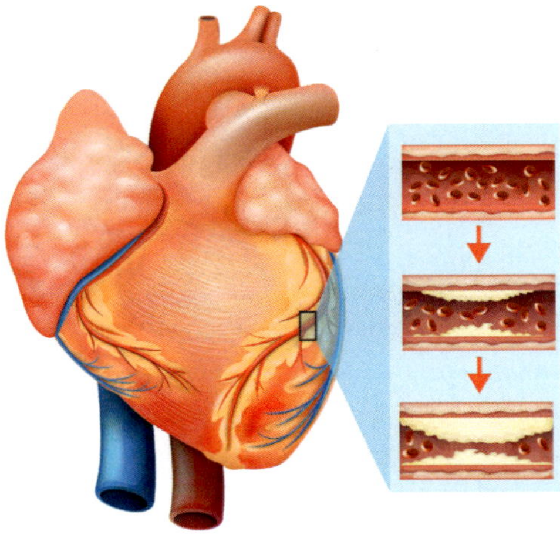

Too much plaque can restrict blood flow in arteries, but it's often hard to diagnose.

Source: http://content.health.harvard.edu/wp-content/uploads/2024/04/b0a19e4e-5eaa-491d-8e0c-1e4ae64c9323.jpg

Even if a person lacks the obvious risk factors or symptoms, the CAC results can help identify their potential risk for a heart attack or stroke, according to the director of preventive cardiology at Brigham and Women's Hospital, which is affiliated with Harvard. For some, it may be a means of receiving the required care ahead of time and potentially preventing a major cardiac incident.

How the test works

A computed tomography (CT) scanner specifically designed for CAC scans is used, such as an electron beam CT or a multidetector CT scanner. Electrodes are positioned on your chest while you lie on your back to track your heart rate. Then, over the course of 20 to 30 seconds, the scanner takes multiple images of your heart. A heart attack is more likely when there is excessive plaque accumulation in the arteries that supply blood to the heart muscle. It's linked to an increased risk of stroke as well. Sometimes, for no apparent reason, the plaque calcifies, causing tiny white spots to appear on the scan. The process of calcification primarily detects the presence of atherosclerosis; however, it may not identify specific regions that are likely to burst and result in a heart attack.

Summary

- Diagnosing Alzheimer's disease involves a thorough assessment encompassing clinical evaluation, cognitive testing, and sometimes neuroimaging. Early diagnosis is critical for initiating appropriate interventions and support.
- An important part of diagnosing Alzheimer's disease includes being able to explain your symptoms. Input from a close family member or friend about your symptoms and their impact on your daily life helps. Tests of memory and thinking skills also help diagnose Alzheimer's disease.
- Alzheimer's disease slowly worsens over time. People living with this disease progress at different rates, from mild Alzheimer's, when they first notice symptoms, to severe, when they are completely dependent on others for daily, routine care such as feeding oneself.
- Diagnosing Alzheimer's disease often involves a combination of clinical assessment, cognitive testing, and neuroimaging. While clinical evaluation and cognitive testing provide valuable insights into cognitive impairment, neuroimaging techniques play a crucial role in supporting the diagnosis and understanding the underlying brain changes associated with Alzheimer's disease.
- Alzheimer's disease (AD) is the most common form of dementia, accounting for about two thirds of all cases globally.
- BBBMs are emerging as important tools to aid in identification of pathology associated with AD; concentrations of Aβ peptides and pTau in the blood have demonstrated associations with the corresponding concentrations in CSF and with PET positivity.
- The intended use of the NIA-AA "ATN" research framework is for research purposes; therefore, there is debate around the use of this framework in clinical practice.
- The process of testing and diagnosing Alzheimer's disease typically involves multiple healthcare professionals working together to provide comprehensive care.
- Alzheimer's disease, a progressive neurological disorder, presents unique challenges in both diagnosis and management. Early detection is crucial, although often challenging due to its subtle onset and progression.
- The diagnosis of AD is essentially a two-stage process. First, a diagnosis of dementia is made, the main conditions from which it should be differentiated being delirium, depression, concomitant physical illness, drug treatment, learning disability, the effects of a severely impoverished environment, and the normal memory loss that accompanies aging.

REFERENCES

1. Altomare, D., Ferrari, C., Caroli, A., Galluzzi, S., Prestia, A., van der Flier, W. M., et al. (2019). Prognostic value of Alzheimer's biomarkers in mild cognitive impairment: The effect of age at onset. *Journal of Neurology, 266*, 2535–2545. https://doi.org/10.1007/s00415-019-09416-1.
2. Arenaza-Urquijo, E. M., & Vemuri, P. (2018). Resistance vs. resilience to Alzheimer disease: Clarifying terminology for preclinical studies. *Neurology, 90*, 695–703. https://doi.org/10.1212/WNL.0000000000005303.

3. Armstrong, M. J., Litvan, I., Lang, A. E., Bak, T. H., Bhatia, K. P., Borroni, B., et al. (2013). Criteria for the diagnosis of corticobasal degeneration. *Neurology, 80*, 496–503. https://doi.org/10.1212/WNL.0b013e31827f0fd1.

4. Ashton, N. J., Benedet, A. L., Pascoal, T. A., Karikari, T. K., Lantero-Rodriguez, J., Brum, W. S., et al. (2022). Cerebrospinal fluid p-tau231 as an early indicator of emerging pathology in Alzheimer's disease. *EBioMedicine, 76*, 103836. https://doi.org/10.1016/j.ebiom.2022.103836.

5. Balasa, M., Gelpi, E., Antonell, A., Rey, M. J., Sánchez-Valle, R., & Molinuevo, J. L., et al. (2011). Clinical features and APOE genotype of pathologically proven early-onset Alzheimer disease. *Neurology, 76*, 1720–1725. https://doi.org/10.1212/WNL.0b013e31821a44df.

6. Beaufils, E., Dufour-Rainfray, D., Hommet, C., Brault, F., Cottier, J. P., Ribeiro, M. J., et al. (2013). Confirmation of the amyloidogenic process in posterior cortical atrophy: Value of the Aβ42/Aβ40 ratio. *Journal of Alzheimer's Disease, 33*, 775–780. https://doi.org/10.3233/JAD-2012-121547.

7. Benedet, A. L., Brum, W. S., Hansson, O., Karikari, T. K., Zimmer, E. R., Zetterberg, H., et al. (2022). The accuracy and robustness of plasma biomarker models for amyloid PET positivity. *Alzheimer's Research & Therapy, 14*, 26. https://doi.org/10.1186/s13195-022-00950-2.

8. Benedet, A. L., Milà-Alomà, M., Vrillon, A., Ashton, N. J., Pascoal, T. A., Lussier, F., et al. (2021). Differences between plasma and cerebrospinal fluid glial fibrillary acidic protein levels across the Alzheimer disease continuum. *JAMA Neurology, 78*, 1471–1483. https://doi.org/10.1001/jamaneurol.2021.3526.

9. Bergeron, D., Gorno-Tempini, M. L., Rabinovici, G. D., Santos-Santos, M. A., Seeley, W., & Miller, B. L., et al. (2018). Prevalence of amyloid-β pathology in distinct variants of primary progressive aphasia. *Annals of Neurology, 84*, 729–740. https://doi.org/10.1002/ana.25333.

10. Bergeron, D., Sellami, L., Poulin, S., Verret, L., Bouchard, R. W., & Laforce, R. Jr. (2020). The behavioral/dysexecutive variant of Alzheimer's disease: A case series with clinical, neuropsychological, and FDG-PET characterization. *Dementia and Geriatric Cognitive Disorders, 49*, 518–525. https://doi.org/10.1159/000512529.

11. Brookmeyer, R., Corrada, M. M., Curriero, F. C., & Kawas, C. (2002). Survival following a diagnosis of Alzheimer disease. *Archives of Neurology, 59*, 1764–1767. https://doi.org/10.1001/archneur.59.11.1764.

12. Bucci, M., Chiotis, K., Nordberg, A., & Alzheimer's Disease Neuroimaging Initiative. (2021). Alzheimer's disease profiled by fluid and imaging markers: Tau PET best predicts cognitive decline. *Molecular Psychiatry, 26*, 5888–5898. https://doi.org/10.1038/s41380-021-01147-w.

13. Chen, Y. F., Ma, X., Sundell, K., Alaka, K., Schuh, K., Raskin, J., et al. (2016). Quantile regression to characterize solanezumab effects in Alzheimer's disease trials. *Alzheimer's & Dementia (New York), 2*, 192–198. https://doi.org/10.1016/j.trci.2016.09.003.

14. Cicognola, C., Janelidze, S., Hertze, J., Zetterberg, H., Blennow, K., Mattsson-Carlgren, N., et al. (2021). Plasma glial fibrillary acidic protein detects Alzheimer pathology and predicts future conversion to Alzheimer dementia in patients with mild cognitive impairment. *Alzheimer's Research & Therapy, 13*, 68. https://doi.org/10.1186/s13195-021-00805-1.

15. Clark, C. M., Pontecorvo, M. J., Beach, T. G., Bedell, B. J., Coleman, R. E., Doraiswamy, P. M., et al. (2012). Cerebral PET with florbetapir compared with neuropathology at autopsy for

detection of neuritic amyloid-β plaques: A prospective cohort study. *The Lancet Neurology, 11*, 669–678. https://doi.org/10.1016/S1474-4422(12)70142-4.

16. Crutch, S. J., Schott, J. M., Rabinovici, G. D., Murray, M., Snowden, J. S., van der Flier, W. M., et al. (2017). Consensus classification of posterior cortical atrophy. *Alzheimer's & Dementia, 13*, 870–884. https://doi.org/10.1016/j.jalz.2017.01.014.
17. Cummings, J., Lee, G., Nahed, P., Kambar, M. E. Z. N., Zhong, K., Fonseca, J., et al. (2022). Alzheimer's disease drug development pipeline: 2022. *Alzheimer's & Dementia (New York), 8*, e12295. https://doi.org/10.1002/trc2.12295.
18. Damoiseaux, J. S. (2012). Resting-state fMRI as a biomarker for Alzheimer's disease? *Alzheimer's Research & Therapy, 4*, 8. https://doi.org/10.1186/alzrt104.
19. de Souza, L. C., Bertoux, M., Funkiewiez, A., Samri, D., Azuar, C., Habert, M. O., et al. (2013). Frontal presentation of Alzheimer's disease: A series of patients with biological evidence by CSF biomarkers. *Dementia & Neuropsychologia, 7*, 66–74. https://doi.org/10.1590/S1980-57642013DN70100011.
20. DeTure, M. A., & Dickson, D. W. (2019). The neuropathological diagnosis of Alzheimer's disease. *Molecular Neurodegeneration, 14*, 32. https://doi.org/10.1186/s13024-019-0333-5.
21. Dubois, B., Feldman, H. H., Jacova, C., Hampel, H., Molinuevo, J. L., Blennow, K., et al. (2014). Advancing research diagnostic criteria for Alzheimer's disease: The IWG-2 criteria. *The Lancet Neurology, 13*, 614–629. https://doi.org/10.1016/S1474-4422(14)70090-0.
22. Dubois, B., Hampel, H., Feldman, H. H., Scheltens, P., Aisen, P., Andrieu, S., et al. (2016). Preclinical Alzheimer's disease: Definition, natural history, and diagnostic criteria. *Alzheimer's & Dementia, 12*, 292–323. https://doi.org/10.1016/j.jalz.2016.02.002.
23. Dubois, B., Villain, N., Frisoni, G. B., Rabinovici, G. D., Sabbagh, M., Cappa, S., et al. (2021). Clinical diagnosis of Alzheimer's disease: Recommendations of the International Working Group. *The Lancet Neurology, 20*, 484–496. https://doi.org/10.1016/S1474-4422(21)00095-7.
24. Engelborghs, S., De Vreese, K., Van de Casteele, T., Vanderstichele, H., Van Everbroeck, B., Cras, P., et al. (2008). Diagnostic performance of a CSF-biomarker panel in autopsy-confirmed dementia. *Neurobiology of Aging, 29*, 1143–1159. https://doi.org/10.1016/j.neurobiolaging.2007.02.010.
25. Fleisher, A. S., Pontecorvo, M. J., Devous, M. D. Sr, Lu, M., Arora, A. K., Truocchio, S. P., et al. (2020). Positron emission tomography imaging with [18F] flortaucipir and postmortem assessment of Alzheimer disease neuropathologic changes. *JAMA Neurology, 77*, 829–839. https://doi.org/10.1001/jamaneurol.2020.0258.
26. Gorno-Tempini, M. L., Hillis, A. E., Weintraub, S., Kertesz, A., Mendez, M., Cappa, S. F., et al. (2011). Classification of primary progressive aphasia and its variants. *Neurology, 76*, 1006–1014. https://doi.org/10.1212/WNL.0b013e31821103e6.
27. Graff-Radford, J., Yong, K. X. X., Apostolova, L. G., Bouwman, F. H., Carrillo, M. C., Dickerson, M. C., et al. (2021). New insights into atypical Alzheimer's disease in the era of biomarkers. *The Lancet Neurology, 20*, 222–234. https://doi.org/10.1016/S1474-4422(20)30447-3.
28. Grothe, M. J., Moscoso, A., Silva-Rodriguez, J., Lange, C., Nho, K., Saykin, A. J., et al. (2023). Differential diagnosis of amnestic dementia patients based on an FDG-PET signature of

autopsy-confirmed LATE-NC. *Alzheimer's & Dementia, 19*, 1234–1244. https://doi.org/10.1002/alz.12695.

29. Hampel, H., Cummings, J., Blennow, K., Gao, P., Jack, C. R. Jr, & Vergallo, A. (2021). Developing the ATX(N) classification for use across the Alzheimer disease continuum. *Nature Reviews Neurology, 17*, 580–589. https://doi.org/10.1038/s41582-021-00548-0.
30. Hansson, O., Seibyl, J., Stomrud, E., Zetterberg, H., Trojanowski, J. Q., Bittner, T., et al. (2018). CSF biomarkers of Alzheimer's disease concord with amyloid-β PET and predict clinical progression: A study of fully automated immunoassays in Bio FINDER and ADNI cohorts. *Alzheimer's & Dementia, 14*, 1470–1481. https://doi.org/10.1016/j.jalz.2018.01.010.
31. Honig, L. S., Barakos, J., Dhadda, S., Kanekiyo, M., Reyderman, L., Irizarry, M., et al. (2023). ARIA in patients treated with lecanemab (BAN2401) in a phase 2 study in early Alzheimer's disease. *Alzheimer's & Dementia (New York), 9*, e12377. https://doi.org/10.1002/trc2.12377.
32. Jack, C. R. Jr, Bennett, D. A., Blennow, K., Carrillo, M. C., Dunn, B., Haeberlein, S. B., et al. (2018). National Institute on Aging and Alzheimer's Association (NIA-AA) Research Framework: Toward a biological definition of Alzheimer's disease. *Alzheimer's & Dementia, 14*, 535–562. https://doi.org/10.1016/j.jalz.2018.02.018.
33. Jack, C. R. Jr, Therneau, T. M., Lundt, E. S., Wiste, H. J., Mielke, M. M., Knopman, D. S., et al. (2022). Long-term associations between amyloid positron emission tomography, sex, apolipoprotein E, and incident dementia and mortality among individuals without dementia: Hazard ratios and absolute risk. *Brain Communications, 4*, fcac017. https://doi.org/10.1093/braincomms/fcac017.
34. Janelidze, S., Zetterberg, H., Mattsson, N., Palmqvist, S., Vanderstichele, H., Lindberg, O., et al. (2016). CSF Aβ42/Aβ40 and Aβ42/Aβ38 ratios: Better diagnostic markers of Alzheimer disease. *Annals of Clinical and Translational Neurology, 3*, 154–165. https://doi.org/10.1002/acn3.274.
35. Jellinger, K. A. (2022). Recent update on the heterogeneity of the Alzheimer's disease spectrum. *Journal of Neural Transmission, 129*, 1–24. https://doi.org/10.1007/s00702-021-02423-3.
36. Josephs, K. A., Tosakulwong, N., Gatto, R. G., Weigand, S. D., Ali, F., Botha, H., et al. (2022). Optimum differentiation of frontotemporal lobar degeneration from Alzheimer disease achieved with cross-sectional tau positron emission tomography. *Annals of Neurology, 92*, 1016–1029. https://doi.org/10.1002/ana.26376.
37. Josephs, K. A., Whitwell, J. L., Boeve, B. F., Knopman, D. S., Petersen, R. C., Hu, W. T., et al. (2010). Anatomical differences between CBS-corticobasal degeneration and CBS-Alzheimer's disease. *Movement Disorders, 25*, 1246–1252. https://doi.org/10.1002/mds.23062.
38. Koga, S., Josephs, K. A., Aiba, I., Yoshida, M., & Dickson, D. W. (2022). Neuropathology and emerging biomarkers in corticobasal syndrome. *Journal of Neurology, Neurosurgery & Psychiatry, 93*, 919–929. https://doi.org/10.1136/jnnp-2021-327007.
39. Leonenko, G., Baker, E., Stevenson-Hoare, J., Sierksma, A., Fiers, M., Williams, J., et al. (2021). Identifying individuals with high risk of Alzheimer's disease using polygenic risk scores. *Nature Communications, 12*, 4506. https://doi.org/10.1038/s41467-021-24773-7.
40. Liu, S., Buch, S., Chen, Y., Choi, H. S., Dai, Y., Habib, C., et al. (2017). Susceptibility-weighted imaging: Current status and future directions. *NMR in Biomedicine, 30*, e3552. https://doi.org/10.1002/nbm.3552.

41. Liu, W., Lin, H., He, X., Chen, L., Dai, Y., Jia, W., et al. (2020). Neurogranin as a cognitive biomarker in cerebrospinal fluid and blood exosomes for Alzheimer's disease and mild cognitive impairment. *Translational Psychiatry, 10*, 125. https://doi.org/10.1038/s41398-020-0800-9.

42. Mattsson-Carlgren, N., Janelidze, S., Palmqvist, S., Cullen, N., Svenningsson, A. L., Strandberg, O., et al. (2020). Longitudinal plasma p-tau217 is increased in early stages of Alzheimer's disease. *Brain, 143*, 3234–3241. https://doi.org/10.1093/brain/awaa286.

43. Mecca, A. P., Chen, M. K., O'Dell, R. S., Naganawa, M., Toyonaga, T., Godek, T. A., et al. (2020). In vivo measurement of widespread synaptic loss in Alzheimer's disease with SV2A PET. *Alzheimer's & Dementia, 16*, 974–982. https://doi.org/10.1002/alz.12143.

44. Mielke, M. M., Hagen, C. E., Xu, J., Chai, X., Vemuri, P., Lowe, V. J., et al. (2018). Plasma phospho-tau181 increases with Alzheimer's disease clinical severity and is associated with tau- and amyloid-positron emission tomography. *Alzheimer's & Dementia, 14*, 989–997. https://doi.org/10.1016/j.jalz.2018.02.013.

45. Milà-Alomà, M., Brinkmalm, A., Ashton, N. J., Kvartsberg, H., Shekari, M., Operto, G., et al. (2021). CSF synaptic biomarkers in the preclinical stage of Alzheimer disease and their association with MRI and PET: A cross-sectional study. *Neurology, 97*, e2065–e2078. https://doi.org/10.1212/WNL.0000000000012786.

46. Minoshima, S., Cross, D., Thientunyakit, T., Foster, N. L., & Drzezga, A. (2022). ^18F-FDG PET imaging in neurodegenerative dementing disorders: Insights into subtype classification, emerging disease categories, and mixed dementia with copathologies. *Journal of Nuclear Medicine, 63*, 2S–12S. https://doi.org/10.2967/jnumed.121.263345

47. Muszyński, P., Groblewska, M., Kulczyńska-Przybik, A., Kułakowska, A., & Mroczko, B. (2017). YKL-40 as a potential biomarker and a possible target in therapeutic strategies of Alzheimer's disease. *Current Neuropharmacology, 15*, 906–917. https://doi.org/10.2174/1570159X14666161216122118.

48. Oeckl, P., Anderl-Straub, S., Von Arnim, C. A. F., Baldeiras, I., Diehl-Schmid, J., Grimmer, T., et al. (2022). Serum GFAP differentiates Alzheimer's disease from frontotemporal dementia and predicts MCI-to-dementia conversion. *Journal of Neurology, Neurosurgery & Psychiatry*. Advance online publication. https://doi.org/10.1136/jnnp-2022-329056.

49. Ossenkoppele, R., Mattsson, N., Teunissen, C. E., Barkhof, F., Pijnenburg, Y., Scheltens, P., et al. (2015). Cerebrospinal fluid biomarkers and cerebral atrophy in distinct clinical variants of probable Alzheimer's disease. *Neurobiology of Aging, 36*, 2340–2347. https://doi.org/10.1016/j.neurobiolaging.2015.04.013.

50. Ossenkoppele, R., Pichet Binette, A., Groot, C., Smith, R., Strandberg, O., Palmqvist, S., et al. (2022). Amyloid and tau PET-positive cognitively unimpaired individuals are at high risk for future cognitive decline. *Nature Medicine, 28*, 2381–2387. https://doi.org/10.1038/s41591-022-01963-5.

51. Ossenkoppele, R., Pijnenburg, Y. A., Perry, D. C., Cohn-Sheehy, B. I., Scheltens, N. M., Vogel, J. W., et al. (2015). The behavioral/dysexecutive variant of Alzheimer's disease: Clinical, neuroimaging and pathological features. *Brain, 138*, 2732–2749. https://doi.org/10.1093/brain/awv191.

52. Ossenkoppele, R., Schonhaut, D. R., Schöll, M., Lockhart, S. N., Ayakta, N., Baker, S. L., et al. (2016). Tau PET patterns mirror clinical and neuroanatomical variability in Alzheimer's disease. *Brain, 139*, 1551–1567. https://doi.org/10.1093/brain/aww027.

53. Pillai, J. A., Bonner-Jackson, A., Bekris, L. M., Safar, J., Bena, J., & Leverenz, J. B. (2019). Highly elevated cerebrospinal fluid total tau level reflects higher likelihood of non-amnestic subtype of Alzheimer's disease. *Journal of Alzheimer's Disease, 70*, 1051–1058. https://doi.org/10.3233/JAD-190461.

54. Rabinovici, G. D., Rosen, H. J., Alkalay, A., Kornak, J., Furst, A. J., Agarwal, N., et al. (2011). Amyloid vs FDG-PET in the differential diagnosis of AD and FTLD. *Neurology, 77*, 2034–2042. https://doi.org/10.1212/WNL.0b013e31823b9c5e.

55. Rasmussen, J., & Langerman, H. (2019). Alzheimer's disease—Why we need early diagnosis. *Degenerative Neurological and Neuromuscular Disease, 9*, 123–130. https://doi.org/10.2147/DNND.S229306.

56. Sabbagh, M. N., Lue, L. F., Fayard, D., & Shi, J. (2017). Increasing precision of clinical diagnosis of Alzheimer's disease using a combined algorithm incorporating clinical and novel biomarker data. *Neurology and Therapy, 6*, 83–95. https://doi.org/10.1007/s40120-017-0074-0.

57. Sarazin, M., Chauviré, V., Gerardin, E., Colliot, O., Kinkingnéhun, S., de Souza, L. C., et al. (2010). The amnestic syndrome of hippocampal type in Alzheimer's disease: An MRI study. *Journal of Alzheimer's Disease, 22*, 285–294. https://doi.org/10.3233/JAD-2010-100184.

58. Sitek, E. J., Barczak, A., Kluj-Kozlowska, K., Kozlowski, M., Barcikowska, M., & Slawek, J. (2015). Is descriptive writing useful in the differential diagnosis of logopenic variant of primary progressive aphasia, Alzheimer's disease and mild cognitive impairment? *Neurologia i Neurochirurgia Polska, 49*, 239–244. https://doi.org/10.1016/j.pjnns.2015.05.001.

59. Snowden, J. S., Stopford, C. L., Julien, C. L., Thompson, J. C., Davidson, Y., Gibbons, L., et al. (2007). Cognitive phenotypes in Alzheimer's disease and genetic risk. *Cortex, 43*, 835–845. https://doi.org/10.1016/S0010-9452(08)70284-2.

60. Stebbins, G. T., & Murphy, C. M. (2009). Diffusion tensor imaging in Alzheimer's disease and mild cognitive impairment. *Behavioral Neurology, 21*, 39–49. https://doi.org/10.1155/2009/548358.

61. Steinacker, P., Semler, E., Anderl-Straub, S., Diehl-Schmid, J., Schroeter, M. L., Uttner, I., et al. (2017). Neurofilament as a blood marker for diagnosis and monitoring of primary progressive aphasias. *Neurology, 88*, 961–969. https://doi.org/10.1212/WNL.0000000000003676.

62. Strikwerda-Brown, C., Hobbs, D. A., Gonneaud, J., St-Onge, F., Binette, A. P., Ozlen, H., et al. (2022). Association of elevated amyloid and Tau positron emission tomography signal with near-term development of Alzheimer disease symptoms in older adults without cognitive impairment. *JAMA Neurology, 79*, 975–985. https://doi.org/10.1001/jamaneurol.2022.1464.

63. Teunissen, C. E., Verberk, I. M. W., Thijssen, E. H., Vermunt, L., Hansson, O., Zetterberg, H., et al. (2022). Blood-based biomarkers for Alzheimer's disease: Towards clinical implementation. *Lancet Neurology, 21*, 66–77. https://doi.org/10.1016/S1474-4422(21)00361-6.

64. Thijssen, E. H., LaJoie, R., Strom, A., Fonseca, C., Iaccarino, L., Wolf, A., et al. (2021). Plasma phosphorylated tau217 and phosphorylated tau181 as biomarkers in Alzheimer's disease and frontotemporal lobar degeneration: A retrospective diagnostic performance study. *Lancet Neurology, 20*, 739–752. https://doi.org/10.1016/S1474-4422(21)00213-1.

65. van der Flier, W. M., Schoonenboom, S. N., Pijnenburg, Y. A., Fox, N. C., & Scheltens, P. (2006). The effect of APOE genotype on clinical phenotype in Alzheimer disease. *Neurology, 67*, 526–527. https://doi.org/10.1212/01.wnl.0000229291.56829.8b.

66. Vemuri, P., & Jack, C. R. Jr. (2010). Role of structural MRI in Alzheimer's disease. *Alzheimer's Research & Therapy, 2*, 23. https://doi.org/10.1186/alzrt47.

67. Villain, N., & Dubois, B. (2019). Alzheimer's disease including focal presentations. *Seminars in Neurology, 39*, 213–226. https://doi.org/10.1055/s-0039-1683376.

68. Vogelgsang, J., Shahpasand-Kroner, H., Vogelgsang, R., Streit, F., Vukovich, R., & Wiltfang, J. (2018). Multiplex immunoassay measurement of amyloid-beta (42) to amyloid-beta (40) ratio in plasma discriminates between dementia due to Alzheimer's disease and dementia not due to Alzheimer's disease. *Experimental Brain Research, 236*, 1241–1250. https://doi.org/10.1007/s00221-018-5205-2.

69. Wattmo, C., Blennow, K., & Hansson, O. (2020). Cerebrospinal fluid biomarker levels: Phosphorylated tau (T) and total tau (N) as markers for rate of progression in Alzheimer's disease. *BMC Neurology, 20*, 10. https://doi.org/10.1186/s12883-020-01603-0.

70. Werry, E. L., Bright, F. M., Piguet, O., Ittner, L. M., Halliday, G. M., Hodges, J. R., et al. (2019). Recent developments in TSPO PET imaging as a biomarker of neuroinflammation in neurodegenerative disorders. *International Journal of Molecular Sciences, 20*, 3161. https://doi.org/10.3390/ijms20133161.

71. Wolk, D. A. (2013). Amyloid imaging in atypical presentations of Alzheimer's disease. *Current Neurology and Neuroscience Reports, 13*, 412. https://doi.org/10.1007/s11910-013-0412-4.

Chapter 6

ALZHEIMER'S DISEASE PRESCRIPTION DRUG TREATMENT

Contents

Introduction 196
6.1. Neurodegenerative Pathways Implicated in Ad 198
6.2. Drug Therapy 200
6.3. Potential Future Drug Treatments 201
6.4. Future Directions 203
6.5. An Update on the Novel and Approved Drugs for Alzheimer's Disease 204
Summary 222
References 222

INTRODUCTION

A decline in cognitive fu0nction severe enough to interfere with day-to-day functioning is referred to as dementia in general. Approximately 75% of dementia cases are caused by Alzheimer's disease (AD). The remaining cases are caused by vascular dementia (VaD), dementia with Lewy bodies, dementia mixed with Alzheimer's and VaD, and frontotemporal dementia.

Many clinicians find it surprising that despite tremendous advancements in the last 20 years in the treatment of a wide range of illnesses—including many cancers treated with targeted therapies like herceptin and HIV treated with ground-breaking combination drug therapies—there has been little progress in the pharmacological management of dementia caused by AD and other causes. But while the former illnesses are nearly always well-defined and limited disease entities, the dementia syndrome is, for the majority of patients, a multifactorial condition. In fact, even within diagnostic entities like AD, there probably exist sub-classifications with therapeutic implications.

There are important treatment implications for both of these findings. Because neurodegenerative illnesses and vascular diseases often coexist in later life, dementia in later life is best understood as a geriatric syndrome. This conceptualization is relevant because pharmacological interventions are likely to be most effective when used as one element of a package that includes other interventions like medication review, exercise and nutrition intervention, and cognitive stimulation/training. This approach is supported by a recent multi-modal intervention study conducted among older individuals at risk of developing dementia. Geriatric syndromes, like falls, rarely respond to single interventions.

Only five medical treatments, involving only two classes of drugs, have been approved for AD to date, despite the serious public health risk that dementia poses. These treatments manage symptoms rather than changing the course of the disease. Furthermore, only a small number of clinical trials pertaining to AD have been conducted in the past 10 years, with a 99.6% failure rate. As long as disease-modifying therapy is limited to symptom management, its ultimate goal will remain unattainable (Hensley, 2010; Salomone et al., 2012; Ansari et al., 2013; Anand et al., 2017; Atri, 2019).

Orientation and Directional Terms

Term	Definition	Illustration
Vascular Dementia	Vascular dementia is caused by decreased blood flow to brain tissue causing memory problems, problems with movement, urinary problems and tremors.	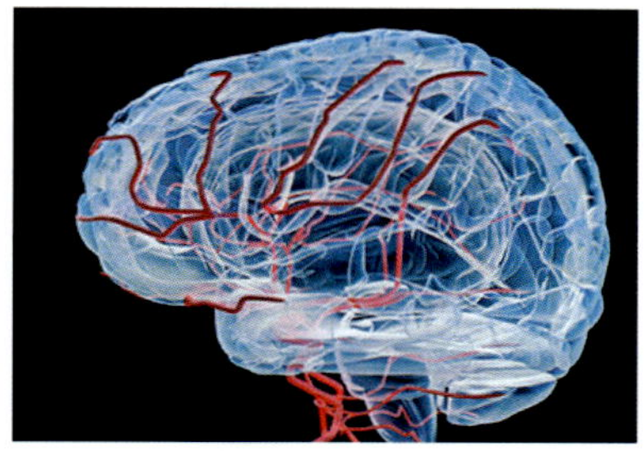
Neurofibrillary Tangles (NFTs)	Neurofibrillary tangles (NFTs) are intracellular aggregates of hyperphosphorylated tau protein that are most commonly known as a primary biomarker of Alzheimer's disease.	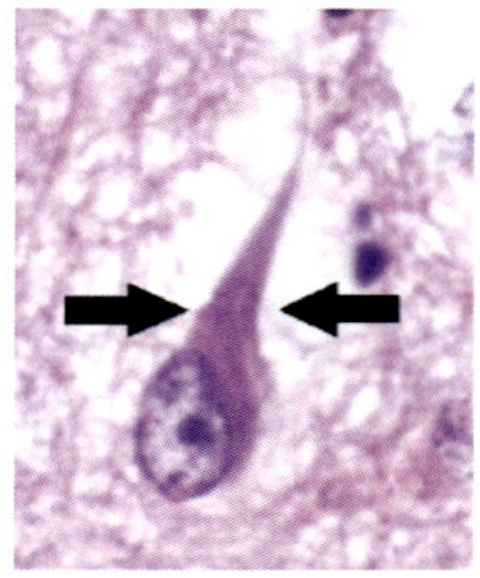
Memantine	Memantine is an antagonist of the N-methyl-D-aspartate receptor (NMDAR) subtype of glutamate receptor. Memantine is used to slow the neurotoxicity involved in Alzheimer's disease and other neurodegenerative diseases.	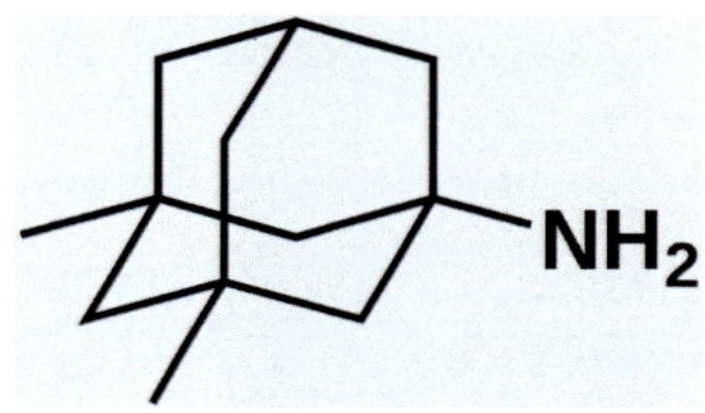
Rivastigmine	Rivastigmine is a cholinesterase inhibitor used for the treatment of mild to moderate Alzheimer's disease. The drug can be administered orally or via a transdermal patch; the latter form reduces the prevalence of side effects, which typically include nausea and vomiting.	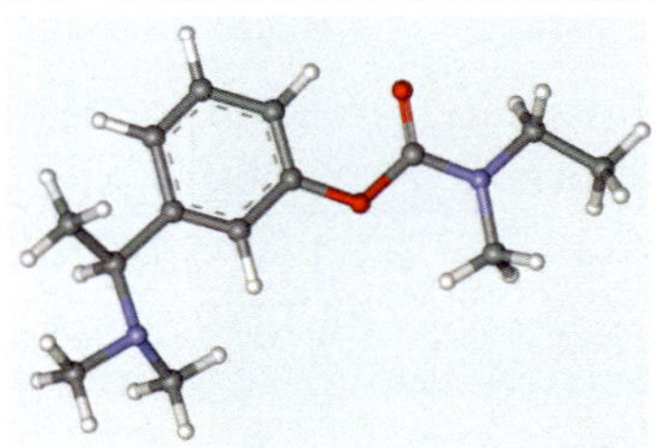
Galantamine	Galantamine is used to treat the symptoms of Alzheimer's disease (AD; a brain disease that slowly destroys the memory and the ability to think, learn, communicate and handle daily activities). Galantamine is in a class of medications called acetylcholinesterase inhibitors.	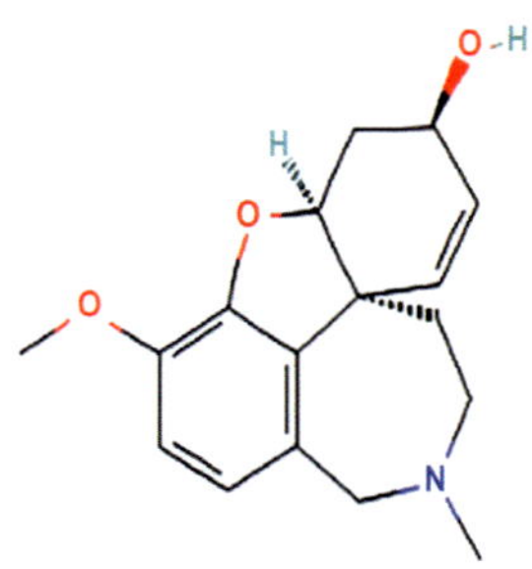

6.1. NEURODEGENERATIVE PATHWAYS IMPLICATED IN AD

The underlying pathology of AD has been explained by several overlapping mechanisms, and both existing and prospective future treatments are predicated on altering these pathways.

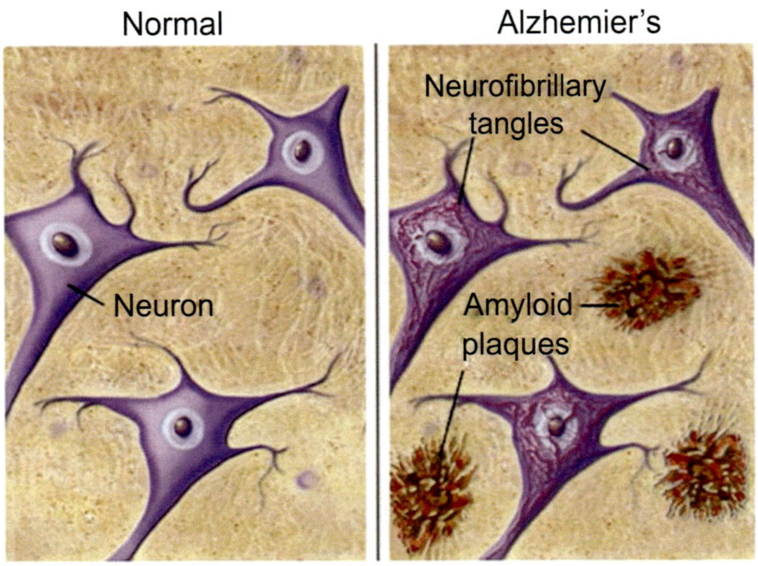

Figure 6.1. *AD-pathogenesis.*

Source: Mitra, A., & Dey, B, (2013). Therapeutic Interventions in Alzheimer Disease. InTech. doi: 10.5772/54915.

6.1.1. Amyloid Cascade Hypothesis

The 1990s saw the emergence of the amyloid hypothesis, which links abnormal processing of the amyloid precursor protein (APP) to the production of amyloid-beta (Aβ). Secretase enzymes cleave amyloid precursor protein (APP), and deviations from this process, particularly in gamma and beta-secretases, can result in aberrant Aβ production. The pathological hallmarks of Alzheimer's disease (AD) include amyloid plaques and neurofibrillary tangles (NFTs), which are made of hyperphosphorylated tau protein and cause neurodegeneration. Aβ can then set off a cascade that results in synaptic damage, neuron loss, and neurodegeneration (Figure 6.1).

6.1.2. Tau Hypothesis

Tau is a neuron-expressed protein that is normally involved in the cytoskeleton of cells in microtubule stabilization. It builds up inside nerve cell bodies as these NFT masses due to hyperphosphorylation. Subsequently, these tangles exhibit anomalous interactions with cellular proteins, impeding their regular functions. Hyperphosphorylation happens after Aβ, and studies indicate that Aβ accumulation could be the catalyst for this process. Furthermore, research indicates that toxic tau can increase the synthesis of Aβ through a feedback loop mechanism.

6.1.3. Cholinergic Hypothesis

The discovery in the 1970s that AD patient brains lacked cholinergic function, which was mediated by deficiencies in the enzyme choline acetyltransferase, marked a significant advance in the field of AD research. This resulted in the cholinergic hypothesis of AD and sparked efforts to therapeutically boost cholinergic activity, along with the realization of the role of acetylcholine in memory and learning. One late stage of the neurodegenerative cascade is cholinergic depletion. Acetyl choline is broken down at the synaptic cleft by the cholinesterase enzyme, which is blocked by cholinesterase inhibitors, enhancing cholinergic transmission.

6.1.4. Excitotoxicity

The progressive loss of neurons in AD is largely attributed to excitotoxicity, which is characterized as excessive exposure to the neurotransmitter glutamate or overstimulation of its N-methyl-D-aspartate (NMDA) receptor. It is believed that this process affects the loss of cholinergic neurons, which causes an excessive inflow of calcium into cells (Hensley, 2010; Salomone et al., 2012; Ansari et al., 2013; Anand et al., 2017; Atri, 2019).

6.1.5. Other Important Etiological Mechanisms

6.1.5.1. Vascular Disease

Vascular disease was once thought to be the primary cause of VaD development, but it is now evident that vascular burden contributes to AD pathogenesis and that there is substantial overlap between the two dementia subtypes. High BMI, smoking, high cholesterol, and high blood pressure are examples of vascular risk factors that have been linked to an increased chance of developing clinical AD. Hypertension is linked to the development of particular neuropathological hallmarks of AD, such as NFTs, and this association seems to be stronger when hypertension is present in midlife as opposed to late life. Vascular lesions, such as cerebral amyloid angiopathy and white matter hyperintensities, are common in patients with AD. Thus, by either increasing the formation of amyloid plaques or NFTs or decreasing their removal from the brain, vascular disease may have a direct impact on them.

These results imply that vascular risk factor management may reduce the rate of cognitive decline in AD patients; however, data from randomized controlled trials do not yet support this theory.

6.1.5.2. Diabetes and Hyperinsulinemia

Diabetes and AD have a well-established correlation, and while vascular burden certainly contributes, it also seems that insulin dysregulation and aberrant insulin metabolism in the central nervous system (CNS) are significant independent risk factors. Both the CNS and blood brain barrier can allow insulin to pass through. While some research has shown that CNS insulin may play a role in regulating tau phosphorylation and preventing Aβ accumulation through the action of an insulin-degrading enzyme, other studies have shown that individuals with AD have reduced insulin levels in their cerebrospinal fluid (CSF). The possible explanation for this is that oversaturation above physiological levels in peripheral hyperinsulinemia leads to a downregulation of insulin uptake across the blood–brain barrier. As a result, the insulin-degrading enzyme is downregulated, which facilitates the removal of amyloid in the brain. Decreased insulin signaling may also increase the activity of the GSK-3 enzyme, which may facilitate the production of tau and NFTs.

Based on promising results from small pilot studies, a study of intranasal insulin as a therapy for AD and mild cognitive impairment

(MCI) is currently underway. These findings have given rise to the theory that medications used to treat diabetes may be able to alter the pathophysiology of AD.

6.1.5.3. Apolipoprotein Gene

The main genetic risk factor for AD has been found to be the apolipoprotein (apo) gene's Apo epsilon 4 (Apoe4) allele, which codes for a protein involved in lipid transport and cholesterol metabolism. People who carry one copy of the e4 allele are three times more likely to develop AD, whereas those who carry two copies have an odds ratio of 14 points nine. Although the exact mechanism by which Apoe4 raises the risk of AD is unknown, it is possible that it does so by influencing Aβ aggregation and clearance, which in turn affects when Aβ deposition starts. Effects on synaptic function, neurotoxicity, tau hyperphosphorylation, and neuroinflammation are some other mechanisms that have been suggested. Although there are currently no clinical trials in this area, it has been suggested that modifying the Apo-related receptor at the blood-brain barrier may provide a therapeutic target to affect Aβ clearance. Other therapeutic options may include modifying Apoe4 levels or converting Apoe4 to Apoe3.

6.1.5.4. Neuroinflammation

An important step in the pathophysiology of AD appears to be the accumulation of glial cells during neuroinflammation, an inflammatory response in the central nervous system. Opinion has since drastically changed from the traditional view that the brain is an "immune-privileged" organ that is isolated from the immune system due to the blood-brain barrier and the immune cells' apparent incapacity to mount an innate immune response. Anti-inflammatory medications may be protective against AD, according to important epidemiological data from the 1990s. Neuroinflammatory cascades are now thought to be a key target for treatment in AD, and NFTs and amyloid plaques may both be immune response drivers.

Unfortunately, meta-analyzes have not shown that non-steroidal anti-inflammatory drugs, aspirin, or steroids are any better than placebo in patients with AD symptoms already present. Nevertheless, there is some evidence that suggests naproxen may be useful in preventing AD in older, healthy individuals. It's possible that the window of opportunity for such treatment is lost by the time symptoms appear because it happens early in the course of the disease (Hensley, 2010; Salomone et al., 2012; Ansari et al., 2013; Anand et al., 2017; Atri, 2019).

6.2. DRUG THERAPY

Nonetheless, the lack of effective disease-modifying medications that resulted from these studies highlights the difficulties in creating a therapeutic agent with the potential to change the course of a disease as complex as AD. A significant portion of research in AD over the past 10 years has been focused on disease-modifying therapy, which will change the course of the disease rather than just treat its symptoms.

6.2.1. Approved Drug Treatments

6.2.1.1. Cholinesterase Inhibitors

The first-generation cholinesterase inhibitor tacrine had hepatotoxic side effects that limited its use. Then came galantamine, rivastigmine, and donepezil, with the former likely being the most often utilized medication.

Efficacy appears similar between these different agents so choice should be based on cost, individual patient tolerance and physician experience.

The starting dose of donepezil is 5 mg in the evening, and if necessary, it can be increased to 10 mg after a month. The patient or caregiver rates improved memory, function, or behavior as the response. Short mental status schedules, like the mini mental state examination, are not intended to detect clinically relevant change, so there is no use in attempting to measure change with these tools. Though opinions on this matter can vary, it is reasonable to consider stopping the medication at that point if there is no improvement after three months of treatment. Before starting a cholinesterase inhibitor, all patients should have an electrocardiogram (ECG) due to the possibility of sick sinus syndrome and other conduction abnormalities. Common side effects include gastrointestinal distress, exhaustion, and cramping in the muscles. When starting a cholinesterase inhibitor in a patient with a history of duodenal or peptic ulcer disease, caution should be exercised. A small percentage of patients may experience agitation or an acute decline in cognition right away after starting the medication; in this case, it should be stopped right away.

Reaction rates vary, with about one-third of patients demonstrating no benefit and a smaller percentage (roughly one-fifth) demonstrating greater benefit. Average effects on cognition and function are typically modest. It is anticipated that cholinesterase inhibitor side effects will prevent approximately one-third of patients from using the medication.

6.2.1.2. Memantine

Memantine uncompetitively inhibits the NMDA receptor, which suggests that it may be neuroprotective by halting the loss of neurons and alleviating symptoms by assisting in the repair of injured neurons (Figure 6.1). Memantine is first prescribed at a dose of 5 mg per day, with weekly dosage increases of 5 mg up to a maximum of 20 mg. Compared to cholinesterase inhibitors, it is usually well tolerated and has fewer side effects, though it can occasionally cause headache, dizziness, sleeplessness, constipation, and hypertension.

There is little evidence to support the use of memantine in milder cases of AD, despite modest benefits being demonstrated in moderate to severe cases. Furthermore, memantine added to donepezil monotherapy may help patients whose cognitive function is declining or who have mid-stage AD. In MCI, neither donepezil nor memantine are helpful.

Despite being the best pharmacological treatments for AD currently available, these drugs have a small average overall effect and don't change the course of the underlying neurodegenerative process. It's possible that therapies like cholinesterase inhibitors won't have the desired effect because the downregulation of cholinergic transmission takes place too far downstream in this process. In light of this, a lot of attention has also been paid to "upstream" targeting of the pathological process (Hensley, 2010; Salomone et al., 2012; Ansari et al., 2013; Anand et al., 2017; Atri, 2019).

6.3. POTENTIAL FUTURE DRUG TREATMENTS

6.3.1. Anti-Amyloid Therapy

Several high-profile clinical trials aimed at altering this amyloid cascade with pharmaceutical agents have been conducted up until recently, but the outcomes have been mainly unsatisfactory. Target sites for these agents typically included APP cleavage-related gamma- or beta-secretase enzymes, as well as directly targeting Aβ.

- **Beta-Secretase Enzyme:** CSF beta-amyloid levels have been shown to be lower in small molecule beta-secretase inhibitors than in controls. Two agents, AZD3293 and MK-8931, are undergoing phase II/III clinical trials, which are scheduled to conclude in 2019.
- **Gamma-Secretase Enzyme:** Semagacestat is a small molecule gamma-secretase inhibitor. Phase III clinical trials involving over 3,000 patients were stopped in 2010 due to worsening cognition at higher doses compared to controls and no improvement in cognition in the study group. In the research group, skin cancer incidence was likewise higher. Tarenflurbil, which is connected to the nonsteroidal anti-inflammatory drug flurbiprofen, has been demonstrated to lower Aβ levels by modifying the gamma-secretase enzyme. However, in phase III trials with nearly 1,700 patients, there was no improvement in cognition or function when compared with placebo.

6.3.2. Immunization

Due to meningoencephalitis cases in 6% of subjects, the first human clinical trial of active immunization against Aβ using the agent AN 1792 was discontinued. Consequently, phase II trials have demonstrated the safety and potential effectiveness of passive immunization with intravenous immunoglobulin containing Aβ antibodies in a small number of patients with mild to moderate AD; however, phase III studies have not found any evidence of slowing the progression of AD.

6.3.3. Monoclonal Antibodies

0Patients with mild to moderate AD participated in a phase III clinical trial from 2007 to 2012 using the monoclonal antibody to Aβ, bepineuzumab. Although it engaged its target, it was demonstrated to lower the rate of amyloid accumulation in Apoe4 carriers without having any effect on cognitive or functional outcomes.

Solanezumab, a different monoclonal antibody, did not meet predetermined end points in patients with mild to moderate AD during the course of two-phase III trials that were concluded in 2012. Pooled analysis then revealed modest benefits in cognitive scores among a subgroup of patients with less severe symptoms, and an extension trial was started in which patients on placebo switched to solanezumab. The two groups' differences in cognitive scores persisted for an additional two years, indicating that solanezumab may have had some disease-modifying effects during the placebo-controlled phase, even though the overall benefit was minimal.

Aducanumab, a different monoclonal antibody, has demonstrated encouraging outcomes in patients with mild to pre-clinical AD. Phase III trials are about to start, and phase Ib studies of 165 patients with pre-clinical/mild AD showed dose-dependent reductions in brain Aβ as well as dose-dependent slowing of the clinical dementia rating and the mini mental state examination at one year.

6.3.4. Tau-Targeted Therapy

Current clinical trials are focused on Tau-targeted strategies, with efforts to prevent hyperphosphorylation and target microtubule stability and aggregation. While agents like lithium and valproic acid may inhibit tau phosphorylation, previous randomized controlled trials of these drugs have shown negative results. However, a recent phase II trial of methylthioninium, a tau aggregation inhibitor, has shown some improvement in cognition in patients with mild and moderate Alzheimer's disease after 50 weeks of therapy. Plans are now underway to proceed to phase III trials (Hensley, 2010; Salomone et al., 2012; Ansari et al., 2013; Anand et al., 2017; Atri, 2019).

6.4. FUTURE DIRECTIONS

Research on potential therapies that could modify diseases has primarily focused on patients with already established and detectable symptoms. However, there is growing evidence indicating that the pathological changes related to dementia actually start occurring years before any clinical signs appear.

This suggests that pharmacological treatments may be more effective when administered during this pre-clinical stage, before the neurodegenerative process is fully developed. To test this theory in clinical trials, early diagnosis techniques are crucial, enabling trials to be conducted during the presymptomatic phases of the disease.

6.4.1. Early Diagnosis

Currently, the primary method for diagnosing Alzheimer's Disease earlier involves examining cerebrospinal fluid and neuroimaging biomarkers, as outlined in the latest research diagnostic criteria for the disease.

6.4.1.1. Cerebrospinal Fluid Biomarkers

CSF tau and amyloid markers reflect the underlying neuropathology of AD and are useful diagnostic markers for dementia. Patients with AD experience a decrease in CSF Aβ42, which may be related to the peptide's plaque deposition. On the other hand, a lower ratio of Aβ42/Aβ40 seems to be a more accurate indicator than Aβ42 on its own. Elevated phosphorylated tau, the main component of NFTs, is more specific than elevated total tau and is also elevated in other dementias, such as VaD and frontotemporal dementia. Elevated total tau is a very sensitive marker for detection of AD. Combinations of these CSF markers have been shown to increase the diagnostic potential in the early stages of AD; for instance, patients with mild cognitive impairment (MCI) who also have high tau levels and low Aβ42 levels have been shown to have a significantly increased risk of AD. Nevertheless, as a stand-alone diagnostic test, the discriminatory power of CSF biomarkers in the differential diagnosis is still not entirely satisfactory, and current presymptomatic evaluation strategies combine results with neuroimaging findings.

6.4.1.2. Neuroimaging

In the past, structural neuroimaging in AD was used to rule out other diagnoses, such as brain tumors, in cases where presentations were unusual. However, by measuring cerebral metabolic rates of glucose metabolism (CMRglc), a surrogate marker for neuronal activity, functional imaging modalities like 18F-fluorodeoxyglucose positron emission tomography (FDG-PET) are now able to detect loss of neuronal function in asymptomatic individuals. Reduced CMRglc is seen in the frontal, posterior, and parietotemporal cingulate cortices in patients with early AD. It has also been demonstrated that these alterations occur in patients with MCI and in people who are genetically predisposed to AD before symptoms manifest. Nonetheless, there is some overlap between the hypometabolic regions of AD and other subtypes of dementia, and the diagnostic accuracy is further enhanced by the additional use of amyloid PET, which measures the surface area of amyloid plaque.

6.4.1.3. Re-evaluating Research Diagnostic Criteria

New research diagnostic criteria have been proposed in response to the need for presymptomatic diagnosis of AD. These criteria formalize the idea that AD is a continuum that progresses from a presymptomatic phase to a symptomatic, pre-dementia phase (MCI), and ultimately to AD. Biomarkers are used in these new criteria to determine whether research subjects with no overt symptoms or very mild overt symptoms have presymptomatic AD. For research purposes, three pre-clinical stages of AD are proposed: subtle cognitive decline, asymptomatic amyloidosis, and asymptomatic amyloidosis with neurodegeneration. These diagnostic standards offer a framework for researching early interventions in AD and will enable a more systematic approach to the diagnosis of presymptomatic AD. Although the definition of presymptomatic AD is helpful and will mostly be applied in the context of research, we also need to consider the moral ramifications of diagnosing a disease with relatively little effective medical treatment at an early stage.

6.4.2. Better Trial Design

More positive clinical outcomes could result from better patient selection for clinical trials. For instance, as demonstrated by the solanezumab trials, the "mild to moderate" AD group may be overly heterogeneous, losing the benefits of treatment within subgroups. Advanced biomarker analysis may help with better study subject selection in addition to earlier diagnosis by enabling the selection of patients with more consistent underlying pathology for focused trials. This customized strategy would resemble a number of cancer treatments in which patients receive customized care based on markers like HER2 (Hensley, 2010; Salomone et al., 2012; Ansari et al., 2013; Anand et al., 2017; Atri, 2019).

6.5. AN UPDATE ON THE NOVEL AND APPROVED DRUGS FOR ALZHEIMER'S DISEASE

Alzheimer's disease (AD) appears to be the most common cause of dementia and one of the biggest issues facing medicine in the twenty-first century. In summary, 40 million people worldwide are anticipated to experience dementia, a number that is expected to double every 20 years until roughly 2050. AD is characterized by progressive memory loss, verbal dysfunction, visual-spatial impairment, and personality abnormalities, all of which require substantial care. Extracellular amyloid plaques and intracellular Tau neurofibrillary tangles are the most common histopathologic lesions in AD. The core component of amyloid or senile plaques (SPs) is exceedingly insoluble and proteolysis-resistant peptide fibrils formed by -amyloid (A) cleavage. After the sequential breakdown of the big precursor protein amyloid precursor protein (APP) by the β- and γ-e -secretase, Aβ peptides with A38, A40, and A42 being the most prevalent forms are generated. β- amyloid (Aβ) cleavage produces highly insoluble and proteolysis-resistant peptide fibrils, which make up amyloid or senile plaques (SPs). However, if APP is first interacted on and broken by the enzyme α-secretase rather than β-secretase, Aβ is not generated. According to the "amyloid hypothesis," Aβ production in the brain sets off a chain of events that leads to the clinical symptoms of AD. The formation of amyloid oligomers is primarily responsible for neurotoxicity and commences the amyloid cascade. Local inflammation, oxidation, production of excess glutamate known as excitotoxicity, and tau hyperphosphorylation are all components of the cascade. Further another theory suggests the mitochondrial dysfunction hypothesis for AD pathogenesis posits that amyloidosis, cell cycle re-entry, and tau phosphorylation are all caused by mitochondrial failure in the AD brain (Figure 6.2 and 6.3)).

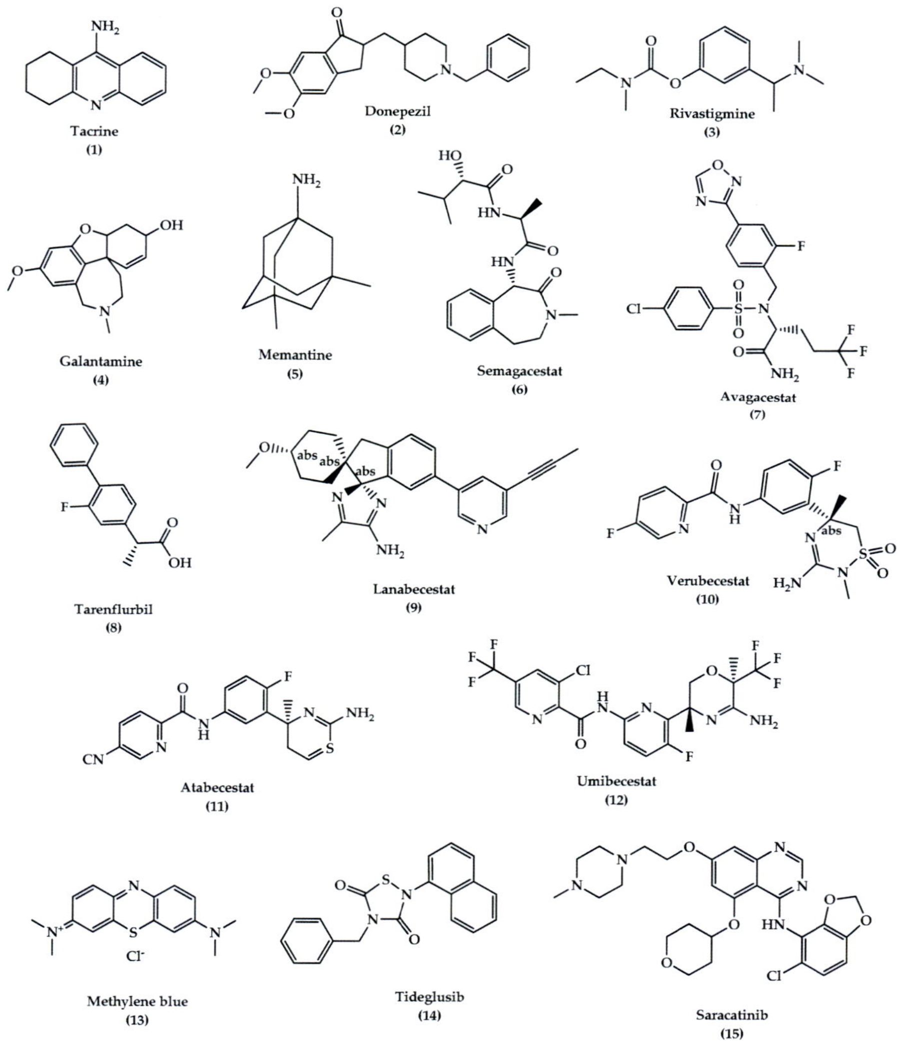

Figure 6.2. *The chemical structures of approved drugs for symptomatic treatment of AD.*

Note: tacrine 1, donepezil 2, rivastigmine 3, galantamine 4, and memantine 5) and disease-modifying compounds that entered clinical trials (semagacestat 6, avagacestat 7, tarenflurbil 8, lanabecestat 9, verubecestat 10, atabecestat 11, umibecestat 12, methylene blue 13, tideglusib 14, and saracatinibin 15).

Source: Breijyeh Z, & Karaman R, (2020). Comprehensive review on Alzheimer's disease: Causes and treatment. Molecules, 25(24), 5789. https://doi.org/10.3390/molecules25245789.

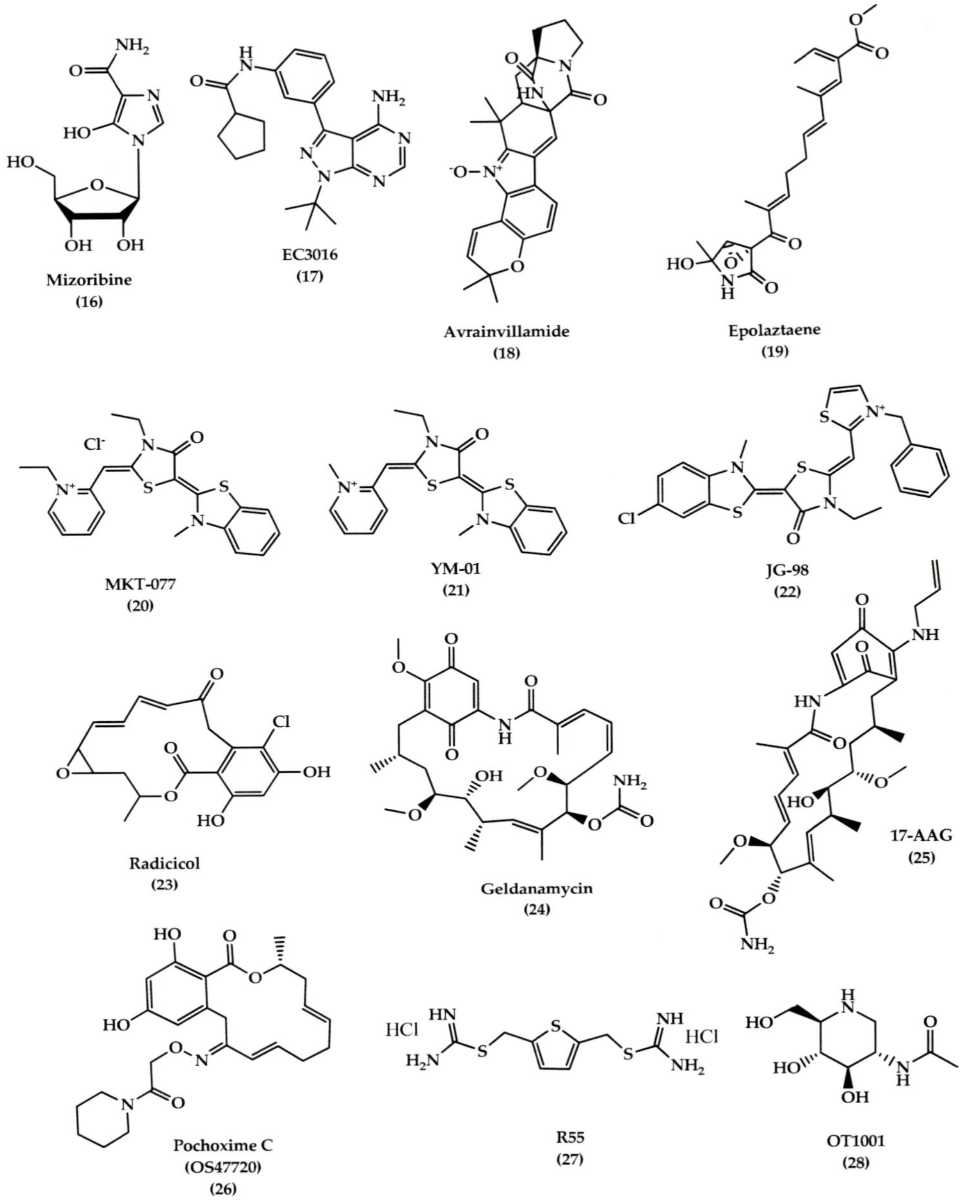

Figure 6.3. *The chemical structures of different chaperone molecules: Mizoribine 16, EC3016 17, Avrainvillamide 18, Epolaztaene 19, MKT-077 20, YM-01 21, JG-98 22, Radicicol 23, Geldanamycin 24, 17-AAG 25, Pochoxime C (OS47720) 26, R55 27, and OT1001 28.*

Source: *Breijyeh Z, & Karaman R, (2020). Comprehensive review on Alzheimer's disease: Causes and treatment. Molecules, 25(24), 5789. https://doi.org/10.3390/molecules25245789.*

Both the glutamatergic and cholinergic neurochemical systems are implicated in the development of AD, according to relevant data. One neurotransmitter that is important for learning and cognitive processes is acetylcholine (ACh). AD patients' brains function and concentration are both compromised. This impairment, along with other presynaptic cholinergic limitations like diminished acetylcholinesterase activity and loss of the cholinergic neural network, support the cholinergic theory of AD. Another neurochemical theory explaining the genesis of AD is the glutamatergic hypothesis mediated by N-Methyl d-aspartate (NMDA). Excitatory neurotransmitter glutamate binds to NMDA receptors, which are critical for learning and memory. On the other hand, glutamate overstimulation of NMDA receptors can occasionally result in neuronal damage due to excitotoxicity.

Given the growing number of individuals suffering from AD, it is clear that finding effective treatments is crucial. NMDA receptor blockers like memantine and acetylcholinesterase inhibitors like donepezil, rivastigmine, and metrifonate are currently used as symptomatic treatments for AD. It is imperative that we find therapies that halt or reduce the progression of disease. Since pathology, genetics, and biochemistry all strongly support the amyloid cascade theory, efforts to explore these therapies have primarily focused on targeting A peptide or clumps in AD.

Together with the pre-clinical research being done by a group of researchers for the treatment of AD, the emergence of various approved drugs and those in the clinical pipeline are elaborated upon with additional insight regarding potential therapies for the disease.

6.5.1. FDA Approved Drugs for AD and Their MOA

A treatment for AD may help to improve cognition and function while slowing the disease's clinical degeneration. There might be other people who can help ease symptoms like disorientation and memory loss. In the US, the Food and Drug Administration (FDA) has approved medications that can be divided into two groups: medications that have the potential to slow down the clinical decline of AD patients and treatments that have the potential to temporarily relieve some of the disease's associated symptoms. Before starting any treatment, it is imperative to consult a healthcare professional to determine its applicability. Patients who use these medications must be closely observed by a healthcare professional who is knowledgeable about them and can ensure that the prescribed protocols are strictly adhered to.

6.5.1.1. Drugs that May Decrease the Evolution of Alzheimer's Disease

Medications in this category may help individuals with Alzheimer's disease to slow down clinical deterioration and enhance cognitive function. Aducanumab was granted accelerated approval by the FDA on June 7, 2021 [FDA Approved Drug Products: Aduhelm (Aducanumab-avwa) Intravenous Injection].

Adrenaline (AduhelmTM) is an intravenous (IV) infusion medication that is an anti-amyloid antibody. Usually, an FDA-approved diagnostic test is advised before the therapy begins. This monoclonal antibody (mAb) is fully human, has a high affinity for aggregated forms of Aβ, and binds parenchymal amyloid more often than vascular amyloid. It was created using a reverse translational medical approach, in which older individuals without AD were given the antibody in the hopes that they would have a particularly strong resistance to the condition. It has been observed that injecting aducanumab intraperitoneally into Tg2576 mice causes parenchymal plaques and aids in their removal without causing microhemorrhages. Additionally, the researchers observed a concentration of brain macrophages surrounding the remaining plaques, indicating that phagocytosis is a likely mechanism of clearance.

The "amyloid cascade hypothesis" states that amyloid-oligopeptide aggregation in the brain is the cause of AD. Aducanumab is a monoclonal IgG1 antibody that attaches itself to amyloid-'s amino acids 3–7.1, 6. The majority of the interaction between amyloid and aducanumab's Fab region is accounted for by the amyloid residues Phe4, His6, Glu3, and Arg5. Animal studies have shown that acetaminophenab treatment reduces amyloid-, although human trials did not show significant improvements in amyloid-40 and amyloid-42 levels.

6.5.1.2. Conventional Pharmacotherapy for AD

The drugs now used to treat AD can be divided into the following categories:

Rivastigmine, Donepezil, Galantamine, and Tacrine are acetylcholinesterase inhibitors.

Memantine is an NMDA antagonist (glutamate inhibitor).

6.5.1.2.1. Acetylcholinesterase Inhibitors

Galantamine has been approved by the FDA for mild and moderate AD, while donepezil and rivastigmine have been approved for mild, moderate, and severe AD, respectively.

Patients with AD have increased acetylcholinesterase activity, which leads to increased acetylcholine breakdown and decreased brain acetylcholine concentrations. Furthermore, the enzyme contributes to the development of neurofibrillary tangles and amyloid plaques. Acylcholinesterase is an additional enzyme that promotes the growth of -amyloid peptide fragments by forming complexes with the expanding fibrillar structures. It has been discovered that individual -amyloid fibrils are more cytotoxic than the resulting complexes. These drugs increase the amount of acetylcholine in the brains of people with mild to moderate AD by inhibiting the enzyme acetylcholinesterase, which is essential for the metabolic breakdown of acetylcholine. These medication classes were found to be well tolerated in the majority of patients.

Typically, diarrhea, nausea, and vomiting are the most common side effects of AChEIs because of their action on the gastro-intestinal tract (git). Hepatic metabolism is thought to be the main method of elimination for donepezil and galantamine, while intestinal and hepatic metabolism are involved in the elimination of rivastigmine. While rivastigmine is a "pseudo-irreversible" acetylcholinesterase and butyrylcholinesterase inhibitor, donepezil and galantamine are known to specifically and reversibly block acetylcholinesterase. Rivastigmine's acetylcholinesterase activity is referred to as "pseudo irreversible" because, following its reaction with the essential active site serine, it forms a covalent carbamoyl-AChE complex, which inhibits the enzyme's ability to catalyze the synthesis of acetylcholine. Galantamine's half-life of elimination is 70 hours, whereas donepezil's is six to eight hours. Rivastigmine has a short half-life for elimination but a long half-life for action.

6.5.1.2.2. Glutamate Inhibitor

Excitotoxicity is a disorder brought on by glutamatergic overstimulation, which increases the calcium load on neurons and damages them. Memantine is a non-competitive NMDA receptor antagonist that is known to mitigate the deleterious effects of elevated brain glutamate concentrations. That said quality has paved the way for it to be used as a beneficial therapeutic drug in AD patients. It has been demonstrated that memantine, an approved medication for the treatment of moderate to severe AD, improves cognitive abilities and the outcomes that follow in AD patients. Most patients tolerate the aforementioned medication well. On the other hand, mild and transient side effects are possible. Its pharmacological makeup may cause it to interact with other drugs. Depending on how each of these drugs works, concurrent treatment with levodopa, other dopamine agonists, and anticholinergics may increase their biological activity.

Because memantine and AChEIs have complementary modes of action, they can be used together. Patients typically benefit from the aforementioned combination therapy, which has no increase in adverse effects and cumulative effects. Better overall functioning and therapeutic outcomes are associated with the duration and durability of monotherapy or combinatorial treatment modalities with higher doses in cases of intermediate or advanced dementia. Pharmacotoxic psychosis can result from mixing memantine with other chemically related NMDA receptor antagonists, such as amantadine, budipine, ketamine, and dextrometorphan. The most frequent side effects observed in clinical trials were fatigue, headaches, agitation, dizziness, and hallucinations. Among the less frequent symptoms that were reported were anxiety, emesis, UTIs, and increased sweating.

6.5.2. Potential Therapeutic Approach for the Treatment of AD

6.5.2.1. Anti-Amyloid Therapy

The amyloid cascade theory links AD to the aggregation of monomeric Aβ. An accumulation of Aβ in the synaptic synapse can lead to the formation of toxic oligomers. These oligomers eventually result in amyloid deposits by forming protobrils. The "Amyloid hypothesis" postulates that the brain's production of Aβ initiates a sequence of pathophysiologic processes that lead to the clinical presentation of Alzheimer's disease. The primary cause of neurotoxicity is thought to be the formation of amyloid oligomers, which in turn set off the amyloid cascade. The cluster's main pathophysiologic pillars are tau hyperphosphorylation, excessive glutamate, inflammation, and oxidation.

Anti-amyloid therapy works through two main mechanisms to avoid the aforementioned condition: either it promotes Aβ clearance or it reduces Aβ42 production and Aβ-plaque burden.

6.5.2.1.1. Reducing of Aβ42 Production

- **α-Secretase Modulators:** According to the current amyloid hypothesis, the breakdown of APP by α-secretase increases the non-amyloidogenic process. Therefore, one important pharmacological approach that has been proposed is the modulation of the enzyme. APH-1105 and ID1201, two -secretase modulators that activate the PI3K/Akt pathway, are currently undergoing clinical trials. APH-1105 is an intranasal treatment for mild to moderate AD, and ID1201 is also an α-secretase activator that is being studied in mild AD subjects.

Another α-secretase modulator that selectively modulates GABA receptors is etazolate (EHT0202). According to reports, the agent has a good tolerance profile in patients with AD.

- **BACE Inhibitors:** Clinical trials with BACE inhibitors, including lanabecestat, verubecestat, and atabecestat, have recently been discontinued due to unforeseen difficulties. The verubecestat and atabecestat trials were also stopped because of inefficacy and safety concerns, respectively, and the lanabecestat phase 3 investigation was stopped because of ineffectiveness. While there were no benefits to cognition or function, all of the treatments decreased cerebrospinal fluid (CSF) Aβ42 in a dose-dependent manner. Moreover, some of the treatments were ineffective and poorly tolerated in individuals with prodromal AD. These results support the theory that inhibiting Aβ production might not be sufficient to stop the disease from getting worse.

Elenbecestat (E2609) and umibecestat (CNP520) are the two agents which are in different phases of clinical trials.

- **γ-Secretase Inhibitors:** Due to significant safety concerns, γ secretase inhibitors are no longer considered a suitable target for the treatment of AD. Further research on this vital enzyme could help to target -secretase therapeutically in a safe manner. As of right now, no γ-secretase effectors are undergoing clinical trials. Semagacestat was associated with worsening daily functioning, increased rates of infections, and skin cancer incidence. Avagacestat was associated with a higher proportion of cognitive decline and negative dose-limiting effects, including an increased risk of skin cancer. Tarenflurbil had minimal blood–brain barrier penetration.

6.5.2.1.2. Reducing Aβ-Plaque Burden

Anti-amyloid aggregation medications interact with the Aβ peptide directly to stop the formation of Aβ42 fibers, which suggests that they may be used as an AD treatment. Scyllo-inositol is an oral medication that inhibits Aβ42 aggregation and has been studied in individuals with AD (ELND005). A phase 2 clinical trial involving AD patients was discontinued due to serious toxicity concerns, and no evidence of ELND005's clinical benefit was found.

KLVFF, a peptide sequence that resembles the hydrophobic center region of the Aβ and eventually replaces natural polypeptides, is another effective treatment. Finally, the KLVFF compound, which is resistant to proteolytic degradation and has a limited capacity to degrade oligomerics, has negligible degrading power over them.

- **Promoting Aβ Clearance:** The two main immunotherapeutic strategies for encouraging Aβ clearance that are currently being studied in various stages of analysis are passive and active immunization.
  - **Passive Immunization:** Passive Ab immunotherapy with monoclonal antibodies is the most effective and promising class. The two main side effects of this medication class are vasogenic edema and cerebral microhemorrhages.

The three main treatments being enrolled for preclinical research or at-risk groups are crenezumab, gantenerumab, and solanezumab; prodromal and very mild AD patients are receiving studies involving these medications. According to the preliminary findings of the BAN2401 trials, patients with AD experienced a decrease in their cerebral amyloid load and a deceleration in their cognitive decline. On the other hand, the gantenerumab preliminary trial in patients with prodromal AD was prematurely stopped because of insufficient therapeutic efficacy; however, the results of the study suggest that a relatively high gantenerumab dosage might be necessary to achieve clinical effectiveness. In order to do this, a double-blind, placebo-controlled study in AD patients is being conducted concurrently with an open-label addition for engaged patients with mild AD. Similarly, solanezumab had not been demonstrated to impede the advancement of brain atrophy until recently.

- **Active Immunization:** A phase 2 study in people with mild or moderate AD episodes is currently being conducted using UB-311, a synthetic peptide used as an Aβ vaccine. In AD patients, it yielded a total response rate during the first phase of the clinical trial. The most frequent adverse effects were agitation and injection site swelling. The rate of cognitive decline was slower in patients with mild AD. Clinical trials are currently testing more potent anti-active immunotherapy drugs that are less likely to activate T cells and more specific to Aβ sites, as a result of the high rate of encephalitis in earlier experiments (AN-1792). As the first active vaccine, ABvac40 is being evaluated. AD patients between the ages of 50 and 85 took part in a phase I trial. No signs of microhemorrhages or vasogenic edema were present. After receiving ABvac40 injections, 92% of the patients produced antibodies specific to Aβ40.

6.5.2.2. Chelation Therapy

One of the main causes of AD is a metal ion imbalance in the brain, so using metal ions in chelation therapy is a suitable approach to treating this condition. As a perfect medication for AD, a metal chelator should have the following characteristics: it should have a moderate metal binding affinity, be able to pass through biological membranes, especially the blood-brain barrier, and have a lower toxicity level. Furthermore, one major complexity is figuring out how selective potential metal chelators are. For the purpose of treating AD, metal chelators must have a strong enough chelating ability to capture free metal ions or metal ions linked to Ab, but not so strong as to interact with metal ions coupled to other metalloproteins that may be important to human health.

A large number of chelating agents exist, but only a small number have favorable pharmacological effects and may find use as AD medications. Given their lower molecular weight and strong scaffolding characteristics, clofidil (CQ) and deferiprone (DFP) have been recognized as promising AD medications.

6.5.2.2.1. Clioquinol (CQ) and its Derivatives

CQ can be used to chelate metal ions, which reduces the aggregation of Aβ. Additionally, it can chelate metal ions from metal–Aβ species in a 2:1 ratio into CQ–Cu(II) or CQ–Zn(II) complexes, preventing metal ions from sticking to Ab and causing brain aggregates to disperse in vitro. These intriguing results shed light on the potential use of metal chelating medications to slow the advancement of AD. In a phase IIa clinical trial involving Alzheimer's patients, CQ showed encouraging results in terms of slowing cognitive decline. As such, possible neurotoxicity and unwanted mutagenic contaminants have prevented CQ from becoming a viable anti-AD medication.

Cu(II), Zn(II), and Fe(III), a bis-8-hydroxyquinoline ligand, significantly increased the potential to protect against the precipitation of b-amyloid peptides in vitro when compared to CQ. It has been demonstrated to prevent Cu–Aβ from producing H2O2, which is connected to detrimental oxidative stress in AD.

Mohamed et al. synthesized (2,20-(1E,10 E)-(1,2- phenylenebis(methan-1-yl-1-ylidene)) bis (azan-1-yl-1-ylidene) dibenzoic acid), which is coordinated to metal ions with the azomethine-N and carboxylate-O as binding sites in a 1: 1 ratio. Magnetic and solid reflectance confirmed the geometrical structure of the formed complexes with the metal ions.

6.5.2.2.2. Deferiprone (DFP) and its Derivatives

Thalassemia is known to be treated with the iron chelator deferiprone (DFP, 3-hydroxy-1,2-dimethylpyridin-4(1H)-one). Within its scaffold, it exhibits a strong positive and significant affinity for metals like iron, copper, and zinc. Due to its low molecular weight and appropriate structure, DFP can be easily optimized. Despite having a C log P value of 1.4, it is too small to cross the blood-brain barrier and has been utilized as a lead compound in the development of multi-target directed ligands (MTDL) for the treatment of AD.

The Zn (II)-curcumin complex and the Cu(II)-curcumin complex can also scavenge free radicals. Furthermore, the Cu(II)-curcumin complex had a higher potential to scavenge free radicals than curcumin and the Zn (II)-curcumin combination. The results may contribute to a better understanding of curcumin's role in AD treatment.

6.5.2.3. Natural Drugs for AD Treatment

Numerous diseases, including AD, have been demonstrated to have their progression and related symptoms slowed down by medication. Many research have been done to examine the advantages of fully extracting plants for AD and to pinpoint the functional elements required to produce the required therapeutic effects. Numerous compounds with anti-inflammatory, anti-amyloidogenic, anticholinesterase, and anti-inflammatory qualities have been demonstrated. These include lignans, flavonoids, tannins, polyphenols, triterpenes, sterols, and alkaloids. People with AD have been treated with a variety of drugs, with encouraging outcomes. (Hensley, 2010; Salomone et al., 2012; Ansari et al., 2013; Anand et al., 2017; Atri, 2019).

A variety of herbal compounds that are being studied for AD are shown in Table 6.1.

Table 6.1. Summary of Clinical Trials Conducted for Anti-Alzheimer's Medicinal Plants

NCT Number	Title	Status	Interventions	Phase	Population	Sponsor	Result
NCT00391833	Effect of *Panax Ginseng* on the Cognitive Performance in AD	Completed	*Panax ginseng*	Phase 1 Phase 2	Enrollment: 97 Age: 40 years to 83 years (adult, older adult)	Seoul National University Hospital, Republic of Korea	Enhanced cognitive metrics observed in Alzheimer's patients. Improvement in memory retention and recall demonstrated significant potential for *Panax ginseng* as a therapeutic agent in cognitive decline associated with AD.

NCT03221894	A Retrospective Study to Investigate the Additive Effectiveness of Chinese Herbal Medicine in AD	Completed	Dietary supplement: GRAPE granules	Not available	Enrollment: 120 Age: 50 years to 85 years (adult, older adult)	Dongzhimen Hospital, Beijing, China; Beijing Hospital, China; Chinese PLA General Hospital, China; Peking University Third Hospital, China	Chinese herbal medicine, specifically GRAPE granules, exhibits supplementary efficacy in mitigating cognitive decline in Alzheimer's patients. Notable improvements in memory consolidation and attentional functions were observed.
NCT04570644	Randomized I/II Phase Study of ALZT-OP1 Combination Therapy in AD and Normal Healthy Volunteers	Completed	ALZT-OP1 (cromolyn and ibuprofen); ALZT-OP1a (cromolyn) and ALZT-OP1b (ibuprofen)	Phase 1	Enrollment: 56 Age: 55 years to 79 years (adult, older adult)	AZ Therapies, Inc., Boston, MA, USA	ALZT-OP1 combination therapy exhibited promising results in both Alzheimer's patients and healthy volunteers. Reduction in neuroinflammatory markers and cognitive enhancement were observed, indicating a potential breakthrough in disease-modifying interventions.
NCT04149860	Study with Lu AF87908 in Healthy Participants and Participants with AD	Recruiting	Lu AF87908; Placebo	Phase 1	Enrollment: 88 Age: 18 years to 65 years (adult, older adult)	H. Lundbeck A/S, Copenhagen, Denmark	Ongoing trial to assess the safety and preliminary efficacy of Lu AF87908 in both healthy individuals and those afflicted with AD. Early indications suggest a potential for cognitive enhancement, warranting further investigation.
NCT02547818	Safety and Efficacy Study of ALZT-OP1 in Subjects with Evidence of Early AD	Completed	ALZT-OP1a; ALZT-OP1b; Placebo ALZT-OP1a; Placebo ALZT-OP1b	Phase 3	Enrollment: 620 Age: 55 years to 79 years (adult, older adult)	AZ Therapies, Inc., Boston, MA, USA	ALZT-OP1 demonstrates safety and substantial efficacy in subjects with early-stage AD. Robust cognitive preservation and a significant reduction in disease progression were observed, supporting its potential as a disease-modifying therapy.

NCT04300569	A Study to Determine the Signs and Symptoms that Impact Daily Life of Participants with Irregular Sleep-Wake Rhythm Disorder	Completed	Non-interventional	Not available	Enrollment: 37 Age: 18 years to 90 years (adult, older adult)	Eisai Inc., Tokyo, Japan	The study delineated the significant impact of irregular sleep–wake rhythm disorder on participants' daily lives. Key indicators affecting cognitive function were identified, shedding light on potential therapeutic avenues.
NCT05591027	Safety and Target Engagement of *Centella Asiatica* in Cognitive Impairment	Not yet recruiting	*Centella asiatica* product; Placebo	Phase 1	Enrollment: 48 Age: 65 years to 85 years (older adult)	Oregon Health and Science University Alzheimer's Association, USA	Anticipated study aims to ascertain safety and efficacy of *Centella asiatica* in cognitive impairment. Preliminary data suggest promising neuroprotective effects, warranting further investigation.
NCT05269173	Efficacy and Safety of *Flos Gossypi*i Flavonoids Tablet in the Treatment of AD	Recruiting	*Flos gossypii* flavonoids tablet	Phase 2	Enrollment: 240 Age: 50 years to 85 years (adult, older adult)	Capital Medical University, China; Xinjiang Uygur Pharmaceutical Co., Ltd., Wuhan, China	Ongoing investigation into the potential of *Flos Gossypii* flavonoids tablet in treating AD. Preliminary data suggest a favorable impact on cognitive function and disease progression.
NCT03286608	Polyphenols and Risk of Dementia	Completed	Observational study (no intervention)	Not available	Enrollment: 1329 Age: 65 years and older (older adult)	Jean-François Dartigues, France; University of Bordeaux, France	Observational study elucidating the relationship between polyphenols and dementia risk. Data underscore a potential protective effect, warranting deeper mechanistic exploration.
NCT00205179	AD: Potential Benefit of Isoflavones	Completed	Novasoy; Placebo	Phase 2	Enrollment: 72 Age: 55 years and older (adult, older adult)	University of Wisconsin, Madison, USA; National Institutes of Health (NIH), USA; National Institute on Aging (NIA), USA	Isoflavones, specifically novasoy, exhibit potential benefits in AD. Significant improvements in cognitive metrics were observed, suggesting a role in disease management.
NCT00500500	Effect of EGb 761® on Patients with Mild to Moderate AD	Terminated	EGb 761® (Tanakan®)	Phase 2	50 years to 85 years (older adult)	Ipsen, Paris, France	Trial exploring the effect of EGb 761® on patients with mild-to-moderate AD. Study discontinued prematurely, with limited conclusive data available.

NCT00164749	A Pilot Study of Curcumin and Ginkgo for Treating AD	Completed	Placebo and ginkgo extract; Curcumin and ginkgo extract	Phase 1 Phase 2	50 years and older	Chinese University of Hong Kong; BUPA Foundation, Hong Kong; Kwong Wah Hospital, Hong Kong	Pilot study investigating the potential benefits of curcumin and ginkgo in AD. Preliminary data suggest a positive impact on cognitive function, warranting further exploration.
NCT00276510	A Study of EGb 761® (Tanakan®) in Dementia of Alzheimer's-Type Onset in Patients Suffering From Memory Complaints	Completed	EGb 761® (Tanakan®); Placebo	Phase 4	70 years and older	Ipsen, Paris, France	Study assessing the impact of EGb 761® in patients with dementia of Alzheimer's-type onset. Data indicate potential cognitive benefits, suggesting a role in early intervention.
NCT00010803	*Ginkgo biloba* Prevention Trial in Older Individuals	Completed	*Ginkgo biloba* Placebo	Phase 3	75 years and older	National Center for Complementary and Integrative Health (NCCIH), USA; Office of Dietary Supplements (ODS); National Institute of Neurological Disorders and Stroke (NINDS), USA; National Institute on Aging (NIA), USA; National Heart, Lung, and Blood Institute (NHLBI), USA	Comprehensive trial investigating the preventive potential of *Ginkgo biloba* in older individuals. No significant cognitive benefits were observed, necessitating further research into alternative interventions.
NCT03090516	Clinical Efficacy of *Ginkgo Bilob*a Extract in the Treatment of AD	Unknown status	*Ginkgo biloba* dispersible tablets; Donepezil; *Ginkgo biloba* dispersible tablets and donepezil	Phase 2 Phase 3	50 years to 85 years	The First Affiliated Hospital with Nanjing Medical University, China	Ongoing investigation into the clinical efficacy of *ginkgo biloba* extract in AD. Preliminary data are pending, with outcomes yet to be determined.

NCT01001637	Efficacy and Safety of Curcumin Formulation in AD	Unknown status	Dietary supplement: Curcumin formulation; Dietary supplement: Placebo	Phase 2	Enrollment: 26 Age: 50 years to 80 years (adult, older adult)	Jaslok Hospital and Research Centre, Mumbai, India; Pharmanza Herbal Pvt Ltd., Gujarat, India; Verdure Sciences; University of California, Los Angeles, USA	Study evaluating the efficacy and safety of curcumin formulation in AD. Preliminary data are pending, with outcomes yet to be determined.
NCT00099710	Curcumin in Patients with Mild to Moderate AD	Completed	Dietary supplement: Curcumin C3 complex	Phase 2	Enrollment: 33 Age: 50 years and older (adult, older adult)	John Douglas French Alzheimer's Foundation, USA; Institute for the study of Aging (ISOA), USA; National Institute on Aging (NIA), USA	Investigation into the potential benefits of curcumin C3 complex in patients with mild-to-moderate AD. Preliminary data suggest positive cognitive effects, warranting further exploration.
NCT01811381	Curcumin and Yoga Therapy for Those at Risk for AD	Unknown status	Curcumin; Behavioral: Aerobic yoga; Behavioral: Non-aerobic yoga; Dietary supplement: Placebo	Phase 2	Enrollment: 80 Age: 50 years to 90 years (adult, older adult)	VA Office of Research and Development, USA	Ongoing trial assessing the combined impact of curcumin and yoga therapy in individuals at risk for AD. Preliminary data are pending, with outcomes yet to be determined.
NCT01716637	Short Term Efficacy and Safety of Perispinal Administration of Etanercept in Mild to Moderate AD	Completed	Etanercept; Dietary supplement: Curcumin, Luteol, Theaflavin, Lipoic Acid, Fish Oil, Quercetin, Resveratrol	Phase 1	Enrollment: 12 Age: 60 years to 85 years (adult, older adult)	Life Extension Foundation Inc., Fort Lauderdale, FL, USA	Study investigating the short-term efficacy and safety of perispinal administration of etanercept in mild-to-moderate AD. Preliminary data indicate a potential for cognitive improvement, warranting further exploration.

NCT04606420	Lifestyle Changes can Reverse Early-Stage AD	Active, not recruiting	Behavioral: Lifestyle medicine	No data available	Enrollment: 51 Age: 45 years to 90 years (adult, older adult)	Preventive Medicine Research Institute; University of California, San Francisco, USA; Harvard Medical School (HMS and HSDM), USA; University of California, SanDiego, USA; The Cleveland Clinic; Renown Health, USA	Ongoing investigation into the potential of lifestyle changes in reversing early-stage AD. Preliminary data are pending, with outcomes yet to be determined.

Source: Nagori K, Nakhate KT, Yadav K, Ajazuddin, & Pradhan M, (2023). Unlocking the therapeutic potential of medicinal plants for Alzheimer's disease: Preclinical to clinical trial insights. Future Pharmacology, 3(4), 877–907. https://doi.org/10.3390/futurepharmacol3040053.

6.5.3. Clinical Trials of Novel Drugs for AD

The development of effective treatments for AD has become a top priority due to the condition's complexity and the growing patient population. The N-methyl-d-aspartate receptor antagonist and cholinesterase inhibitors are two examples of the current treatments for AD that can temporarily lessen mental symptoms but cannot reverse or stop the disease's progression. From an amyloid standpoint, a large number of multinational pharmaceutical companies have carried out a number of clinical trials involving amyloid cleansing as a treatment, but none of them have proven effective. Numerous therapies have been created and tested by researchers, such as behavioral submission, neurotransmitter mutations, anti-amyloid and anti-tau interventions, anti-inflammation and neuroprotection interventions, cognitive enhancement, and behavioral submission. Numerous novel therapies are currently undergoing various stages of clinical trials (Table 6.2).

Table 6.2. Disease Modifying Agents for the Treatment of Alzheimer's Disease in Clinical Trials

Disease Modifying Agents	Mechanism of Action
Phase 3 Clinical Trials	
Aducanumab	Monoclonal antibody—targets β-amyloid and removes it.
Gantenerumab	Monoclonal antibody—binds and removes β-amyloid.
CAD106b	Amyloid vaccine—stimulates production of antibodies against β-amyloid.
BAN2401	Monoclonal antibody—reduces protofibrillar β-amyloid.
TRx0237 (LMTX)	Tau protein aggregation inhibitor.
AGB101	Low-dose levetiracetam—improves synaptic function and reduces amyloid-induced neuronal hyperactivity

ALZT-OP1 (cromolyn + ibuprofen)	Mast cell stabilizer and anti-inflammatory—promotes microglial clearance of amyloid
Azeliragon	RAGE (Receptor for Advanced Glycation End-products) antagonist—reduces inflammation and amyloid transport into the brain
BHV4157 (troriluzole)	Glutamate modulator—reduces synaptic levels of glutamate and improves synaptic functioning
Masitinib	Tyrosine kinase inhibitor—modulates inflammatory mast cell and reduces amyloid protein and tau phosphorylation
Phase 2 Clinical Trials	
Crenezumab	Monoclonal antibody—targets soluble oligomers and removes β-amyloid
ABBV-8E12	Monoclonal antibody—prevents tau propagation
ABvac40	Active immunotherapy—targets β-amyloid and removes it
BAN2401	Monoclonal antibody—removes amyloid protofibrils and reduces amyloid plaques
BIIB092	Monoclonal antibody—removes tau and reduces tau propagation
LY3002813 (donanemab)	Monoclonal antibody—removes amyloid by recognizing aggregated pyroglutamate form of Aβ
LY3303560 (zagotenemab)	Monoclonal antibody—neutralizes soluble tau aggregates
Semorinemab (RO7105705)	Monoclonal antibody—removes extracellular tau
APH-1105	Alpha-secretase modulator—reduces amyloid
Daratumumab	Monoclonal antibody—immunomodulatory that targets CD38 and regulates microglial activity
Dasatinib + Quercetin	Tyrosine kinase inhibitor (dasatinib) + flavonoid (quercetin)—reduces senescent cells and tau aggregation
IONIS MAPTRx (BIIB080)	Epigenetic, Tau Antisense oligonucleotide—reduces tau production
Lithium	Neurotransmitter receptors ion channel modulator—improves neuropsychiatric symptoms
Nilotinib	Tyrosine kinase inhibitor—promotes clearance of amyloid and tau proteins
Posiphen	Selective inhibitor of APP—reduces amyloid, tau, and α-synuclein production
PTI-125	Filamin A protein inhibitor—reduces tau hyperphosphorylation, synaptic dysfunction, and stabilizes soluble amyloid and the α7 nicotinic acetylcholine receptor interaction
PQ912	Glutaminyl cyclase (QC) enzyme inhibitor—reduces amyloid plaques and pyroglutamates Aβ production
Riluzole	Glutamate receptor antagonist—reduces glutamate-mediated excitotoxicity
Thiethylperazine (TEP)	Activates ABCC1 (ATP binding cassette subfamily C member 1 transport protein)—removes amyloid
Phase 1 Clinical Trials	
BIIB076	Monoclonal antibody—removes tau and reduces tau propagation
Lu AF87908	Monoclonal antibody—removes tau

anle138b	Aggregation inhibitor—reduces tau aggregation
RO7126209	Monoclonal antibody—removes amyloid
TPI-287	Stabilizes tubulin-binding, microtubule, and reduces cellular damage mediated by tau

Source: Breijyeh Z, & Karaman R, (2020). Comprehensive review on Alzheimer's disease: Causes and treatment. Molecules, 25(24), 5789. https://doi.org/10.3390/molecules25245789.

The first monoclonal antibody to target Aβ in AD through passive immunotherapy was bepineuzumab. Trials were stopped after the first two studies were completed and showed no treatment efficacy on cognitive or functional outcomes. A phase 2b study of the BACE-1 inhibitor E2609 (elenbecestat) in amyloid-PET patients with mild AD, prodromal AD, or MCI found that CSF A levels were reduced in a dose-dependent manner. Nothing major has changed with AD. Score Composite, also known as CDR-SB score. The therapeutic efficacy of elenbecestat was examined in a 24-month study to assess its safety and efficacy in studies on Alzheimer's disease (MISSION AD1) and MISSION AD2 trials of prodromal AD. The aforementioned trials are anticipated to continue until December 2023. Sodium oligo-mannurarate, or GV-971, attaches to multiple amyloid sites, further destabilizes, stops Aβ synthesis, and speeds up Aβ elimination. In a phase 3 trial that began in April 2014, the effects of GV-971 on mild to severe forms of AD were examined. The findings of this study demonstrated the substantial cognitive benefits of GV-971. The neuroprotective and anti-inflammatory properties of the dihydropyridine calcium channel blocker nilvadipine, which can decrease Aβ production and increase Aβ clearance, were assessed (Hensley, 2010; Salomone et al., 2012; Ansari et al., 2013; Anand et al., 2017; Atri, 2019).

The NILVAD trial, which took place in 2013, examined the effectiveness of nilvadipine in people with AD. ADAS-Cog was the main outcome measure, but there was no difference in the primary or secondary end point measures according to a published report.

In a phase 3 trial, the efficacy of suvorexant for treating insomnia in patients with mild to severe AD was investigated. Merck noted that the case's first and second goals had been achieved. Thus, it can be concluded that suvorexant may be a useful medication for treating the psychological and behavioral symptoms of AD. A key player in controlling the release of different neurotransmitters is EVP-6124, an agonist of the 7 nicotinic acetylcholine receptor and an antagonist of the 5-HT3 receptor. Cholinergic neurotransmission is improved, leading to an increase in cognitive function. Due to a gastrointestinal side effect, the FDA placed a clinical hold on the trial, which was started as a phase 3 evaluation of safety.

The dopamine system is stabilized by apiprazole (DSSs). It enhances the reduction of neuropathy caused by neurites. This treatment may be able to eliminate the neurotoxicity caused by Aβ in AD-related psychosis. In a phase 3 clinical trial, aripiprazole's efficacy at varying doses was investigated in agitated AD patients. The attempt was abandoned in March 2016 due to the difficulty in finding volunteers.

Two phase 3 clinical trials involving azeliragon for patients with mild AD were started in the year 2018, and a phase 3 study in people with AD who have poor glucose tolerance began in 2019 and is anticipated to be finished in 2023.

Planning is necessary to ensure that experiments involving different drugs, such as those that target neurotransmitter flexibility and neuroprotective effects, mental enhancement, anti-amyloid and anti-tau, can yield promising outcomes, given the scarcity of anti-AD drugs (Hensley, 2010; Salomone et al., 2012; Ansari et al., 2013; Anand et al., 2017; Atri, 2019).

6.5.4. Significance of Research

There are currently a number of AD treatment options under investigation. Nutraceuticals and phytopharmaceuticals are becoming more and more well-liked in the fight against Alzheimer's. Drugs undergoing clinical trials have the potential to improve the quality of life for AD patients and pave the way for new, effective treatment options (Hensley, 2010; Salomone et al., 2012; Ansari et al., 2013; Anand et al., 2017; Atri, 2019).

A Closer Look

Rivastigmine in Alzheimer's Dementia

Rivastigmine is a medication commonly prescribed for the treatment of Alzheimer's dementia, a progressive neurodegenerative disorder characterized by cognitive decline, memory loss, and impaired daily functioning. As a cholinesterase inhibitor, rivastigmine works by increasing the levels of acetylcholine, a neurotransmitter involved in memory and learning, in the brain. By doing so, it helps to improve cognitive function and slow down the progression of symptoms in individuals with Alzheimer's dementia.

One significant aspect of rivastigmine's mechanism of action is its ability to inhibit both acetylcholinesterase and butyrylcholinesterase enzymes. By inhibiting these enzymes, rivastigmine prevents the breakdown of acetylcholine, allowing it to accumulate in the synaptic clefts between neurons. This increased availability of acetylcholine enhances cholinergic neurotransmission, which is often impaired in Alzheimer's disease due to the loss of cholinergic neurons.

Clinical studies have demonstrated the efficacy of rivastigmine in improving cognitive function and activities of daily living in patients with mild to moderate Alzheimer's dementia. It has been shown to have beneficial effects on memory, attention, language, and executive function, as well as reducing behavioral symptoms such as agitation and aggression.

Rivastigmine is available in various formulations, including oral capsules, oral solution, and transdermal patches, providing flexibility in dosing and administration. The transdermal patch, in particular, offers the advantage of continuous drug delivery, minimizing fluctuations in plasma concentration and reducing gastrointestinal side effects commonly associated with oral administration.

While rivastigmine can provide symptomatic relief and improve quality of life for individuals with Alzheimer's dementia, it is important to note that it does not alter the underlying course of the disease or reverse the neurodegenerative process. Therefore, its benefits may be limited, and its effectiveness tends to diminish over time as the disease progresses. Additionally, like all medications, rivastigmine may cause side effects, including nausea, vomiting, diarrhea, dizziness, and insomnia, which should be monitored and managed by healthcare providers (Hensley, 2010; Salomone et al., 2012; Ansari et al., 2013; Anand et al., 2017; Atri, 2019)

SUMMARY

- Dementia is a general term for a decline in cognitive ability severe enough to interfere with daily life. Alzheimer's disease (AD) accounts for almost three-quarters of cases of dementia, with the remainder accounted for by vascular dementia (VaD), mixed Alzheimer's and VaD, dementia with Lewy bodies, and frontotemporal dementia.
- Rivastigmine is a medication used to manage and treat neurodegenerative disease, specifically dementia, in patients with Alzheimer's and Parkinson disease. It is in the cholinesterase inhibitor class of drugs. This activity reviews the indications, action, and contraindications for rivastigmine as a valuable agent in managing dementia (and other disorders when applicable).
- Memantine is an antagonist of the N-methyl-D-aspartate receptor (NMDAR) subtype of glutamate receptor. Memantine is used to slow the neurotoxicity involved in Alzheimer's disease and other neurodegenerative diseases.
- Donepezil hydrochloride, a piperidine derivative, is a centrally acting, rapid, and reversible acetylcholinesterase inhibitor primarily utilized for treating Alzheimer's disease. Acetylcholinesterase is an enzyme that breaks down acetylcholine after its release from the presynapse. By binding reversibly to acetylcholinesterase, donepezil inhibits acetylcholine hydrolysis, thereby increasing acetylcholine availability at the synapses and enhancing cholinergic transmission.
- Galantamine is a medication used in the management and treatment of Alzheimer's disease. It is in the acetylcholinesterase inhibitor class of drugs. This activity reviews the indications, mechanism of action, contraindications, adverse event profile, and other key factors of galantamine therapy pertinent for healthcare team members in the care of patients with dementia, mainly Alzheimer's disease and other conditions.

REFERENCES

1. Abdallah, S. M., Zayed, M., & Mohamed, G. G. (2010). Synthesis and spectroscopic characterization of new tetradentate Schiff base and its coordination compounds of NOON donor atoms and their antibacterial and antifungal activity. *Arabian Journal of Chemistry, 3*, 103–113. https://doi.org/10.1016/j.arabjc.2010.04.019.
2. Ahmed, M., Malik, M., Teselink, J., Lanctôt, K. L., & Herrmann, N. (2019). Current agents in development for treating behavioral and psychological symptoms associated with dementia. *Drugs & Aging, 36*(7), 589–605. https://doi.org/10.1007/s40266-019-00677-2.
3. Anand, A., Patience, A. A., Sharma, N., & Khurana, N. (2017). The present and future of pharmacotherapy of Alzheimer's disease: A comprehensive review. *European Journal of Pharmacology, 815*, 364–375. https://doi.org/10.1016/j.ejphar.2017.08.013.
4. Ansari, N., & Khodagholi, F. (2013). Natural products as promising drug candidates for the treatment of Alzheimer's disease: Molecular mechanism aspect. *Current Neuropharmacology, 11*(4), 414–429. https://doi.org/10.2174/1570159X13804999475.
5. Areosa, S. A., & Sherriff, F. (2003). Memantine for dementia. *Cochrane Database of Systematic Reviews, 3*, CD003154. https://doi.org/10.1002/14651858.CD003154.

6. Arndt, J. W., Qian, F., Smith, B. A., et al. (2018). PH: Structural and kinetic basis for the selectivity of aducanumab for aggregated forms of amyloid-beta. *Scientific Reports, 8*(1), 6412. https://doi.org/10.1038/s41598-018-24899-1.

7. Atri, A. (2019). Current and future treatments in Alzheimer's disease. *Seminars in Neurology, 39*, 227–240. https://doi.org/10.1055/s-0039-1685506.

8. Atri, A., Molinuevo, J. L., Lemming, O., et al. (2013). Memantine in patients with Alzheimer's disease receiving donepezil: New analyses of efficacy and safety for combination therapy. *Alzheimer's Research & Therapy, 5*, 6. https://doi.org/10.1186/alzrt160.

9. Bandegi, A. R., Rashidy-Pour, A., Vafaei, A. A., & Ghadrdoost, B. (2014). Protective effects of Crocus sativus L. extract and crocin against chronic-stress induced oxidative damage of brain, liver and kidneys in rats. *Advances in Pharmacological Sciences, 2014*, 493-499. https://doi.org/10.1155/2014/493-499.

10. Banks, W. A., Jaspan, J. B., Huang, W., & Kastin, A. J. (1997). Transport of insulin across the blood-brain barrier: Saturability at euglycemic doses of insulin. *Peptides, 18*(10), 1423–1429. https://doi.org/10.1016/S0196-9781(97)00200-X.

11. Bendova, P., Mackova, E., Haskova, P., et al. (2010). Comparison of clinically used and experimental iron chelators for protection against oxidative stress-induced cellular injury. *Chemical Research in Toxicology, 23*(6), 1105–1114. https://doi.org/10.1021/tx100118t.

12. Biasibetti, R., Tramontina, A. C., Costa, A. P., et al. (2013). Green tea (-) epigallocatechin-3-gallate reverses oxidative stress and reduces acetylcholinesterase activity in a streptozotocin-induced model of dementia. *Behavioral Brain Research, 236*, 186–193. https://doi.org/10.1016/j.bbr.2012.08.032.

13. Bihaqui, S. W., Singh, A. P., & Tiwari, M. (2012). Supplementation of Convolvulus pluricaulis attenuates scopolamine-induced increased tau and Amyloid precursor protein (AβPP) expression in rat brain. *Indian Journal of Pharmacology, 44*(5), 593. https://doi.org/10.4103/0253-7613.100375.

14. Birks, J. S., & Harvey, R. (2003). Donepezil for dementia due to Alzheimer's disease. *Cochrane Database of Systematic Reviews, 3*, CD001190. https://doi.org/10.1002/14651858.CD001190.

15. Bishop, G. M., & Robinson, S. R. (2004). Physiological roles of amyloid-beta and implications for its removal in Alzheimer's disease. *Drugs & Aging, 21*(10), 621–630. https://doi.org/10.2165/00002512-200421100-00001.

16. Bloom, G. S. (2014). Amyloid-β and tau: The trigger and bullet in Alzheimer's disease pathogenesis. *JAMA Neurology, 71*(4), 505–508. https://doi.org/10.1001/jamaneurol.2013.5847.

17. Bondi, M. W., Edmonds, E. C., & Salmon, D. P. (2017). Alzheimer's disease: Past, present, and future. *Journal of the International Neuropsychological Society, 23*(9–10), 818–831. https://doi.org/10.1017/S1355617717000984.

18. Brayne, C., & Davis, D. (2012). Making Alzheimer's and dementia research fit for populations. *The Lancet, 380*(9851), 1441–1443. https://doi.org/10.1016/S0140-6736(12)61803-0.

19. Breitner, J. C., Baker, L. D., Montine, T. J., et al. (2011). Extended results of the Alzheimer's disease anti-inflammatory prevention trial. *Alzheimer's & Dementia, 7*(4), 402–411. https://doi.org/10.1016/j.jalz.2010.12.014.

20. Budimir, A. (2011). Metal ions, Alzheimer's disease, and chelation therapy. *Acta Pharmaceutica, 61*(1), 1–14. https://doi.org/10.2478/v10007-011-0001-6.

21. Calvó-Perxas, L., Turró-Garriga, O., Vilalta-Franch, J., et al. (2017). Trends in the prescription and long-term utilization of antidementia drugs among patients with Alzheimer's disease in Spain: A cohort study using the registry of dementias of Girona. *Drugs & Aging, 34*(4), 303–310. https://doi.org/10.1007/s40266-017-0456-6.

22. Carson, M. J., Doose, J. M., Melchior, B., Schmid, C. D., & Ploix, C. C. (2006). CNS immune privilege: Hiding in plain sight. *Immunological Reviews, 213*(1), 48–65. https://doi.org/10.1111/j.1600-065X.2006.00441.x.

23. Chakravarthi, K. K., & Avadhani, R. (2013). Beneficial effect of aqueous root extract of Glycyrrhiza glabra on learning and memory using different behavioral models: An experimental study. *Journal of Natural Science, Biology, and Medicine, 4*(2), 420–425. https://doi.org/10.4103/0976-9668.117025.

24. Chang, X., Rong, C., Chen, Y., Yang, C., Hu, Q., & Mo, Y. (2015). (−)-Epigallocatechin-3-gallate attenuates cognitive deterioration in Alzheimer's disease model mice by upregulating neprilysin expression. *Experimental Cell Research, 334*, 136–145. https://doi.org/10.1016/j.yexcr.2015.04.009.

25. Cho, W. H., Park, J. C., & Kim, D. H. (2014). ID1201, the ethanolic extract of the fruit of *Melia toosendan* ameliorates impairments in spatial learning and reduces levels of amyloid beta in 5XFAD mice. *Neuroscience Letters, 583*, 170–175. https://doi.org/10.1016/j.neulet.2014.09.032.

26. Clarke, E. T., & Martell, A. E. (1992). Stabilities of 1,2-dimethyl-3-hydroxy-4-pyridinone chelates of divalent and trivalent metal ions. *Inorganic Chimica Acta, 191*, 57–63. https://doi.org/10.1016/0020-1693(92)80037-W.

27. Coleman, P. J., Gotter, A. L., Herring, W. J., Winrow, C. J., & Renger, J. J. (2017). The discovery of suvorexant, the first orexin receptor drug for insomnia. *Annual Review of Pharmacology and Toxicology, 57*, 509–533. https://doi.org/10.1146/annurev-pharmtox-010715-103308.

28. Corder, E. H., Saunders, A. M., Strittmatter, W. J., et al. (1993). Gene dose of apolipoprotein E type 4 allele and the risk of Alzheimer's disease in late onset families. *Science, 261*(5123), 921–923. https://doi.org/10.1126/science.8346443.

29. Coric, V., Salloway, S., & Van Dyck, C. H. (2015). Targeting prodromal Alzheimer's disease with avagacestat: A randomized clinical trial. *JAMA Neurology, 72*, 1324–1333. https://doi.org/10.1001/jamaneurol.2015.0604.

30. Craft, S., Baker, L. D., Montine, T. J., et al. (2012). Intranasal insulin therapy for Alzheimer's disease and amnestic mild cognitive impairment: A pilot clinical trial. *Archives of Neurology, 69*(1), 29–38. https://doi.org/10.1001/archneurol.2011.233.

31. Craft, S., Peskind, E., Schwartz, M. W., et al. (1998). Cerebrospinal fluid and plasma insulin levels in Alzheimer's disease: Relationship to severity of dementia and apolipoprotein E genotype. *Neurology, 50*(1), 164–168. https://doi.org/10.1212/WNL.50.1.164.

32. Cummings, J. L., Morstorf, T., & Zhong, K. (2014). Alzheimer's disease drug-development pipeline: Few candidates, frequent failures. *Alzheimer's Research & Therapy, 6*, 37. https://doi.org/10.1186/alzrt269.

33. Cummings, J., Lee, G., Ritter, A., Sabbagh, M., & Zhong, K. (2019). Alzheimer's disease drug development pipeline: 2019. *Alzheimer's & Dementia, 5*, 272–293. https://doi.org/10.1016/j.trci.2019.06.005.
34. Defeudis, F. V. (2002). Bilobalide and neuroprotection. *Pharmacological Research, 46*, 565–568. https://doi.org/10.1016/S1043-6618(02)00233-5.
35. Deraeve, C., Pitíe, M., Mazarguil, H., & Meunier, B. (2007). Bis-8-hydroxyquinoline ligands as potential anti-Alzheimer's agents. *New Journal of Chemistry, 31*, 193–195. https://doi.org/10.1039/B614589A.
36. Doody, R. S., Raman, R., & Farlow, M. (2013). A phase 3 trial of semagacestat for treatment of Alzheimer's disease. *New England Journal of Medicine, 369*, 341–350. https://doi.org/10.1056/NEJMoa1210951.
37. Dunstan, R., Bussiere, T., Engber, T., et al. (2011). The role of brain macrophages on the clearance of amyloid plaques following the treatment of Tg2576 with BIIB037. *Alzheimer's & Dementia, 7*(4), S700. https://doi.org/10.1016/j.jalz.2011.05.1819.
38. Egan, M. F., Kost, J., & Voss, T. (2019). Randomized trial of verubecestat for prodromal Alzheimer's disease. *New England Journal of Medicine, 380*, 1408–1420. https://doi.org/10.1056/NEJMoa1812840.
39. Farrer, L. A., Cupples, L. A., Haines, J. L., et al. (1997). Effects of age, sex, and ethnicity on the association between apolipoprotein E genotype and Alzheimer's disease: A meta-analysis. *JAMA, 278*(16), 1349–1356. https://doi.org/10.1001/jama.1997.03550160069041.
40. Farris, W., Mansourian, S., Chang, Y., et al. (2003). Insulin-degrading enzyme regulates the levels of insulin, amyloid beta-protein, and the beta-amyloid precursor protein intracellular domain in vivo. *Proceedings of the National Academy of Sciences of the United States of America, 100*(7), 4162–4167. https://doi.org/10.1073/pnas.0230450100.
41. Ferrada, V., Arancibia, B., Loeb, E., Norambuena, C., Olea-Azar, Huidobro-Toro, J. P. (2007). Neurotoxicology, 28, 445–449. https://doi.org/10.1016/j.neuro.2007.02.004.
42. Ferrero, J., Williams, L., Stella, H., Leitermann, K., Mikulskis, A., O'Gorman, J., & Sevigny, J. (2016). First-in-human, double-blind, placebo-controlled, single-dose escalation study of aducanumab (BIIB037) in mild-to-moderate Alzheimer's disease. *Alzheimer's & Dementia: Translational Research & Clinical Interventions, 2*(3), 169–176. https://doi.org/10.1016/j.trci.2016.04.002.
43. Francis, P. T. (2005). The interplay of neurotransmitters in Alzheimer's disease. *CNS Spectrums, 10*(S18), 6–9.
44. Galimberti, D., & Scarpini, E. (2017). Pioglitazone for the treatment of Alzheimer's disease. *Expert Opinion on Investigational Drugs, 26*(1), 97–101. https://doi.org/10.1080/13543784.2017.1265778.
45. Hardy, J., & Selkoe, D. J. (2002). The amyloid hypothesis of Alzheimer's disease: Progress and problems on the road to therapeutics. *Science, 297*(5580), 353–356. https://doi.org/10.1126/science.1072994.
46. Hasnain, M., & Vieweg, W. V. (2014). Possible role of vascular risk factors in Alzheimer's disease and vascular dementia. *Current Pharmaceutical Design, 20*(38), 6007–6013. https://doi.org/10.2174/1381612820666140410201855.

47. He, Q., Sun, J., Wang, Q., Wang, W., & He, B. (2014). Neuroprotective effects of ginsenoside Rg1 against oxygen-glucose deprivation in cultured hippocampal neurons. *Journal of the Chinese Medical Association, 77*, 142–149. https://doi.org/10.1016/j.jcma.2013.12.004.

48. Heneka, M. T., Carson, M. J., El Khoury, J., et al. (2015). Neuroinflammation in Alzheimer's disease. *The Lancet Neurology, 14*(4), 388–405. https://doi.org/10.1016/S1474-4422(15)70016-5.

49. Henley, D., Raghavan, N., Sperling, R., Aisen, P., Raman, R., & Romano, G. (2019). Preliminary results of a trial of atabecestat in preclinical Alzheimer's disease. *New England Journal of Medicine, 380*, 1483–1485. https://doi.org/10.1056/NEJMc1900861.

50. Hensley, K. (2010). Neuroinflammation in Alzheimer's disease: Mechanisms, pathologic consequences, and potential for therapeutic manipulation. *Current Alzheimer Research, 7*(1), 1–14. https://doi.org/10.2174/156720510790274414.

51. Herring, W. J., Roth, T., Krystal, A. D., & Michelson, D. (2019). Orexin receptor antagonists for the treatment of insomnia and potential treatment of other neuropsychiatric indications. *Journal of Sleep Research, 28*(2), e12782. https://doi.org/10.1111/jsr.12782.

52. Hoi, C. P., Ho, Y. P., Baum, L., & Chow, A. H. L. (2010). Neuroprotective effect of honokiol and magnolol, compounds from *Magnolia officinalis*, on beta-amyloid-induced toxicity in PC12 cells. *Phytotherapy Research, 24*, 1538–1542. https://doi.org/10.1002/ptr.3126.

53. Huang, H. C. C., & Jiang, Z. F. F. (2009). Accumulated amyloid-beta peptide and hyperphosphorylated tau protein: Relationship and links in Alzheimer's disease. *Journal of Alzheimer's Disease, 16*(1), 15–27. https://doi.org/10.3233/JAD-2009-0924.

54. Huang, L. K., Chao, S. P., & Hu, C. J. (2020). Clinical trials of new drugs for Alzheimer's disease. *Journal of Biomedical Science, 27*, 18.

55. Huang, M., Jiang, X., Liang, Y., Liu, Q., Chen, S., & Guo, Y. (2017). Berberine improves cognitive impairment by promoting autophagic clearance and inhibiting production of β-amyloid in APP/tau/PS1 mouse model of Alzheimer's disease. *Experimental Gerontology, 91*, 25–33.

56. Hull, M., Sadowsky, C., & Arai, H. (2017). Long-term extensions of randomized vaccination trials of ACC-001 and QS-21 in mild to moderate Alzheimer's disease. *Current Alzheimer's Research, 14*, 696–708.

57. Jaturapatporn, D., Isaac, M. G. E. K. N. G., McCleery, J., & Tabet, N. (2012). Aspirin, steroidal and non-steroidal anti-inflammatory drugs for the treatment of Alzheimer's disease. *Cochrane Database of Systematic Reviews, 2*, CD006378. https://doi.org/10.1002/14651858.CD006378.pub2.

58. Jeong, E. J., Hwang, L., Lee, M., Lee, K. Y., Ahn, M. J., & Sung, S. H. (2014). Neuroprotective biflavonoids of *Chamaecyparis obtusa* leaves against glutamate-induced oxidative stress in HT22 hippocampal cells. *Food and Chemical Toxicology, 64*, 397–402.

59. Kalaria, R. N., & Ballard, C. (1999). Overlap between pathology of Alzheimer's disease and vascular dementia. *Alzheimer's Disease and Associated Disorders, 13*(Suppl 3), S115–S123. https://doi.org/10.1097/00002093-199900133-00020.

60. Kim, J., Basak, J. M., & Holtzman, D. M. (2009). The role of apolipoprotein E in Alzheimer's disease. *Neuron, 63*(3), 287–303. https://doi.org/10.1016/j.neuron.2009.06.026.

61. Kishita, N., Backhouse, T., & Mioshi, E. J. (2020). Nonpharmacological interventions to

improve depression, anxiety, and quality of life (QoL) in people with dementia: An overview of systematic reviews. *Geriatric Psychiatry and Neurology, 33*(1), 28–41.

62. Krishnankutty, John, V. (2003). Synthesis, characterization, and antitumor studies of metal chelates of some synthetic curcuminoids. *Synthetic Communications, 33*, 343–358.
63. Lautenschläger, M., Sendker, J., Hüwel, S., Galla, H. J., Brandt, S., & Düfer, M. (2015). Intestinal formation of trans-crocetin from saffron extract (*Crocus sativus* L.) and in vitro permeation through intestinal and blood brain barrier. *Phytomedicine, 22*, 36–44.
64. Lawlor, B., Segurado, R., Kennelly, S., Rikkert, M. G. O., Howard, R., & Pasquier, F. (2018). Nilvadipine in mild to moderate Alzheimer's disease: A randomized controlled trial. *PLoS Medicine, 15*(9), e1002660.
65. Lee, J. W., Lee, Y. K., Ban, J. O., Ha, T. Y., Yun, Y. P., & Han, S. B. (2009). Green tea (-)-epigallocatechin-3-gallate inhibits β-amyloid-induced cognitive dysfunction through modification of secretase activity via inhibition of ERK and NF-κB pathways in mice. *The Journal of Nutrition, 139*, 1987–1993.
66. Lim, G. P., Chu, T., Yang, F., Beech, W., Frautschy, S. A., & Cole, G. M. (2001). The curry spice curcumin reduces oxidative damage and amyloid pathology in an Alzheimer's transgenic mouse. *Journal of Neuroscience, 21*, 8370–8377.
67. Lipton, S. A. (2005). The molecular basis of memantine action in Alzheimer's disease and other neurologic disorders: Low-affinity, uncompetitive antagonism. *Current Alzheimer Research, 2*(2), 155–165. https://doi.org/10.2174/1567205053585882.
68. Liu, C. C., Kanekiyo, T., Xu, H., & Bu, G. (2013). Apolipoprotein E and Alzheimer's disease: Risk, mechanisms and therapy. *Nature Reviews Neurology, 9*(2), 106–118. https://doi.org/10.1038/nrneurol.2012.263.
69. Lu, F. P. P., Lin, K. P. P., & Kuo, H. K. K. (2009). Diabetes and the risk of multi-system aging phenotypes: A systematic review and meta-analysis. *PLoS ONE, 4*(1), e4144. https://doi.org/10.1371/journal.pone.0004144.
70. Luchsinger, J. A., Tang, M. X. X., Shea, S., & Mayeux, R. (2004). Hyperinsulinemia and risk of Alzheimer's disease. *Neurology, 63*(7), 1187–1192. https://doi.org/10.1212/01.WNL.0000140293.63683.2A.
71. Mandelkow, E. M., & Mandelkow, E. (1998). Tau in Alzheimer's disease. *Trends in Cell Biology, 8*(11), 425–427. https://doi.org/10.1016/S0962-8924(98)01348-3.
72. Manning, F. C. (1994). Tacrine therapy for the dementia of Alzheimer's disease. *American Family Physician, 50*, 819–826.
73. Martinez, A., Gil, C., & Perez, D. I. (2011). Glycogen synthase kinase 3 inhibitors in the next horizon for Alzheimer's disease treatment. *International Journal of Alzheimer's Disease, 2011*, 280502. https://doi.org/10.4061/2011/280502.
74. McGeer, P. L., Schulzer, M., & McGeer, E. G. (1996). Arthritis and anti-inflammatory agents as possible protective factors for Alzheimer's disease: A review of 17 epidemiologic studies. *Neurology, 47*(2), 425–432. https://doi.org/10.1212/WNL.47.2.425.
75. Morales, I., Guzmán-Martínez, L., Cerda-Troncoso, C., Farías, G. A., & Maccioni, R. B. (2014). Neuroinflammation in the pathogenesis of Alzheimer's disease: A rational framework for the

search of novel therapeutic approaches. *Frontiers in Cellular Neuroscience, 8*, 112. https://doi.org/10.3389/fncel.2014.00112.

76. Mufson, E. J., Counts, S. E., Perez, S. E., & Ginsberg, S. D. (2008). Cholinergic system during the progression of Alzheimer's disease: Therapeutic implications. *Expert Review of Neurotherapeutics, 8*(11), 1703–1718. https://doi.org/10.1586/14737175.8.11.1703.

77. Murphy, M. P., & LeVine, H. (2010). Alzheimer's disease and the amyloid-beta peptide. *Journal of Alzheimer's Disease, 19*(1), 311–323. https://doi.org/10.3233/JAD-2010-1221.

78. National Institute for Health and Care Excellence. (2011). Donepezil, galantamine, rivastigmine and memantine for the treatment of Alzheimer's disease. London: NICE. Retrieved from: https://www.nice.org.uk/guidance/ta217/chapter/3-The-technologies (accessed on 29 June 2024).

79. Ngandu, T., Lehtisalo, J., Solomon, A., et al. (2015). A 2-year multidomain intervention of diet, exercise, cognitive training, and vascular risk monitoring versus control to prevent cognitive decline in at-risk elderly people (FINGER): A randomized controlled trial. *The Lancet, 385*(9984), 2255–2263. https://doi.org/10.1016/S0140-6736(15)60461-5.

80. O'Brien, J. T., & Markus, H. S. (2014). Vascular risk factors and Alzheimer's disease. *BMC Medicine, 12*, 218. https://doi.org/10.1186/s12916-014-0218-y.

81. Petrovitch, H., White, L. R., Izmirilian, G., et al. (2000). Midlife blood pressure and neuritic plaques, neurofibrillary tangles, and brain weight at death: The HAAS. Honolulu-Asia Aging Study. *Neurobiology of Aging, 21*(1), 57–62. https://doi.org/10.1016/S0197-4580(00)00087-2.

82. Ravona-Springer, R., Davidson, M., & Noy, S. (2003). Is the distinction between Alzheimer's disease and vascular dementia possible and relevant? *Dialogues in Clinical Neuroscience, 5*(1), 7–15. https://doi.org/10.31887/DCNS.2003.5.1/rravona-springer.

83. Robinson, D. M., & Keating, G. M. (2006). Memantine: A review of its use in Alzheimer's disease. *Drugs, 66*(11), 1515–1534. https://doi.org/10.2165/00003495-200666110-00012.

84. Salomone, S., Caraci, F., Leggio, G. M., et al. (2012). New pharmacological strategies for treatment of Alzheimer's disease: Focus on disease modifying drugs. *British Journal of Clinical Pharmacology, 73*(3), 504–517. https://doi.org/10.1111/j.1365-2125.2011.04074.x.

85. Serrano-Pozo, A., Frosch, M. P., Masliah, E., & Hyman, B. T. (2011). Neuropathological alterations in Alzheimer's disease. *Cold Spring Harbor Perspectives in Medicine, 1*(1), a006189. https://doi.org/10.1101/cshperspect.a006189.

86. Tolppanen, A. M. M., Solomon, A., Soininen, H., & Kivipelto, M. (2012). Midlife vascular risk factors and Alzheimer's disease: Evidence from epidemiological studies. *Journal of Alzheimer's Disease, 32*(3), 531–540. https://doi.org/10.3233/JAD-2012-120725.

87. Valenti, R., Pantoni, L., & Markus, H. S. (2014). Treatment of vascular risk factors in patients with a diagnosis of Alzheimer's disease: A systematic review. *BMC Medicine, 12*, 160. https://doi.org/10.1186/s12916-014-0160-z.

88. Whitehouse, P. J. (1998). The cholinergic deficit in Alzheimer's disease. *The Journal of Clinical Psychiatry, 59*(Suppl 13), 19–22.

89. Yarchoan, M., & Arnold, S. E. (2014). Repurposing diabetes drugs for brain insulin resistance in Alzheimer's disease. *Diabetes, 63*(7), 2253–2261. https://doi.org/10.2337/db14-0288.

Chapter 7

NONDRUG TREATMENT FOR ALZHEIMER'S DISEASE

Contents

Introduction 230
7.1. Need For Non-Drug Treatment for Alzheimer's Disease 232
7.2. Non-Pharmacological Treatment of Alzheimer's 234
7.3. Cognitive-Oriented Interventions 246
7.4. Physical Exercise Interventions 251
7.5. Brain Stimulation 254
7.6. Nutrition Supplementations 257
Summary 262
References 262

INTRODUCTION

Alzheimer's disease, a progressive neurodegenerative disorder, presents a formidable challenge to individuals affected by the condition, their families, and healthcare providers alike. While pharmacological interventions can help manage symptoms to some extent, there is growing recognition of the importance of nondrug treatments in improving the quality of life for those living with Alzheimer's disease.

Nondrug treatments encompass a wide range of interventions aimed at addressing the diverse needs and challenges faced by individuals with Alzheimer's disease. These interventions focus on enhancing cognitive function, promoting emotional well-being, maintaining functional independence, and supporting overall quality of life. Importantly, nondrug treatments are often used in conjunction with pharmacological therapies to provide comprehensive care tailored to the individual's unique needs and preferences.

One of the cornerstones of nondrug treatment for Alzheimer's disease is cognitive stimulation therapy. This approach involves engaging individuals in structured activities and exercises designed to stimulate cognitive function, memory, and problem-solving skills. Cognitive stimulation therapy may include reminiscence therapy, reality orientation, puzzle games, arts and crafts, and music therapy, among other activities. These interventions not only provide cognitive benefits but also foster social interaction, emotional expression, and a sense of purpose and accomplishment.

Physical exercise is another key component of nondrug treatment for Alzheimer's disease. Regular physical activity has been shown to improve cardiovascular health, promote neuroplasticity, and reduce the risk of cognitive decline. Exercise programs tailored to the individual's abilities and interests can help maintain mobility, strength, and balance, while also enhancing mood, sleep quality, and overall well-being.

In addition to cognitive and physical interventions, psychosocial support and caregiver education are essential components of nondrug treatment for Alzheimer's disease. Counselling, support groups, and educational programs can help individuals and their caregivers better understand the disease process, develop coping strategies, and access community resources. By providing emotional support, practical guidance, and a sense of connection, these interventions play a vital role in promoting resilience and improving the caregiving experience.

Overall, nondrug treatments offer a holistic approach to managing Alzheimer's disease, addressing the multifaceted needs of individuals affected by the condition and optimizing their quality of life. By combining cognitive stimulation, physical exercise, psychosocial support, and caregiver education, healthcare providers can empower individuals with Alzheimer's disease to live as fully and independently as possible, while also supporting their caregivers in providing compassionate and effective care.

Orientation and Directional Terms

Term	**Definition**	**Illustration**
Nonpharmacological Intervention	Non-pharmacological interventions (NPIs) are science-based, non-invasive actions that can help prevent, treat, or cure health problems.	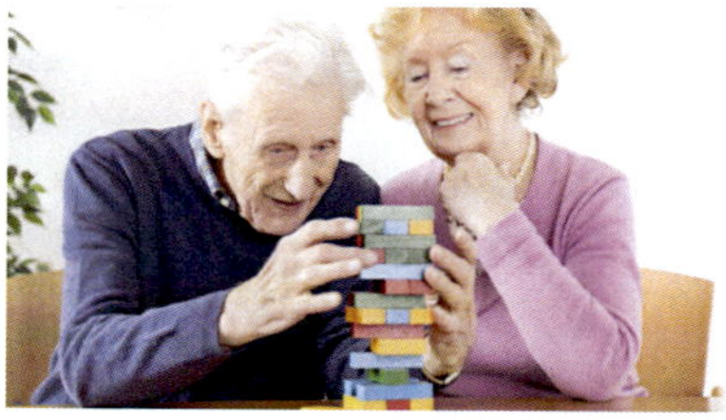
Sleep disordered breathing	Sleep disordered breathing (SDB) refers to a wide spectrum of sleep-related conditions including increased resistance to airflow through the upper airway, heavy snoring, marked reduction in airflow (hypopnea), and complete cessation of breathing (apnea).	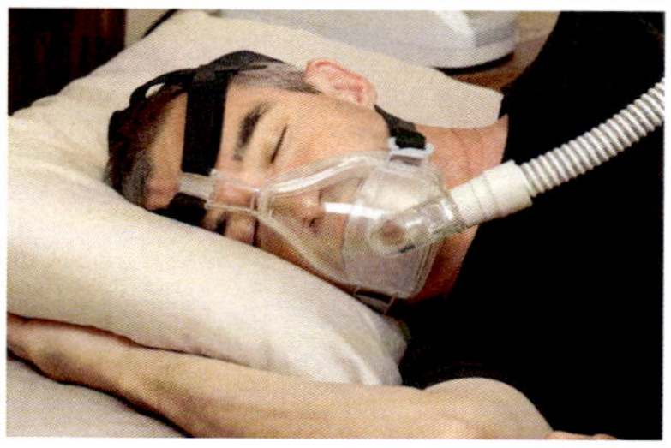
Snoezelen therapy	Snoezelen therapy, also known as controlled multisensory environment, is a therapy that uses a stimulating environment to help people with autism, dementia, or brain injury feel safe and in control.	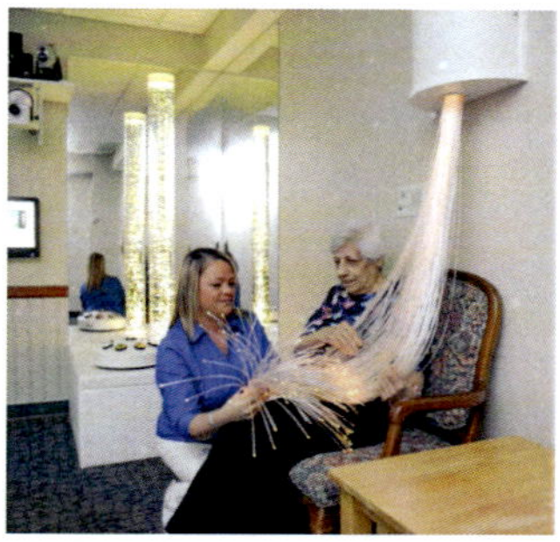
Reminiscence therapy	Reminiscence therapy is a treatment that helps people recall past events, emotions, and thoughts to improve their psychological well-being.	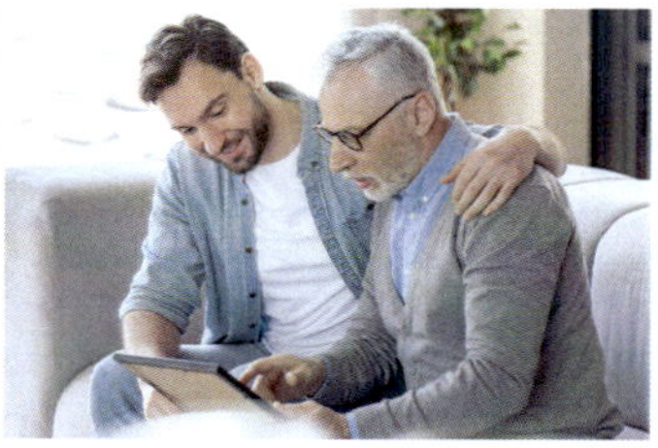
Insomnia	Insomnia is a sleep disorder that makes it difficult to fall asleep, stay asleep, or get quality sleep.	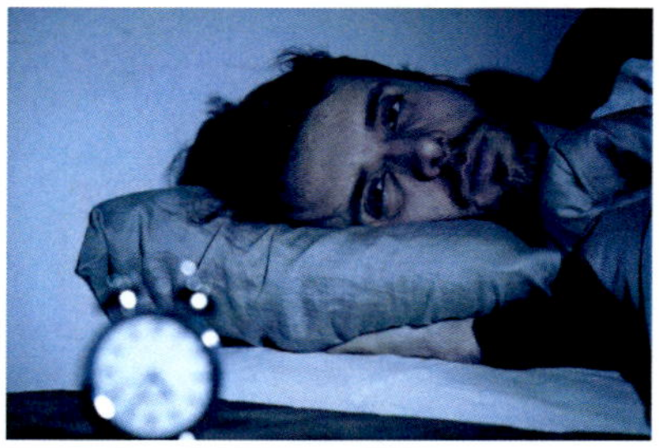

7.1. NEED FOR NON-DRUG TREATMENT FOR ALZHEIMER'S DISEASE

Alzheimer's disease is a neurological condition in which memory loss and cognitive decline are brought on by the death of brain cells. Cognitive decline, memory loss, and sleep issues are common symptoms that accompany the disease's progression. This brief message explains the importance of using nonpharmacological intervention to treat sleep problems that arise from Alzheimer's disease and its advantages. Alzheimer's is a kind of dementia characterized by a steady decline in intellectual function and memory, thinking, and behavior issues.

Typically, symptoms start out slowly and get worse over time, eventually becoming severe enough to make daily tasks difficult. Individuals who have Alzheimer's disease frequently experience insomnia, which throws off their sleep schedule. There isn't a known scientific reason why sleep disturbances associated with dementia occur. Nonetheless, memory loss, behavioral abnormalities, and altered sleep patterns all affect the brains of those with Alzheimer's disease. There are two approaches to treating Alzheimer's disease symptoms (Figure 7.1).

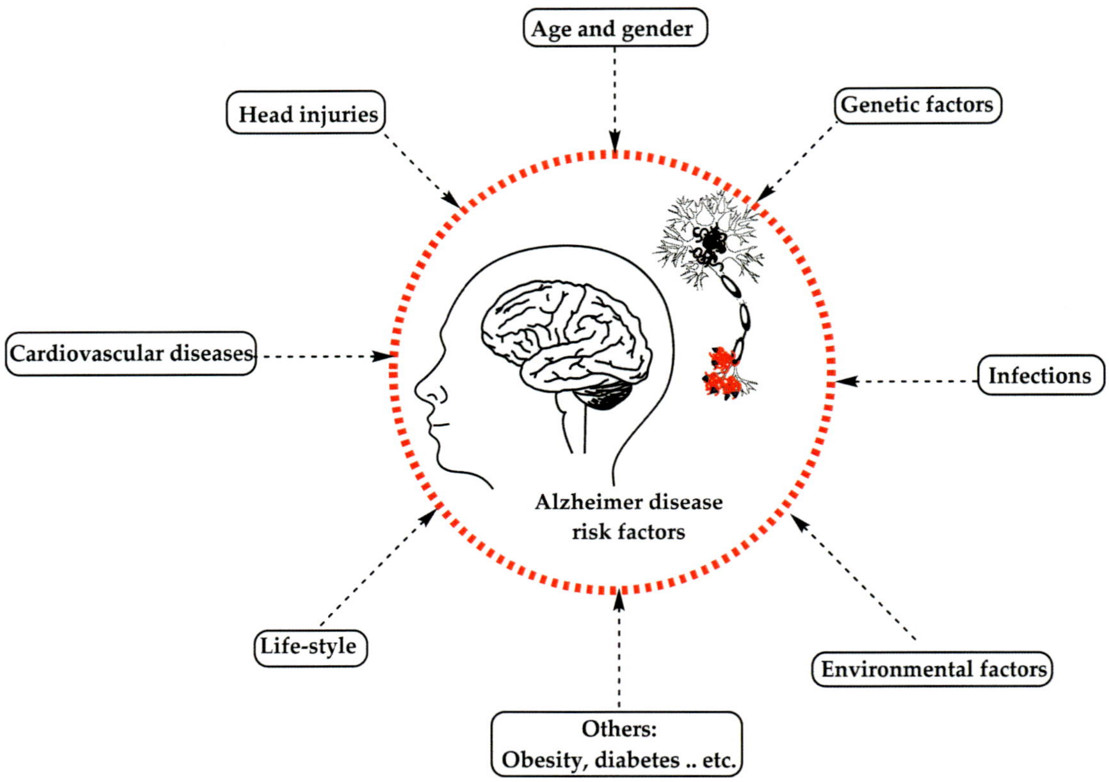

Figure 7.1. *Alzheimer's dementia.*

Source. Breijyeh Z, & Karaman R, (2020). Comprehensive review on Alzheimer's disease: Causes and treatment. Molecules, 25(24), 5789. https://doi.org/10.3390/molecules25245789.

When it comes to treating sleep issues in patients with Alzheimer's disease, non-pharmacological therapeutic interventions should take precedence. Alzheimer's patients frequently experience changes in their sleep patterns, even though the cause of their insomnia is still well understood. The effects of Alzheimer's brain are somehow responsible for the alterations in the patient's behavior, memory, and sleep patterns. Sleep disturbances are also common in older adults without dementia, but they tend to be more severe and occur more frequently in those with Alzheimer's. Though some studies have also discovered them in the early stages, there is evidence that sleep abnormalities are more prevalent in the later stages of Alzheimer's disease.

Alzheimer's patients frequently experience sleep-related issues, such as staying up later at night, wandering at night and disturbing their carers' sleep, napping during the day, and becoming agitated in the early evening and experiencing sundown. A medical examination is crucial to rule out any curable illnesses that might be exacerbating sleep issues. Sleep apnea, restless legs syndrome, and depression are common medical comorbidities. A higher chance of cognitive decline due to sleep disturbances in breathing is associated with the genetic predisposition that also manifests in Alzheimer's disease. The study, which was also endorsed by the American Thoracic Society, showed that millions of neurons firing throughout the cerebral cortex during deep sleep—a process known as slow waves—help to consolidate memory. Low attention and memory are linked to sleep apnea syndrome.

There are two approaches to treating the sleep disturbance associated with Alzheimer's disease: non-pharmacological and pharmaceutical. The National Institutes of Health (NIH) strongly advises against using pharmaceutical interventions in favor of non-pharmacological ones. It has been discovered that providing medication to patients with Alzheimer's disease does not usually improve their overall quality of sleep. Moreover, there are risks associated with using medications to treat sleep issues, which may outweigh the advantages of receiving medical care.

The non-pharmacological interventions for sleep disturbance caused by Alzheimer's disease should take precedence. Given that certain sleep aids may have detrimental side effects. Using non-pharmacological interventions to create a welcoming sleeping environment and encourage rest for an individual with Alzheimer's disease not only helps the patient with sleep issues but also slows down the progression of memory loss.

Non-pharmacological treatments included creating a sleeping environment that was appropriate for the patient, monitoring the patient to minimize midday naps, and improving the patient's sleep routine. The goal of therapeutic intervention is to keep the patient active during the day to reduce sleep disturbances.

Teaching and assisting patients with different behavioral disciplines, such as regularizing their mealtimes, bedtimes, and wake-up times, can be a part of non-pharmacological supportive therapy. The patient will be assisted in seeking out a morning sun bath and engaging in regular exercise before four hours of bedtime. The phase relationships between melatonin rhythm, the circadian rest-activity cycle, and core body temperature are all largely regulated by light. Exposure to morning light has been found to be advantageous for those who experience phase delays, meaning that their bedtime and wake-up times are delayed. Bright light therapy guidelines for sleep and circadian rhythm disorders have been published by the American Academy of Sleep Medicine.

Encouraging them to eat a balanced diet and abstain from nicotine, caffeine, and alcohol. preventing the patient from developing additional medical conditions, such as managing any pain. If donepezil, tacrine, rivastigmine, or any other cholinesterase inhibitor is currently being taken by the patient. that you shouldn't give them right before bed. Aside from these patients, the temperature-controlled bedroom lights provide comfort and a sense of security. Make sure he should only use the bed for sleeping, and assist and encourage him to sleep in a baby-like manner. Discourage him from remaining in bed while awake. It is preferable for them to avoid watching television when they are awake.

It has been discovered that sleep issues are linked to cognitive decline and memory loss in Alzheimer's disease, even though the precise relationships between Alzheimer's disease and sleep issues are unclear. The nonpharmacological medical treatment for sleep problems in dementia patients is valued and has opened the door for further research in this area to prevent adverse effects (Casey et al., 2010; O'Neil et al., 2011; Siebern et al., 2012).

7.2. NON-PHARMACOLOGICAL TREATMENT OF ALZHEIMER'S

The number of people receiving new diagnoses for dementia syndrome, including Alzheimer's disease, is rising in tandem with the aging population. The price of treatment is rising concurrently. This has caused specialists to concentrate on less expensive, non-pharmacological dementia treatment.

The scientific investigation of non-pharmacological interventions for dementia patients and family caregivers is not as established or historical as the investigation of pharmacological interventions. Undoubtedly, scientists have always assumed that in addition to medication, it is helpful to reassure, activate, and modify the surroundings and other procedures that non-medical staff members specifically encounter. For a long time, these practices have been regarded as appropriate and helpful, but not particularly fascinating or stimulating for additional scientific study. Nonetheless, research on non-pharmacological methods for treating dementia patients and their families has surfaced in the past 10 years.

Maintaining or enhancing one's capacity for walking, self-sufficiency, gross and fine motor skills, and cognitive abilities is the aim of nonpharmacological treatment. Simultaneously, an additional objective is to effectively occupy leisure time, impact dementia symptoms and day-to-day activities, and enhance both spoken and nonspoken communication between the patient and their caregiver or nurse.

The activities we select need to be suitable for the sufferer's condition. There are several non-pharmacological approaches; the therapist chooses from a range of options, considering the patient's age, disease stage, and gender; for this reason, the individual approach must be emphasized.

Comprehensive activities that suitably impact both the physical and mental aspects as well as the psychosocial interactions are required. The patient's strengths should always be highlighted in activities. The patient must be in a setting they are familiar with. It matters how the activities are carried out. Failure to complete an activity successfully does not indicate a loss. A patient with dementia should incorporate this kind of treatment into their daily routine.

Non-pharmacological approaches to dementia management focus on the following problem areas:

- Early diagnosis and patient support in the initial phase of the disease.
- Providing information, preserving or improving cognitive functions.
- Preservation or improvement of the patient's self-sufficiency.

- Mitigating or eliminating problematic behavior and the psychological symptoms of dementia.
- Improving the quality of life for the patient with dementia.
- Improving the communication between the patient and the doctor treating them.
- Improving the quality of life of patients in the terminal stages of dementia.
- Support for carers

Because patients benefit from a certain regularity of the daily routine in the advanced stages of dementia, a regular daytime routine is an essential component of care for a patient with dementia. An innate rhythm arises from the timing of meals, leisure pursuits, or personal grooming. By providing a range of options and scheduling individual activities on particular days, we can effectively occupy the patient's time and avert periods of distress. We place a strong emphasis on treating each patient as an individual and respecting their abilities because overly engaging or excessively busy activities can have the opposite effect.

In the comprehensive treatment of dementia patients, nutritional support plays a significant role as a component of comprehensive therapy. Treatment outcomes can be enhanced with proper nutrition. International epidemiological and clinical research has demonstrated that dietary supplements can significantly improve the course of cognitive impairment and lower its risk. Omega-3 fatty acids, gingko biloba, fish products, and adequate fish consumption (two to three servings per week) have an impact on cognitive function and can delay the onset of cognitive impairments in older adults. A dementia patient's diet should include a lot of walnuts. Protein, vitamins, omega-3 fatty acids, trace minerals, lecithin, and oils are abundant in them. Walnuts are a significant component of the diet when it comes to brain function. Walnuts are particularly high in polyunsaturated fatty acids when compared to other nuts, which typically have a high concentration of monounsaturated fatty acids. They are cholesterol-free and contain a very small amount of sodium. They also have a sufficient amount of thiamine, folic acid, and tocopherol, a form of vitamin E. They are rich in iron, phosphorus, magnesium, and manganese. According to a folktale, walnuts are said to support brain health because they resemble brains.

Enhancing brain activity and having a preventive effect are apples, spinach, extra virgin olive oil, grape juice, red wine, salmon, curry powder and curcumin, cinnamon, coffee, and hot chocolate. We tend to gravitate toward substances that cause nervous system irritation when we are trying to stretch our thinking or memory. They go by the name "memory poisons" occasionally. These drugs enhance concentration and memory while stimulating the brain. These kinds of substances include alcohol, caffeine, nicotine, and tranquilizers (tranquilizers).

One of the most crucial aspects of caring for a patient with dementia is helping them become self-sufficient. Caretakers ought to possess the necessary qualifications and patience to guide patients toward self-care through gradual steps, instruction, and support. This strategy must also be used carefully; it is important to understand the patient's condition and abilities because you cannot expect a patient to perform tasks that they are no longer capable of performing. In the mild and moderate stages of the illness, this course of action is advised.

By giving them varied tasks, patients can maintain and improve their capabilities. This is known as patient activation. Specifically, pet therapy is more of a home-based form of treatment when taking care of a pet keeps the dementia patient active.

Actually, one of the earliest methods of treating patients is orientation. Only a few aspects of orientation are used in reality at the moment. When used consistently and completely, this strategy enhances patient orientation, but at the expense of extreme discomfort. These days, when a patient has transient memory loss, orientation in reality is primarily used in the early stages of Alzheimer's disease. When experiencing a temporary loss of memory, the patient can use a calendar that shows the day, month, and year as well as their name, address, and other details to help them come back to reality. Appropriate methods include using pictograms to help patients with their spatial orientation and color-coding rooms. When a patient has memory loss in the early to moderate stages of their illness, orientation in reality is crucial, and assistive technology can help them get situated in the actual environment.

Activities that are programmed are appropriate for patients with advanced dementia. Patients require the most specialized care as their disease worsens and their overall condition worsens. If the patient feels overburdened by the individual activities, we stop attempting to coerce them into actively participating and instead adjust to their unique needs, abilities, and pace. It can be argued that planning activities is largely a specific requirement at this point in the disease and is an essential component of care in the advanced stages.

Another name for milieu therapy is environmental manipulation. In the mild and moderate stages of Alzheimer's disease, its use is appropriate. It involves taking a thorough, one-on-one approach to each patient and customizing their working environment to make them feel comfortable and enable them to better navigate the abundance of sensory input available to them. Certain senior living facilities that cater specifically to dementia patients acknowledge this idea beforehand. The patient's ease of orientation within the facility is especially crucial. One issue might be, for instance, the patient being unaware of the unusual toilet flushing design or the taps/faucets. In order to prevent the patient from being tempted to leave the ward, it is sometimes advisable to conceal the entrance door, for example, with wallpaper. There should be minimal movement and stability in the area.

7.2.1.1. Practical Demonstration

The patient rooms in the ward of gerontological psychiatry were assigned numbers. It was more difficult for patients to get around in this area, and they frequently did not go back to their room. Upon hanging fruit-themed door signs—bananas, oranges, pears, apples, and plums—it became apparent that the patient had an easier time getting situated in the room.

Information sharing is a component of the lifestyle approach for caregivers. It's important to accept that patients with dementia may have unique habits. These consist of the patient's daily schedule, routines, dressing style, toileting habits, activities they can do on their own, and those for which they require assistance. Respect for long-standing customs and rituals by the medical team will make treatment easier. Failing to do so frequently results in hostility, disturbances, and other circumstances that exacerbate the patient's condition. To this end, some facilities use entry interviews and questionnaires with the goal of gathering as much information as possible. The patient's tendency toward aggression typically increases if the attending personnel rejects the patient's regular routines and rituals. Experienced family caregivers can provide invaluable support in the treatment of the ill, according to practice.

7.2.1.2. Practical Demonstration

A patient in an elderly social care facility would always evacuate onto the floor rather than the toilet. The medical staff's repeated instructions and the toilet's pictogram labeling were ineffective. Such unpleasant and perplexing circumstances happened. A more thorough investigation into the reasons behind the patient's refusal to evacuate into the toilet revealed that he was raised in a socially isolated household and only started using a toilet as an adult. The patient was taught where to flee with a straightforward intervention that involved taking down the colored curtain at the entrance to the toilet and the toilet door. Another way to handle the situation might be to have the patient wear a disposable diaper, which would make them uncomfortable but make the work of the attending staff easier. A seemingly straightforward situation can also have an easy solution when approached individually.

7.2.1. Cognitive Training

Targeted brain stimulation with an emphasis on various cognitive capacities is known as cognitive training. It is primarily used by people with early to intermediate stages of Alzheimer's who wish to independently train their cognitive abilities. It enhances life quality and delays the progression of the illness. Depending on the patient's attitude, it may also be enjoyable or a daily activity. Research has indicated that cognitive training can cause adverse effects, including depression and frustration, in certain patients who are in the moderate to severe stages of the illness. The methods of cognitive training are applicable to daily life. For instance, we can complete math problems without a calculator, go shopping without a shopping list, and occasionally even learn something "by heart," like a poem or song, or even mimic the lead actors after a movie has finished. Preventing cognitive decline, boosting self-worth and confidence, encouraging self-sufficiency in daily tasks, supporting social interactions, preserving quality of life, and improving welfare and enjoyment of accomplishment are all areas in which cognitive training is particularly significant. The two worst things for memory are inactivity and a deficiency of processing stimuli. Like any other organ or muscle, the memory becomes "lazy" and functions worsens if it is not regularly stimulated.

7.2.1.1. Practical Demonstration

- **Example 1:** Over the course of several years, the 81-year-old patient has noticed that her memory is failing and that she forgets things easily. She loses track of everything she wants to buy, everything she wants to take out of the fridge, and birthdays and other important occasions for her relatives. She needs to write down every appointment and piece of information in a diary or calendar. She goes shopping alone for shorter trips, but she must always prepare a shopping ticket. The customer has a busy life. She walks for thirty minutes each day, which supports memory functions and increases brain oxygenation. She meets people and regains her enthusiasm by going to the retirees' club and university of the third age. She watches television quizzes, solves crossword puzzles, and reads books every day. These routine activities are a normal part of an engaged senior's life and help to train the brain in an organic way while stimulating cognitive functions.

- **Example 2:** Seniors practiced their memory skills in a retirement community. They decided to take part in food preparation. Patients recalled numerous recipes, particularly for pancakes, while being closely monitored by their therapist. They had to consider recipes more carefully because they are not cooking for themselves and are in a social care facility. They came to an agreement on a recipe together, which they cooked while the therapist watched.

This activation serves as an illustration of how cognitive training can be applied covertly and integrated into an institutionalized senior citizen's daily routine.

7.2.2. Snoezelen Therapy

The multifunctional technique known as Snoezelen therapy is carried out in a setting that is especially comfortable and suitable. With the ability to become aware of their surroundings, this therapy provides appropriate alternative solutions for patients suffering from dementia. It enables them to react to their surroundings more effectively. The stimulating environment can create inner balance and peace by calming the body and mind, which in turn helps to reduce aggression and improve mood. It stimulates the senses outside the body, including hearing, sight, touch, smell, and taste, using stimuli like light and sound effects, soothing music, tactile surfaces, and the alluring aroma of essential oils. It not only helps to stimulate and activate old habits, but it also creates an environment that evokes pleasant and pleasant memories.

The name of a multisensory room that uses technology to elicit sensual reactions and responses from its patrons is Snoezelen. It offers stunning sensory experiences. This space awakens and stimulates the senses, releases tension, and makes one feel good. In addition, it elicits memories, focuses and harmonizes stimuli, eliminates fear, provides security, and lessens aggressiveness, self-destruction, and violent behavior.

It is not possible to predict a patient's response in advance when using Snoezelen therapy. Even though it makes us feel at ease, we should also be prepared for the opposite response. To keep the patient from becoming overstimulated, multisensory stimulation is advised once or twice a week, separated by at least thirty minutes. All stages of dementia are suitable for Snoezelen therapy, but if we are interested in a patient who is in a severe stage, we can stimulate their mind and elicit positive emotions.

7.2.2.1. Practical Demonstration of a Negative Reaction

The patient, an 86-year-old man suffering from a severe case of Alzheimer's dementia, is unable to recognize his family members, has trouble moving, speaks incoherently, sleeps during the day, and becomes restless at night. The patient averted his eyes and started scanning the area as he approached the Snoezelen room entrance. The patient was positioned in the wheelchair in the middle of the space, and we started the lighting effects—bubble cylinders, a starry sky, and soft music. We went past interactive optical fibers that he touched with his hands while he was on his knees. For roughly 10 minutes, the patient remained quiet, taking in his surroundings and fiddling with the interactive fibers in his hands. After some time, the patient started to show signs of anxiety. He fidgeted, lowered his eyes, and whispered something inaudibly. He eventually began to yell incoherently. He was combative. The Snoezelen therapy is now complete.

Since the patient responded in the same way to repeated therapies, we will select a different non-pharmacological approach instead of using this multisensory stimulus for that particular patient.

7.2.3. Reminiscence Therapy

A technique called reminiscence therapy makes use of memories and their recall through a variety of stimuli. Of course, because of its preventive and activating qualities, it is also appropriate for seniors in good health. Patients with dementia, who suffer from short-term memory problems, benefit most from it; on the other hand, they frequently have surprisingly good recall of past events.

Reminiscence therapy generally involves a therapist having a conversation about the elderly person's (or group's) life up to that point, including past activities, events, and experiences. Appropriate tools, such as old photos, objects, tools, and appliances for the home, as well as fashion accessories, movies, folk or dance music, and so on, are frequently used in these conversations. The activity can be mostly planned, but it can also be entirely unplanned and spontaneous, with the therapeutic element occasionally taking center stage. When it comes to reliving past experiences—especially those that are positively and personally significant, like family gatherings, holidays, weddings, celebrations, etc.—reminiscence therapy is particularly helpful for those who are suffering from dementia.

This kind of therapy makes use of memories and employs a variety of stimuli to encourage recall. Its objectives are to uphold human dignity, advance communication, and better the general situation. Individual or group, it can take many different forms. Some of the techniques include looking through photo albums, watching vintage movies, narrating old stories, and engaging in other activities like reciting or singing.

There are also memory rooms available for clients in certain facilities; these rooms have interior furnishings and environmental modifications that reflect the clients' younger years.

- **Practical Recommendations:** Reminiscence therapy can involve a variety of scenarios that elicit both happy and sad feelings, such as memories of parents, siblings, and lost time. We do not need to be concerned about the patient's feelings of sadness or anger, and we should try to avoid them at all costs. An individualized approach is crucial because, while emotional expression may relieve some people, it may also exacerbate depression in others. It is sometimes necessary to guide the patient toward accepting aging as a natural cycle of life that needs to be respected. It is better to avoid using this method if thinking back on memories brings up extremely painful and unpleasant ones.

7.2.4. Validation Therapy

One of the earliest targeted non-pharmacological treatments for dementia patients is thought to be validation therapy.

We give the theoretical foundation more thought in light of the procedure's specifications, which should be more beneficial to the reader. Naomi Feil was the one who developed the validation method. Born in Munich in 1932, Naomi Feil was raised in a retirement community where her father served as the director. In addition, her mother, who headed the social department, had a job there. Following her social work studies, she began working with the elderly and was granted a Master's degree in social work. Her displeasure with the strategies and practices of long-term care for the elderly led her to start creating her own therapeutic approach. Between 1963 and 1980, this therapy underwent its entire development. She mainly used her own experience to build her model in addition to the theoretical underpinnings. She had a great deal of experience because she had lived among the elderly for practically her entire life. She spent seven years working with the seniors and was raised among them as a child. Afterwards, she worked with elderly and confused people over 80 for more than 40 years.

The Naomi Feil Validation Concept is now acknowledged as a technique based on the most recent findings in the treatment of elderly patients suffering from dementia, Alzheimer's disease, or other related illnesses. Both gerontology and palliative medicine endorse this approach. A type of communication and treatment called validation is applied to elderly patients with dementia syndrome or other conditions characterized by mental disorientation. Its foundations include various psychological concepts, therapeutic modalities, and biographical elements. We can help a senior with dementia syndrome by using the validation method, which is regarded as high moral support. But in order to provide it, staff members must be willing to approach the situation from a completely different angle, make an effort to determine the true reason behind the disoriented seniors' behavior, and consistently apply new techniques with the patient.

By definition, validation is a delicate generalization made by professionals who work with dementia patients. Respect for individuals is its central tenet. We neither actively oppose nor condone the false beliefs that people with dementia hold. Acknowledging someone's feelings and letting them know they are real is known as validating them. When feeling is suppressed, uncertainty results.

Helping elderly people stay in their homes for as long as possible, regaining confidence, lowering stress, coping with unresolved conflicts from the past, enhancing verbal and nonverbal communication, preventing a return to vegetation, improving walking ability and general physical health, bringing joy and energy to the caregiver, and assisting families in communicating with their bewildered relatives are all goals of validation.

There are several principles that a user of validation must consider if they want to perform validation therapy on old, disoriented people. One must realize a few facts:

- Even poorly oriented or disoriented seniors are unique and have their value.
- Do not try to change them at all costs, accept them as they are.
- We must be able to listen; empathic listening creates an environment conducive to confiding, reduces their anxiety and, above all, brings dignity.
- Expressed, accepted and validated painful feelings become weaker. But if ignored and suppressed they remain strong.
- There are reasons for the behavior the poorly oriented and disoriented old people.
- The behavior of these people can be rooted in one or more human needs. Processing

unresolved task for a peaceful and balanced death, the need to live in peace, the need to regain their balance, as mobility memory and senses are lost, the need to give meaning to a gloomy reality, to find a place where they can feel happy, the need for status, recognition, self-sufficiency, the need to be productive and useful, the need to be respected and to belong, the need to express their feelings and be heard, the need for human contact, the need for certainty and security, not limitation, the need for any stimulation, and finally the need to reduce pain and complications.

- In the case of failure of verbal expression and short-term memory, old learned patterns of behavior return.
- Things, persons, or objects of the past are replaced by personal symbols that represent them and have an emotional charge.
- Disoriented or partially oriented seniors live at different levels of consciousness, often at the same time.
- By weakening the five senses, these seniors can stimulate and use their own 'inner meaning,' seeing through their inner vision and hearing the tones from the past.
- Various emotions, colors, sounds, coincidences, smells, tastes and images can now awaken emotions that recall similar emotion from the past.

When we validate an elderly person, we do not argue with them, we do not present an opposing viewpoint, and we do not attempt to change their orientation unless the elderly person expresses interest in doing so. Neither group nor individual therapy sets strict guidelines to address it over time. The person who uses validation is seen as a conscientious helper rather than an authority.

7.2.4.1. Forms of Validation Therapy

The basic forms of validation therapy include individual and group forms. In the individual form, the therapist works in three steps.

- In the first step, they collect all available information that is needed for the validation itself, but also for evaluating its effectiveness. The therapist gets information on things 'here and now' and about 'things then and there.'
- The second step involves determining the phase in which the person is. In this step, they compare the information obtained with the individual's statements and determines the stage or phase in which the old person is located.
- The third step is the validation therapy itself. A therapist should come regularly and use validation techniques that can help them at different stages.

In order for each member of the group to be able to express their feelings, communicate both verbally and nonverbally, solve problems, participate in certain social roles, learn the maximum amount of control, and, most importantly, develop a sense of self-worth, mutual trust must be built. Reducing fear, lowering the need for restraint and calming techniques, and preventing vegetative states in elderly dementia patients are the objectives of group validation. For family members and employees, getting validation will also lessen the likelihood that they will experience burnout syndrome.

For optimal utilization of the validation team, all employees can be involved, including cleaning, kitchen, office, social work, and physiotherapy staff in addition to the nursing staff. Forming a validation team to apply the same validation techniques to the client or patient is the best course of action.

The therapy itself in the group consists of seven steps.

- Acquainting yourself with the person is the first step. At this point, it's also important to assess the disorientation phase or stage in terms of personal validation. The "Life story and basic behavior" form or the questionnaire "Selecting members of the validation group" can be used to get the right evaluation. All of this is required since getting to know the other members of the group is essential to its success.
- Choosing the group's members is the second step. Due to the group's diversity, it must be put together such that each member has a specific role. A former cleric might lead singing, and a former voice instructor could lead prayer. Naomi Feil provides a detailed description of the ideal member composition and state of disorientation. 5 to 10 people should be in the group: two people in the third stage who could respond to the validation therapist, one person with a leader personality, one person who is wise and hospitable, four or five people who enjoy discussion, and two people who do not feel threatened by people who are disoriented.
- Assigning each member a role is the third step. A person should take on the same role at every meeting since it gives him a sense of security and upholds his dignity. Naomi Feil provides several examples, including an emcee who opens and closes the meeting, a singer who leads the group in song, a group reader, a chair and flower preparer, a secretary, and a host.
- It is appropriate to include every employee in the validation process in the fourth step. This can aid in planning and carrying out the plan. They can offer a space and/or refreshments, bring specific group members, and make suggestions for new participants or discussion topics.
- Together with the conversation, movement, and eating comes the fifth step: music. One song should be played at the beginning and end of the session. It's a good idea to choose the discussion topics ahead of time: missing a loved one, moving, becoming bored, or trying to find a new meaning in life.
- The sixth action item is to set up a meeting. This step includes creating a meeting schedule, as well as setting up the space and materials, creating a schedule, and gathering all the information needed for the meeting.
- Step seven involves meeting oneself on its own. It ought to be completed at the same time and location every week at the very least. The introduction, life, conclusion, and planning for the next meeting make up its four sections. Validation

meetings are based on an individual with dementia expressing what they truly want to say, even if it does not align with reality, and providing a suitable and appropriate response.

7.2.4.2. Practical Demonstration

The psychiatric ward received a patient, 82 years old, who was admitted with a severe case of Alzheimer's disease. Time and space disorientation plagued the patient. The patient's advanced age and restricted mobility made him more vulnerable to falls. The patient took sedatives and antipsychotics. Hospitalization was required because the patient in the home was constantly disappearing, refusing to follow instructions from caregivers, becoming agitated at night, and yelling. In spite of the psychopharmaceuticals, the patient's behavior did not alter while they were in the hospital. He was fidgety during the day and would frequently run out of the room to go home. The patient's behavior was challenging to manage, so the medical staff made sure he was reminded that he was hospitalized, could not go home, and had to lie in bed all the time. The Naomi Feil validation concept states that we do not argue with him or present him with an opposing viewpoint, nor are we attempting to change his orientation. In our interactions with the patient, we made an effort to follow these suggestions. In the event that the patient asked to return home, we diverted the conversation and did not inform him of his whereabouts or the reasons he was unable to do so. The patient started talking about what he used to do at home and where he worked when we asked him why he wanted to go home, what he would do there, what he used to do outside in the garden, and who he met. This does not imply that the patient was getting better, but he did communicate more softly and without yelling, and following a group walk through the department, the patient was quiet in the chair and could be directed.

7.2.5. Doll Therapy

Patients with different types and degrees of dementia, mental retardation, physical disability, and various psychiatric disorders can benefit greatly from doll therapy as a comprehensive therapeutic approach. It is renowned for being easily accessible and having little financial burden. The size and appearance of the therapeutic dolls are similar to those of small children. Natural materials, which are also hypoallergenic, are used to make dolls. It is soft, pleasant to touch, and it gives the patient a positive sensory boost. For easier handling, each body part has been carefully balanced. Because the legs are pliable, you can wrap them around the patient and promote hugs. Basal stimulation includes this kind of manipulation. All of the dolls intentionally maintain a neutral gaze by not looking forward with their eyes. The patients report that it makes them feel calm and doesn't make them feel bad. The basis of doll therapy is the long-term memory pathways. It is common for these patients—women in particular—to want to look after someone or something and to search for their children.

Increasing welfare, eliciting happy feelings, sound sleep, enhancing eating habits, decreasing agitation, irritability, anxiety episodes, apathy, depression, aggression, and tension by diverting attention to a substitute, as well as enhancing communication and sociability are just a few advantages linked to using dolls with patients. Despite the advantages, using therapeutic dolls has drawbacks as well, such as infantilizing the elderly and violating ethical standards. These reasons mean that under no circumstances can we generalize their mass use; instead, we must emphasize the individual approach.

It is essential to train caregivers or family members before using therapeutic dolls with an Alzheimer's patient. Understanding the advantages as well as any potential drawbacks in the future is crucial. Employee attitude is another factor that affects success. Success is rare when employees have a bad attitude or are not dedicated to the task at hand. It is important to learn some basic information about one's role as a parent before beginning doll therapy, as the patient's past traumas may make the use of doll therapy inappropriate. This could include a child's passing, their serious illness, or their lack of interest in their parent.

Every patient ought to have a doll of their own. It is advised to find out if the patient is a mother or a father, as well as to determine the patient's hair type and color. To reduce confusion, dolls should differ from one another in terms of their faces, heights, and attire. The patient's preferences may be followed when choosing clothes, or appropriate accessories like a cap, socks, gloves, boots, blankets, and the like may be added. Our goal is to keep them tidy. In order to prevent issues that could manifest as the patient acting negatively or as aversion to the therapist or therapy, we start doll therapy slowly and gradually. We only leave the doll for a brief period of time; leaving it out all day may cause the feelings we are trying to rekindle in a patient who has dementia.

We offer the patient the doll in an unforced way, letting them choose whether or not to pay attention. It is appropriate to put it in a visible, easily accessible location where people can see it, inquire about it, or take it. When a patient is bedridden or has low vision, we hold the doll in our arms, take a seat next to them, and begin conversing with it. We closely observe the patient's reactions, and we provide it to them when they express interest. We do not forbid men or women from showing interest in the doll, as both genders may find it intriguing. We keep an eye on the patient and pay close attention to how they address their doll when they are speaking to her. To reassure them that we see things the same way they do, we make sure to use their preferred method of address.

We only leave the doll for a brief period of time because some patients treat it like their baby and expect feelings and surprises. We only take it with their consent, providing a reasoned explanation and specifics about where we are taking it and when we plan to return it. The patient will lose interest in the doll if we leave it with them all day. We never try to coerce or compel the patient to do anything with the doll. They may develop an emotional attachment to it, which may lead to negative behavior (aggression, agitation, and anxiety). It can serve as a bridge for other interactions, like working, talking, and taking walks.

In doll therapy, unfavorable circumstances can also arise. One of these is the patient's ability to recall unpleasant experiences from their past. The therapist's job in these cases is to pinpoint these incidents and provide the patient with the necessary pacification.

7.2.5.1. Practical Example

A patient with a moderate diagnosis of Alzheimer's disease was treated with doll therapy. She is reserved when discussing herself because she knows she has a medical condition. The most vivid memories she has of her past are of the rural areas surrounding her hometown. After a pause, and often for an extended period of time, she answered each question. She doesn't express her feelings clearly enough on the outside. She blames aging for her memory loss. She experiences attention problems and hallucinations occasionally. She occasionally speaks gibberish. She looks away when she is speaking. We made the decision to treat the patient with a therapeutic doll. We got off to a naturally relaxed start. After we showed the patient the therapeutic doll we were holding in our hands one morning, she started to ask who it was and expressed a desire to hold it in her arms. She started chatting to her while humming her childhood favorites. She even gave her the name of her daughter at other meetings. Depending on the baby's level of interest, we left him for one or two hours. To prevent therapy from becoming stale and instead provide the patient with a joyful emotional experience that revitalizes their mind, we did not use the baby on a daily basis.

7.2.6. Ervin Böhm's Psychobiographic Model

The psychobiographic model developed by Ervin Böhm is a globally recognized nursing paradigm that is currently the most used in German-speaking nations for geriatric and gerontological psychiatric care. By igniting the seniors' interest and revitalizing their psyche, the model seeks to support the ability of old and confused people to care for themselves, as well as ways to retain or restore this ability for as long as possible. The goal of the psychobiographic model is to broaden the patient's perspective, particularly with regard to the elderly, for whom care needs to shift away from the "caring mother" role and toward tolerance. Previous approaches to care, in which all tasks were handled by the attending staff, did not take into account the client's retained skills and knowledge, were primarily concerned with meeting needs, and led to the client becoming dependent on the care.

Böhm puts the following goals at the forefront of care:

- reviving the human psyche,
- reviving the interest of the carers, and
- broadening the perception of social normality.

Reviving the Human Psyche: Böhm's ultimate objective in providing care for the elderly is to bring back their soul, also known as the "elan vital," which is the primal source of human action and motivation. Increasing their expertise can help revive the professional interest of caregivers and revitalize the interest of carers.

According to Böhm, his care model is an all-encompassing systemic theory meant to enhance medical care. Therapeutic treatment, even in the absence of psychopharmaceuticals, should be based on a patient's thymopsychic biography and should improve both the patient's physical and mental well-being.

When we prioritize a patient's biography over their medical and nursing diagnoses, we treat dementia as a personality disorder rather than viewing the patient as a human being with a soul.

7.2.6.1. Practical Demonstration

A 67-year-old patient suffering from severe Alzheimer's disease is admitted to the psychiatric ward due to behavioral issues, physical and verbal aggression, and sleeplessness. 62 years of age, he suffered a stroke. Along with increased irritability and impulsivity, the patient is disoriented. The patient's behavior is challenging to control and their cooperation is minimal even with medication. We concentrated on the patient's life story and, in collaboration with the patient's spouse, we searched for possibilities that might affect the patient's conduct. We chose to utilize the patient's sentimental blanket during their hospital stay because the patient's wife started talking about it. The blanket was a wedding present that the patient had received. The patient showed interest in his blanket and recognized it right away. Although the patient did not immediately change his behavior, we were able to influence cooperation and lessen his aggressive behavior by using an empathic approach (Casey et al., 2010; O'Neil et al., 2011; Siebern et al., 2012).

7.3. COGNITIVE-ORIENTED INTERVENTIONS

0The three primary categories of cognitive-oriented interventions are customized cognitive rehabilitation, cognitive stimulation, and cognitive training. These therapies have drawn more attention lately as potential preventative measures or ways to improve AD treatment. Table 7.1 provides an overview of the cognitive-oriented interventions randomized controlled trials (RCTs) on AD patients that have been published in the past 10 years.

Table 7.1. Reversing AD-Associated Cognitive Health Requires Addressing Potential Contributors to Cognitive Decline with a Personalized, Multi-Therapeutic Approach. Each of the Strategies Mentioned in the Table has the Ability to Improve Cognition and Brain Health, and When Practiced Together, they Create a Powerful Synergy with Sustained Improvement

Multi-Therapeutic Strategies	**Goals**
Nutrition	Improves cognition and supports brain health by • creating insulin sensitivity • promoting metabolic flexibility/ ketosis • reducing inflammation • improving vascular health • promoting autophagy
Exercise	• increases brain-derived neurotrophic factor (BDNF) that stimulates neuroplasticity • increases cerebral blood flow and oxygenation • mitigates overall stress • optimizes body mass index (BMI) • improves insulin sensitivity • reduces inflammation • stabilizes brain volume and decreases white matter lesions
Sleep	• enhances ability to focus, learn, and memorize • reduces stress • promotes neuroplasticity • improves waste-clearing capacity

Stress Management	• activates parasympathetic arm of HPA axis and balances stress hormones • increases cerebral blood flow and oxygenation • improves insulin sensitivity • reduces inflammation • boosts cognitive acuity
Mental Exercise (Brain Stimulation)	• promotes neural connectivity in response to new learning • improves mood, thinking, hearing, problem-solving, reasoning, and memory • lowers risk of cognitive decline and dementia • improves activities of daily living
Detoxification	Improves cognition and supports brain health by • treating dementogen exposure and limiting ongoing exposure • reducing systemic and brain inflammation • optimizing gut, oral and nasal microbiome • upregulating the immune system and mitochondrial energetics
Herbs & Supplements	Improve cognition and support brain health by • promoting neural connectivity and effective synaptic support • optimizing trophic support • upregulating the immune system and gut health • reducing inflammation • boosting cognitive acuity • improving vascular health • neutralizing free radicals

Source: Rao RV, Subramaniam KG, Gregory J, Bredesen AL, Coward C, Okada S, Kelly L, & Bredesen DE, (2023) Rationale for a multi-factorial approach for the reversal of cognitive decline in Alzheimer's disease and MCI: A review. International Journal of Molecular Sciences, 24(2), 1659. https://doi.org/10.3390/ijms24021659.

The first recognized nonpharmacological intervention for dementia that targets a specific cognitive function is cognitive training. e.g., executive functions, such as language, memory, and attention. By completing a few theoretically motivated standard tasks, it enhances dementia-associated cognition by attempting to preserve or restore the targeted cognitive domains' normal functioning for as long as feasible. Chunking-based cognitive training may help maintain cognitive functions in the early stages of Alzheimer's disease (AD). For example, it has been reported that adaptive chunking training for patients with mild AD has significantly improved verbal working memory performance. This improvement was demonstrated by reduced task-related activation of the lateral prefrontal and parietal cortex on functional magnetic resonance imaging (fMRI). In addition, prospective memory can also mean recalling to carry out a planned action in the future (e.g., even in extremely mild or preclinical stages), as well as deficiencies in prospective memory. Examples of these activities include turning off an oven, taking medication, and so forth.

In elderly people and those with very mild AD, a straightforward perspective memory encoding technique has been shown to be beneficial in regaining prospective memory function. Furthermore, after interventions, there was enhanced activation of the right lentiform nucleus, the thalamus, and the bilateral superior temporal gyrus, according to fMRI echo planar with blood oxygenation level dependent (BOLD) contrast. Cognitive assessment changes were correlated with the degree of activation in the left superior gyrus, precuneus, and left thalamus. The idea that multidimensional stimulation targeting cognition, behavior, and motor functioning significantly improved the cognitive-behavioral status of patients with AD at least partially by restoring neural functioning is supported by the strong correlation these fMRI data showed with the neuropsychological and neurobehavioral measures. Patients with early AD who received a culture-specific picture-based cognitive training also showed improvements in language, memory, and attention. The functional effectiveness of the cognitive training correlated well with the fMRI data, suggesting that fMRI could be included as an observing outcome for this kind of clinical study. Overall, the cognitive training appeared to be effective to the targeted cognitive domains. Nevertheless, no registered RCTs or publications comparing the benefits of donepezil and cognitive training could be located. There could be drawbacks to cognitive training, like insufficient training providers, a limited group of AD patients who could benefit from the program, and the brief duration of training-induced effects. Furthermore, it's possible that no patient will benefit from the same training regimen, necessitating customized patient care. Furthermore, due to a lack of standardized protocols, it is challenging to compare the effects of cognitive training across studies for further optimization. Standardized methodologies and longitudinal studies are needed to resolve or improve these issues.

7.3.1. Cognitive Stimulation

The Cochrane Review of Reality Orientation database's theories and data serve as the foundation for the cognitive stimulation therapy (CST) model. Reminiscence therapy and reality orientation therapy are two examples of group activities and discussions that fall under the umbrella of cognitive stimulation. The goal of these approaches is to improve an individual's overall social and cognitive functioning. Based on the finding that this method was at least as effective as cholinesterase inhibitors (ChEIs) in reducing cognitive decline, the 2006 NICE guideline recommended using this approach as a routine procedure for patients with mild-to-moderate dementia. Additionally, CST supports dementia patients by improving memory, orientation, language comprehension, coping and adaptation skills, communication, sustainability, lowering anxiety and depression, and ultimately raising quality of life. Furthermore, compared to the CST-only group, the combination of CST and emotion recognition rehabilitation has produced better results in emotion identification as well as accuracy and processing speed.

Reminiscence therapy employs all of the senses as memory triggers, using them as a non-specific stimulation method (e.g., audiovisual resources) to aid dementia patients in recalling things from their former lives—either orally or nonverbally, in a group setting or alone—to improve their ability to adjust to the present. This is due to the fact that people suffering from dementia frequently maintain distant memories, meaning they typically remember things from their early years or even childhood, but not from earlier in the same day (ecmnesia). Reminiscence therapy strongly suggests happy memories, focused topics for sessions, and a broad summary and assessment for the final session. Patients with mild-to-moderate AD who received a 12-week reminiscence therapy showed improved cognitive function (measured by the standardized Mini Mental Test) but decreased depressive symptoms (measured by the Geriatric Depression Scale, GDS).

Furthermore, in patients with mild AD, computerized process-based cognitive training in conjunction with reminiscence therapy has shown promising results on cognitive functioning (measured by the Mini-Mental State Examination, MMSE) and functional abilities (measured by instrumental activities of daily living, ADL). Reminiscence therapy is currently being tested clinically on a Chinese cohort. Audiovisual materials are frequently used in reminiscence therapy to facilitate the retrieval of autobiographical memories. Musical memory appears to be a relative preservation in AD, and familiar music appears to be a privileged stimulus to influence emotions and memory in patients with AD or dementia. Based on this evidence, clinical trials have actively studied music-based therapies alone or in conjunction with visual stimulation, with positive outcomes in behavior, emotion, and cognition. Furthermore, it has been found that employing 40 Hz for rhythmic sensory stimulation significantly improves the emotions and behaviors of mild-to-moderate AD cases.

However, it is important to note that while CST includes positive elements of reality orientation therapy, such as providing continuous memory and orientation information regarding personal matters and living surroundings through repeated stimulation, studies have shown that the benefits may only be short-term. For example, in one study, mindfulness stimulation was found to maintain cognitive function in Alzheimer's patients receiving donepezil treatment, comparable to cognitive stimulation and superior to muscle relaxation. Additionally, a separate study found that combining reality orientation with AChEIs improved cognitive outcomes over AChEIs alone, indicating the potential of reality orientation as a complementary intervention for AD-related dementia. Ongoing research is being conducted to determine the long-term benefits of CST for patients with early and mild-stage dementia.

7.3.2. Individualized Cognitive Rehabilitation

Originally developed with younger brain-injured patients, cognitive rehabilitation is now being increasingly used in the treatment of dementia. It involves a personalized program that addresses specific functional challenges and sets realistic goals to assist patients and their families in daily life. The focus is on developing strategies to compensate for impairments and improve daily performance, rather than solely on cognitive ability. Caregivers are often involved in these programs. Measures such as instrumental ADL, goal achievement, patient satisfaction, and caregiver burden are typically used to evaluate the effectiveness of this intervention. In a study comparing cognitive training, reminiscence therapy, and personalized cognitive rehabilitation, only personalized rehabilitation significantly reduced functional disability and delayed institutionalization. Additionally, manual-guided cognitive rehabilitation was found to be more effective than standardized cognitive training in improving quality of life. This individualized approach also provides mental and psychological support to patients and their caregivers. In a preliminary open trial, a cognitive-behavioral intervention was found to decrease depression in patients and reduce distress in caregivers simultaneously.

These effects were still present three months after the intervention, but more research is needed due to the small sample size and lack of controls. Future cognitive rehabilitation studies need to focus on aberrant motor behaviors in patients with Alzheimer's disease, as these behaviors can lead to early institutionalization and increased burden on caregivers. In a separate trial, patients with Alzheimer's disease who underwent cognitive rehabilitation for learning or relearning instrumental activities of daily living showed increased aberrant motor behaviors, warranting further investigation in larger studies. Different methods of intervention may be effective, as positive outcomes were seen in groups using Memo+ and SenseCam, but not in those using written diaries. While early diagnosis and intervention are recommended for Alzheimer's disease, early psychosocial interventions did not appear to slow disease progression or delay institutionalization compared to controls.

7.3.3. Assessments of Outcomes

Evaluating and re-evaluating the status of various cognitive domains should be a key component of outcome assessments. MMSE, ADAS-Cog, and CAMCOG are common cognitive assessments used for this purpose. MMSE tests multiple cognitive domains such as orientation, attention, memory, language, and visual-spatial skills. ADAS-Cog is the FDA-approved measure for drug RCTs, while CAMCOG is a standardized instrument for assessing cognitive impairment or dementia. In addition to these broad measures, specific cognitive domains like attention, memory, language, executive function, and processing speed should also be carefully assessed. For example, the Trail Making A&B tests are used to evaluate visual scanning, processing speed, and executive functions.

Second, because behavioral disturbances impact up to 90–98% of AD patients at all stages of the disease and frequently lower the quality of life for both patients and their caregivers, measuring them in addition to traditional assessments for cognitive domains is crucial for assessing trial outcomes. As a result, changes in behavioral and psychological symptoms of dementia (BPSD), particularly AMB, must be evaluated when planning clinical trials of cognitive rehabilitation for AD. AMB was found to deteriorate in contrast to other BPSD, such as depression and delusions, which were found to improve following cognitive interventions. According to many studies, AMB symptoms tend to worsen as AD progresses and are connected with the degree of cognitive impairment. Patients with AD frequently experience it, which increases the burden on caregivers and early institutionalization.

It is necessary to incorporate calming elements into cognitive intervention programs, such as aromatherapy and relaxing music to help patients better handle stress brought on by the disease or the intervention, as the worsening of AMB observed in AD patients may be at least partially explained by increased anxiety during intervention. The increased AMB during the cognitive intervention for AD has been explained by several theories, the most likely of which is the reduced stress-threshold model. Other helpful instruments, such as the Neuropsychiatric Inventory (NPI) or assessments tailored to anxiety and depression, can also be used to evaluate the psychological symptoms using the Hamilton Depression Rating Scale (HDRS) and the Cornell Scale for Depression in Dementia (CSDD).

Thirdly, the quality of life (QoL) of AD patients and their caregivers is also important to consider, as the disease is chronic and progressive and requires long-term clinical management. In addition to the caregiver's burden and QoL questionnaire, other variables that could impact QoL should be assessed. These variables include the Barthel Index (BI) for daily activities, ADL, and the delay of institutionalization (Casey et al., 2010; O'Neil et al., 2011; Siebern et al., 2012).

7.3.4. Limitations

One of the main issues with implementing these cognitive-based techniques into clinical practice is the inconsistent nature of the outcomes. The main causes of the discrepancies were sample size variations, methodological heterogeneity across studies, and most significantly, bias in intervention protocols, follow-up plans, and outcome measures, all of which make it difficult to draw conclusive findings. Furthermore, it is not entirely clear if severe AD cases will benefit in any way from this kind of nonpharmacological intervention.

Consequently, we must draw attention to the necessity of more carefully thought-out RCTs, with larger sample sizes and outcome measures that go beyond the direct cognitive outcomes that are concurrently assessed. An overview of the overall duration of the intervention sessions and the outcome metrics (1. mental categories; 2. neurological evaluations; 3. QoL and ADL) of the examined studies (Figure 7.2).

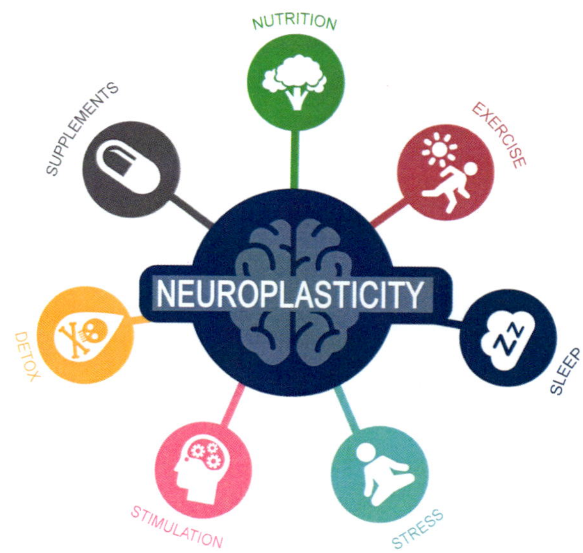

Figure 7.2. *Identifying and addressing potential contributors to cognitive decline with a personalized, multi-therapeutic approach is supportive of cognitive health. Image depicts the various core strategies for the reversal of AD and MCI and for optimizing brain health.*

Source: Rao RV, Subramaniam KG, Gregory J, Bredesen AL, Coward C, Okada S, Kelly L, & Bredesen DE, (2023). Rationale for a multi-factorial approach for the reversal of cognitive decline in Alzheimer's disease and MCI: A review. International Journal of Molecular Sciences, 24(2), 1659. https://doi.org/10.3390/ijms24021659.

7.4. PHYSICAL EXERCISE INTERVENTIONS

It is commonly known that individuals with dementia also have low levels of muscle strength and physical function, which can lead to a variety of unfavorable outcomes, including aberrant gait patterns, a higher risk of falling, fractures from falls, increased vulnerability to injuries, and other comorbidities. Furthermore, new research indicates that walking may be viewed as a cognitive function and that gait abnormalities and subsequent falls in AD patients are linked to cognitive dysfunction, including executive dysfunction. Based on observational evidence that lower levels of physical activity and cardiorespiratory fitness are strongly associated with less brain atrophy, less detrimental effects of cerebral amyloid on cognition, and a lower risk of dementia, physical exercises have therefore been proposed as an effective type of intervention for improving the physical health and well-being of patients with dementia. One study found that a 12-month exercise program effectively prevented falls in both mild and advanced AD, though the exact mechanisms are still mostly unknown. Exercise helps patients with AD not only physically but also psychologically by lowering blood pressure and improving performance on activities of daily living. Additionally, exercise training may be a nonpharmacological means of protecting against AD, as suggested by epidemiological research, which is supported by alterations in brain anatomy, including enlarged hippocampi and increased brain neurogenesis.

A specific exercise program, usually consisting of aerobic exercise at a moderate-to-high intensity, or exercise based on an individual's own exercise habits at a low intensity can be used as a physical exercise intervention for AD. The intervention can take place at home or in a group setting and can involve single-task, dual-task, or multitask training. Table 7.2 provides an overview of the RCTs of physical exercise interventions on AD patients that have been published in the past 10 years.

Table 7.2. Criteria for a Perfect AD Drug

Increase/Optimize	**Decrease/Prevent/Optimize**
APP α-cleavage	homocysteine
Neprilysin	APP β-cleavage
IDE	APP γ-cleavage
Aβ clearance	Caspase-6 cleavage
Autophagy	Caspase-3 cleavage
BDNF	APP b-oligomerization
NGF	P-tau and PHF
Netrin-1	Oxidative damage and ROS production
ADNP	NFkB
SIRT1	Glial scarring
PP2A activity	Inflammation
Phagocytosis	Synaptoclastic signaling
Insulin sensitivity	Neuronal cell death
Axoplasmic transport	
Mitochondrial function	
Cholinergic neurotransmission	
Long-term potentiation	
Vit D, B12, and Zinc	

Resolvins	
Detoxification	
Vascularization	
cAMP	
Glutathione	
Estradiol, progesterone, pregnenolone, DHEA, GABA, free T3, free T4, TSH	

A perfect drug is one that increases and optimizes all parameters on the left as they tend to be lowered or down-regulated in AD. The same drug decreases, lowers, or reduces the parameters on the right side, as these tend to be elevated in AD. The highlighted items indicate the targets of preference for most pharmaceutical companies. While some drugs are designed to target amyloid, others are focused on tau. However, here again, it is a mono-therapeutic strategy, and past single target-based failures have cast doubts on this approach.

Source. Rao RV, Subramaniam KG, Gregory J, Bredesen AL, Coward C, Okada S, Kelly L, & Bredesen DE, (2023). Rationale for a multi-factorial approach for the reversal of cognitive decline in Alzheimer's disease and MCI: A review. International Journal of Molecular Sciences, 24(2), 1659. https://doi.org/10.3390/ijms24021659.

7.4.1. Different Types of Physical Exercise Interventions

A widely accessible, low-risk, and inexpensive intervention that may have the ability to modify disease is aerobic exercise. While a 16-week aerobic exercise program with moderate-to-high intensity outperformed usual care in improving cardiorespiratory fitness, single-task and dual-task physical performance, and exercise self-efficacy in patients with mild AD who attended regularly, neither program significantly improved cognitive domains. A 26-week aerobic exercise program with moderate intensity also improved functional ability in older adults with probable AD. Two additional trials yielded different results, showing that a 3-month aerobic exercise program improved their quality of life and cognitive function, even in cases of mild AD. The enhanced Stroop color naming test and Trail Making AandB tests, which show improved cognitive function, were probably the result of improved brain energy metabolism, which increased ketone utilization while preserving brain glucose uptake. Vascular biomarkers for cardiorespiratory fitness will be measured concurrently with a large-scale RCT that aims to determine the impact of a 6-month, moderate-intensity cycling intervention on the global cognition of mild-to-moderate Alzheimer's disease.

Exercise decreased the number of falls in older adults with advanced AD as well, not just in those without cognitive decline. Exercise at home that combines cognitive and physical stimuli has been shown to improve ADL, cognitive function, and physical performance in AD patients. More significantly, though, home exercise seems to improve executive function more than group exercise. Patients with AD who participated in a 12-week dual-task training program saw improvements in a variety of areas, such as aerobic fitness, depressive state, and cognitive abilities., which were linked to improvements in cerebral blood flow, cognitive function, and occipital gray matter density as well as an increase in brain oscillation (the electrical activity of the cerebral cortex as measured by EEG) and a decrease in theta/alpha ratio. Furthermore, the same study's findings on enhanced muscle strength and balance are particularly significant because balance and mobility issues in AD patients are linked to a lower quality of life and an increased risk of falling. Patients with AD can benefit from physical intervention in a simpler, safer, and more practical way by exercising according to their own habits. For example, sundown syndrome (defined as the emergence or exacerbation of neuropsychiatric symptoms in the late afternoon, evening, or at night; approximately 66% of community-dwelling AD patients experience this condition) can be effectively treated with regular walking. For older patients with mild-to-moderate AD, even lower weekly energy expenditure levels may be linked to health benefits, but not to improvements in cognition.

7.4.2. Intensity and Duration of Intervention

For patients with mild AD, physical exercise intervention is a promising strategy to maintain or mprove functional ability and body fitness. This could enhance quality of life and performance on ADLs, as well as lower the risk of falls. It is still unclear, though, if exercise helps with cognition in AD patients. A number of the published clinical trials reported beneficial cognitive outcomes, many of which persisted for the duration of the intervention but not over time. Due to the variety of documented training techniques, e.g., it is challenging to come to a firm conclusion about the best protocols for this kind of intervention due to a variety of factors, including the small sample size that limits the power to detect significant group effects, aerobic training on a treadmill, cycling, and home-based physical activities; training intensities ranging from mild to high; durations ranging from three to twelve months; and outcome measures involving global cognition and specific domains. Large-scale comparative studies are therefore required to investigate the best kind of exercise intervention, the recommended quantity of exercise, the most sensitive and meaningful outcome measures, and the compelling evidence that physical activity has an impact on patients' cognitive abilities. Furthermore, cohorts with early-onset familial AD or severe AD should be examined in order to determine whether this kind of intervention can be used.

7.5. BRAIN STIMULATION

Many neuropsychiatric disorders can be controlled by brain stimulation methods such as transcranial direct current stimulation (tDCS), transcranial pulse stimulation (TPS), repetitive transcranial magnetic stimulation (rTMS), deep brain stimulation (DBS), and intermittent theta burst stimulation (iTBS). Prior research has indicated that brain stimulation may have some promising benefits in the management of AD (Casey et al., 2010; O'Neil et al., 2011; Siebern et al., 2012).

Table 7.3 provides an overview of the RCTs of brain stimulation on AD patients that have been published in the past 10 years.

Table 7.3. A Selection of Conditions in Which DBS is Being Actively Researched as a Viable Treatment Option

Condition	Area of Stimulation	First Author	Year of Publication
Parkinson's Disease	Subthalamic nucleus (STN)	Deuschl, Xie	2006, 2015
	Globus Pallidus internus (GPi)	Bloomstedt, Baker	2018, 2010
	Zona Incerta	Bloonstedt, Ossowska	2018, 2020
	Pedunculopontine nucleus	Thevathasan	2018
Essential Tremor	Ventral intermediate thalamus	Baizabal-Carvallo	2014
	Zona incerta	Fytagoridis	2012
Dystonia	GPi	Vidailhet	2013
Alzheimer's Disease	Fornix		
	Ventromedial prefrontal cortex	Mao, Lozano	2018, 2016
	Hippocampus	Scharre, Chakravarty	2018, 2016
	Nucleus Basalis Meynert	Kuhn	2014
Huntington's Disease	GPi	Velez-Lago	2013
Obsessive Compulsive Disorder (OCD)	Anteromedial GPi	Nair	2014
	Nucleus Accumbens	Huff, Denys	2010, 2010
	Anterior limb of the internal capsule (ALIC)	Denys, Kammen	2020, 2022
	Ventral Capsule/Ventral Striatum (VC/VS)	Park, Kammen, Greenburg	2019, 2022, 2008
	STN	Kammen, Li, Chabardes	2022,2020, 2013
	Inferior thalamic peduncle	Germann, Lee, Kammen	2022,2019, 2022
	Bed nucleus of the stria terminalis	Luyten, Mosley, Raymaekers, Kammen	2015, 2021, 2016, 2022
Epilepsy	Anterior nucleus of thalamus	Salanova	2018
Depression	VC/VS	Malone	2009
	Nucleus Accumbens	Bewernick	2010

Source: Senevirathne DKL, Mahboob A, Zhai K, Paul P, Kammen A, Lee DJ, Yousef MS, & Chaari A, (2023). Deep brain stimulation beyond the clinic: Navigating the future of Parkinson's and Alzheimer's disease therapy. Cells, 12(11), 1478. https://doi.org/10.3390/cells12111478.

7.5.1. Deep Brain Stimulation (DBS)

DBS is an invasive neurosurgical method that uses internal pulse generators attached to electrodes in particular brain regions to modify neuron activity. During a 12-month observation period, DBS of the fornix or nucleus basalis of Meynert appeared to be safe and well tolerated in AD patients, with no discernible adverse effects on nutrition. Although mean hippocampal atrophy was significantly slower within 12 months of implantation, there was no significant difference in cognitive functions between the positive-treated and sham-treated groups, and cerebral glucose metabolism increased only at 6 months but not at 12 months.

7.5.2. Transcranial Direct Current Stimulation (tDCS)

The non-invasive tDCS method functions by creating a small direct current in the targeted cortical region. Little electrodes are applied to the scalp above the targeted brain region during the procedure. Cortical excitability is facilitated by this stimulation, which leads to neuroplasticity. When it comes to administering tDCS, it is comparatively easy, safe, portable, and affordable when compared to other brain stimulation techniques. These benefits are crucial for the long-term at-home administration of tDCS. A growing body of clinical research has demonstrated that tDCS can improve the cognitive function of people who suffer from cognitive impairment. While stimulation at the dorsolateral prefrontal cortex for a longer duration (6 months) improved language function and global cognition, stimulation at the left temporal cortex for a shorter period of time (10 days) did not significantly improve verbal memory function. Notably, both for the short-term (10 days) and long-term (more than 8 months) interventions, anodal tDCS seemed to be able to preserve the degree of neuropsychological performance and slow down the progression of AD in advanced AD cases.

7.5.3. Repetitive Transcranial Magnetic Stimulation (rTMS)

It has been stated that the rTMS method is a risk-free, non-invasive way to control and modulate neural cell activity. Repeated application of rTMS can either stimulates (e.g., employing 5–20 Hz stimulation) or inhibits (e.g., excitability of cortical neurons by creating magnetic fields to alter the synaptic activities of neuronal circuits within particular brain networks (using stimulation at frequencies ≤ 1 Hz). Because of its neuroplasticity and vital role in cognition, the dorsolateral prefrontal cortex (DLPFC) has been the target brain region in the majority of studies. Particularly in the mild stage of AD, a 6-week rTMS intervention markedly enhanced global cognitive functions, memory, and language levels. Following left lateral parietal rTMS, improved visual recognition memory functions and clock drawing scores were linked to increased peripheral BDNF levels and antioxidant capacity. rTMS is frequently given in conjunction with cognitive training. According to earlier research, patients with mild-to-moderate AD who received both cognitive training and real rTMS therapy demonstrated superior cognitive benefits, a high adherence rate, and an excellent safety profile compared to those who received only cognitive training and sham rTMS (Casey et al., 2010; O'Neil et al., 2011; Siebern et al., 2012).

7.5.4. Transcranial Pulse Stimulation (TPS)

TPS, a new ultrasonication method for medical use, uses single ultrasound pulses (3 µs) that are repeated every 200–300 ms. The first method that enables reliable targeting and non-invasive DBS is ultrasound. Additionally, this permits the targeted brain region to be stimulated in a controlled manner without affecting other brain regions. Following TPS treatment, neuropsychological scores improved significantly in patients with probable AD. This improvement was linked to upregulation of the memory network and could last for up to three months. Pre-to-post analysis of the follow-up study's neuropsychological test battery showed a significant improvement, which was linked to less cortical atrophy in the critical brain regions of AD. Standardizing local skull thickness for inclusion criteria and developing a standard brain sonication concept are necessary for future research on the use of TPS in AD patients. Future research should take into account cognitive training in addition to TPS as a treatment.

7.5.5. Intermittent Theta Burst Stimulation (iTBS)

Although iTBS is a novel brain stimulation method that produces increased cortical excitability faster than traditional rTMS, there hasn't been much research done on its potential use in the treatment of AD. Only one pilot study, which was published during the review period, demonstrated that iTBS of the left DLPFC of patients with AD improved memory, attention, executive function, language, and association memory (AM), all of which were negatively correlated with connectivity of the DLPFC and right precuneus. Larger sample size blinded RCTs are required to validate these findings and determine the ideal treatment parameters.

7.5.5.1. Limitations and Future Research Directions of Brain Stimulation in Patients with AD

More research is obviously valuable in order to quantify the long-term effects of brain stimulation on the cognitive performance of patients with AD, as these effects are still largely unclear. To find out how long the effects last and to investigate the efficacy's time course, future research could concentrate on tracking those who benefit from this kind of treatment for up to a year following the intervention course. Further studies on patients with more severe conditions might also be beneficial, as they may need more stimulation intensity in relation to motor threshold in order to be more effective. Ultimately, more research is needed to fully understand the precise neurobiological processes underlying brain stimulation (Casey et al., 2010; O'Neil et al., 2011; Siebern et al., 2012).

7.6. NUTRITION SUPPLEMENTATIONS

A nutrient intervention in mild cognitive impairment (MCI) demonstrated positive effects on brain atrophy, indicating that diet is a significant modifiable risk factor for dementia and MCI. Since it is unlikely that the nutrient intervention will have a noticeable effect quickly, clinical trials in this field frequently take months or even years to see results (Table 7.4).

Table 7.4. A Summary of Clinical Studies Examining Vegetarian Diet Impact on ADRD

Study Design	Country	Population	Follow-Up	Exposure	Outcome	Results	Covariates	References
NS	US and Canada	Vegetarian, n= 72 (32 M 40 F) (62 white, 10 non-white) Age: 76.6 ± 8.3 years Non-vegetarian, n = 60 (24 M 36 F) (44 white, 16 non-white) Age: 73.5 ± 7.7 years	10 years	FFQ, historic dietary habits survey instrument	Verbal learning, memory, attention, processing speed, executive function, visuospatial abilities, language, global cognitive functioning, MMSE, AMNART, and GDS	Vegetarian diet not associated with lower mild memory impairment likelihood. More stable diet associated with better memory/ language.	Age, education	[Gatto, N.M.; et al. 2021]
Prospective cohort study	Taiwan	Buddhist Tzu Chi Foundation volunteers Non-vegetarian, n = 3154 (1345 M 1809 F) Age: 57.8 ± 6.3 years Vegetarian, n = 1737 (461 M 1276 F) Age: 58.1 ± 6.5 years	Average 9.2 years	Baseline questionnaires to assess dietary pattern, overall plant-based diet index	MCI and dementia diagnosis	Vegetarians associated with less risk of dementia compared with non-vegetarians after adjusting for covariates.	Gender, age, smoking, drinking, education level, marital status, regular exercise, comorbidities	[Tsai, J.H.; et al. 2022]
Longitudinal	US	n = 3337 (1200 M 2137 F) Age: 73.7 ± 5.72 years African American (AA), n = 2012; white, n = 1325	NS	FFQ	Episodic memory, perceptual speed, and MMSE	↗ plant-based diet associated with slower ↘ in GC, PS, and EM in AA but not in white participants. AA in the highest quintile of high plant-based diet had significantly slower rates of GC, PS, and EM than individuals in the lowest quintile.	Age, gender, presence of apolipoprotein E4 (APOE ε4) allele, lifestyle factors (education, cognitive activities, smoking, calorie intake, risk factors for cardiovascular disease, time and interaction time × each covariate)	[Liu, X.; et al. 2022]

AMNART: American National Adult Reading Test; APOE: apolipoprotein E; EM: episodic memory; FFQ: Food Frequency Questionnaire; GC: global cognition; GDS: Geriatric Depression Scale; MCI: mild cognitive impairment; MMSE: Mini-Mental State Examination; NS: not specified; PS: perceptual speed; VIQ: estimated verbal intelligence; ↘: decline; ↗: increase.

Source. Ellouze I, Sheffler J, Nagpal R, & Arjmandi B, (2023). Dietary patterns and Alzheimer's disease: An Updated review linking nutrition to neuroscience. Nutrients; 15(14), 3204. https://doi.org/10.3390/nu15143204.

A combined formula containing docosahexaenoic acid (DHA), eicosapentaenoic acid (EPA), vitamin B12, B6, C, E, folic acid, and other nutrients would be administered for a duration of 24 months for prodromal AD patients had positive effects on hippocampal atrophy measurements, cognition, and function, but not on the neuropsychological test battery, which was the primary outcome. Along with good tolerability, safety, and high intake adherence, administering a nutrient supplementation (Souvenaid) of similar ingredients resulted in a significant increase in the exploratory memory outcome. Additionally, in a different large-scale trial using a combined formula, the active-treated group's behavioral and cognitive performance improved over the course of three to six months and was sustained during open-label extensions. These essential nutritional components have also undergone independent testing in various investigations. In the OmegAD study, for example, patients with mild-to-moderate AD showed preserved cognitive function with higher plasma levels of omega-3 fatty acid (ω3 FA).

Additionally, a 6-month dietary DHA supplementation resulted in higher plasma concentrations of DHA and EPA as well as an upregulated global DNA hypomethylation in peripheral blood leukocytes (PBLs), which may have an impact on inflammatory and other critical processes during the progression of AD. For those with dementia or cognitive impairment, daily EPA-and DHA-enriched omega-3 polyunsaturated fatty acid (PUFA) supplements did not appear to have any discernible positive effects on mood or cognition. Because low blood folate levels can change AD patients' inflammatory responses, folic acid supplements are helpful for AD patients at various stages of the disease. Only ApoE4 noncarriers showed signs of improved cognition following a three-month feeding of food high in medium-chain triglycerides. In AD patients, supplementing with Macushield (which contains meso-zeaxanthin, lutein, and zeaxanthin) has only improved visual function—not cognitive function. In mild AD, supplementing with purified plasmalogen derived from scallops has improved cognitive function; supplementing with soy isoflavones has not. Probiotics have been added to nutritional supplements because of the gut-brain axis link between altered microbiota and cognitive behaviors. These changes have been shown to positively impact cognitive performance, as evidenced by elevated MMSE scores and altered metabolic statuses, which suggests that probiotics may be useful as a nonpharmacological intervention for patients with mild AD. Amino acids are being used to treat cognitive impairment in addition to the nutrients mentioned above or their essential components. Seven essential amino acids (Leu, Phe, Lys, Ile, His, Val, Trp) have been shown to have positive effects on improving cognitive and psychosocial functioning in a clinical trial involving middle-aged and older adults. Oral administ has become more popular.

In addition to supplementing with nutrient formula, nutritional guidance is another kind of intervention that is crucial for maintaining appropriate nutritional status, enhancing quality of life, and preventing falls in home-dwelling patients with AD and their families. These researched AD families have changed their diets and attitudes toward nutrition and diet-related behaviors because of the highly feasible advice, which has improved their quality of life and decreased their risk of falling without affecting their body weight.

Future clinical trial designs for nonpharmacological interventions need to take several factors into account. First, similar to pharmacological treatments, certain confounding factors may also tend to influence non-drug interventions, such as he "everyday" and "clinical day" variables of the participants, as well as variations in culture. These unrecognized factors could potentially skew perceptions of an intervention's effectiveness. To reduce the possible impact of confounding variables, some statistical techniques like multivariate modeling and stratification are used; however, in order to achieve adequate statistical power, these techniques need large sample sizes. As an alternative, using case-controlled, pair-matched research may help lessen the impact of confounders. To remove the distorted effects, therefore, large sample trials or well planned pair-matched studies might be required.

Second, because neurodegeneration or aging dystrophy causes cognitive impairment in dementia to worsen over time, assessing efficacy in the short term may highlight the initial, surface-level outcomes. For example, after a thorough intervention, improvements in short-term cognition were observed; however, these benefits vanished over the course of a 24-month long-term follow-up. At a 2-year follow-up visit, cognition (as measured by the MMSE) did not improve in the case of physical exercise interventions. In relation to the nutritional interventions, positive cognitive outcomes were seen during follow-ups that lasted less than six months, but they frequently vanished during longer follow-ups. The overwhelming reality here should cause us to reconsider how we approach creating non-pharmacological interventional strategies for AD patients. Consequently, the effects of interventions should be verified over an extended period of time using placebo or sham stimulations when planning future research.

Thirdly, it is important to note that certain nonpharmacological treatments for reactive neuropsychiatric symptoms against transient psychosocial conflicts may result in a time-dependent dilution (also known as placebo effects), which may subsequently enhance the quality of life for dementia patients. Therefore, it is imperative to critically reevaluate these invisible hidden effects in order to prevent making a mistaken conclusion. The placebo response may also depend on other elements like the length of the study, sample size, and study design. Placebo-controlled studies should be carried out whenever possible in the future because time-dependent effects are important when determining the effectiveness of an intervention, and data from ongoing clinical trials may not be sufficient to draw a firm conclusion. To assess placebo response, it may also be possible to use a control database that has model predictions conditioned for baseline severity. I hope more research is done on these non-pharmacological treatments for AD (Casey et al., 2010; O'Neil et al., 2011; Siebern et al., 2012).

A Closer Look

Transcranial Direct Current Stimulation (tDCS)

Transcranial Direct Current Stimulation (tDCS) is a non-invasive neuromodulation technique that involves delivering low-intensity electrical currents to specific regions of the brain through electrodes placed on the scalp. This technique has gained attention in neuroscience research and clinical practice for its potential to modulate neuronal activity, enhance cognitive function, and treat various neurological and psychiatric conditions.

The mechanism of action of tDCS involves the application of a weak direct current (typically between 1 to 2 milliamperes) through electrodes positioned over targeted brain areas. The electrical current passes through the scalp and underlying tissues, influencing the resting membrane potential of neurons and altering their excitability. Depending on the polarity of the electrodes, tDCS can either enhance or inhibit neuronal activity in the stimulated brain region.

Research has demonstrated that tDCS can induce changes in cortical excitability that outlast the duration of stimulation, a phenomenon known as "aftereffects." These aftereffects are thought to be mediated by modifications in synaptic efficacy, neurotransmitter release, and neuroplasticity mechanisms within the stimulated brain circuits. By modulating neuronal activity and synaptic plasticity, tDCS holds promise as a tool for enhancing cognitive functions such as attention, memory, learning, and decision-making.

In addition to cognitive enhancement, tDCS has been investigated as a potential treatment for various neurological and psychiatric disorders. Clinical studies have explored its efficacy in conditions such as depression, schizophrenia, chronic pain, stroke rehabilitation, Parkinson's disease, and Alzheimer's disease. While research in these areas is ongoing and results are mixed, tDCS shows potential as an adjunctive or alternative therapy for individuals who may not respond to conventional treatments or who experience intolerable side effects.

One of the key advantages of tDCS is its relatively low cost, ease of use, and portability compared to other neuromodulation techniques such as transcranial magnetic stimulation (TMS) or deep brain stimulation (DBS). However, challenges remain in optimizing stimulation parameters, ensuring reproducibility of effects, and identifying patient populations most likely to benefit from tDCS therapy. As research in this field continues to evolve, tDCS holds promise as a versatile tool for modulating brain function and treating neurological and psychiatric disorders (Casey et al., 2010; O'Neil et al., 2011; Siebern et al., 2012).

SUMMARY

- Nondrug treatments encompass a wide range of interventions aimed at addressing the diverse needs and challenges faced by individuals with Alzheimer's disease.
- Alzheimer's disease is a neurological disorder in which the death of brain cells causes memory loss and cognitive decline which commonly progress with cognitive deterioration, memory loss, and sleep problems.
- The management patent with Alzheimer's disease for their sleep problems should be given preference to non-drug therapeutic intervention.
- A regular daytime routine is an important part of care for a patient with dementia because in the advanced stages of dementia, patients benefit from a certain regularity of the daily routine.
- Cognitive training is targeted stimulation of brain functions with a focus on multiple cognitive abilities. It is mainly used in initial and middle stage Alzheimer's patients who want to train their cognitive skills by themselves.
- Snoezelen therapy is a multifunctional method that is performed in a particularly pleasant and adapted environment.
- Reminiscence therapy is a method that uses memories and their recall using various stimuli. Of course, it is also suitable for healthy seniors, for its preventive and activating significance.
- Validation therapy is considered to be one of the first specific non-pharmacological approaches to patients affected by dementia.
- Doll therapy is a very effective form of comprehensive therapy in patients with various forms and degrees of dementia,
- Physical exercise intervention for AD can be performed by specific exercise program (often aerobic exercise) with moderate-to-high intensity, or exercise based on individuals own exercise habits with low intensity; the intervention can be either home-based or group-based, either single-task, dual-task, or multitask training.
- Brain stimulation techniques, including deep brain stimulation (DBS), transcranial direct current stimulation (tDCS), repetitive transcranial magnetic stimulation (rTMS), transcranial pulse stimulation (TPS), and intermittent theta burst stimulation (iTBS), can regulate cognitive functions in a variety of neuropsychiatric diseases.

REFERENCES

1. Aging Options. (2017). Studies appear to link disrupted sleep and Alzheimer's disease. Retrieved from: https://agingoptions.com/news/studies-appear-to-show-a-link-between-disrupted-sleep-and-alzheimers/.
2. Alzheimer's Association. (2017). Treatments for sleep changes. Retrieved from: http://www.alz.org/alzheimers_disease_10429.asp (accessed on 29 June 2024).

3. Alzheimer's Society. (2021). Sleep and night-time disturbance. Retrieved from: https://www.alzheimers.org.uk/info/20064/symptoms/107/sleep_and_night-time_disturbance (accessed on 29 June 2024).

4. American Thoracic Society. (2017). Genetic susceptibility to Alzheimer's may increase sleep-disordered breathing cognitive impairment. Retrieved from: https://www.newswise.com/articles/genetic-susceptibility-to-alzheimer-s-may-increase-sleep-disordered-breathing-cognitive-impairment.

5. Amieva, H., Robert, P. H., Grandoulier, A. S., et al. (2016). Group and individual cognitive therapies in Alzheimer's disease: The ETNA3 randomized trial. *International Psychogeriatrics, 28*(5), 707–717. https://doi.org/10.1017/S1041610215001830.

6. Becker, W. C., Dorflinger, L., Edmond, S. N., Islam, L., Heapy, A. A., & Fraenkel, L. (2017). Barriers and facilitators to use of non-pharmacological treatments in chronic pain. *BMC Family Practice, 18*, 41. https://doi.org/10.1186/s12875-017-0605-7.

7. Bonmati-Carrion, M. A., Arguelles-Prieto, R., Martinez-Madrid, M. J., et al. (2014). Protecting the melatonin rhythm through circadian healthy light exposure. *International Journal of Molecular Sciences, 15*(12), 23448–23500. https://doi.org/10.3390/ijms151223448.

8. Brueggen, K., Kasper, E., Ochmann, S., et al. (2017). Cognitive rehabilitation in Alzheimer's disease: A controlled intervention trial. *Journal of Alzheimer's Disease, 57*(4), 1315–1324. https://doi.org/10.3233/JAD-160771.

9. Brunelle-Hamann, L., & Thivierge, S. M. (2015). Impact of a cognitive rehabilitation intervention on neuropsychiatric symptoms in mild to moderate Alzheimer's disease. *Neuropsychological Rehabilitation, 25*(5), 677–707. https://doi.org/10.1080/09602011.2014.964731.

10. Burns, J. M., Cronk, B. B., Anderson, H. S., et al. (2008). Cardiorespiratory fitness and brain atrophy in early Alzheimer's disease. *Neurology, 71*(3), 210–216. https://doi.org/10.1212/01.wnl.0000317094.86209.cb.

11. Casey, D. A., Antimisiaris, D., & O'Brien, J. (2010). Drugs for Alzheimer's disease: Are they effective? *Pharmacy and Therapeutics, 35*(4), 208–211.

12. Castellano, C. A., Paquet, N., Dionne, I. J., et al. (2017). A 3-month aerobic training program improves brain energy metabolism in mild Alzheimer's disease: Preliminary results from a neuroimaging study. *Journal of Alzheimer's Disease, 56*(4), 1459–1468. https://doi.org/10.3233/JAD-161163.

13. Craig, D., Mirakhur, A., Hart, D. J., et al. (2005). A cross-sectional study of neuropsychiatric symptoms in 435 patients with Alzheimer's disease. *American Journal of Geriatric Psychiatry, 13*(6), 460–468. https://doi.org/10.1097/00019442-200506000-00004.

14. De la Rosa, A., Olaso-Gonzalez, G., Arc-Chagnaud, C., et al. (2020). Physical exercise in the prevention and treatment of Alzheimer's disease. *Journal of Sport and Health Science, 9*(5), 394–404. https://doi.org/10.1016/j.jshs.2020.01.004.

15. De Oliveira, A. M., Radanovic, M., de Mello, P. C. H., et al. (2015). Nonpharmacological interventions to reduce behavioral and psychological symptoms of dementia: A systematic review. *BioMed Research International, 2015*, 218980. https://doi.org/10.1155/2015/218980.

16. Deschenes, C. L., & McCurry, S. M. (2009). Current treatments for sleep disturbances in individuals with dementia. *Current Psychiatry Reports, 11*(1), 20–26. https://doi.org/10.1007/s11920-009-0004-7.

17. Erickson, K. I., Voss, M. W., Prakash, R. S., et al. (2011). Exercise training increases size of hippocampus and improves memory. *Proceedings of the National Academy of Sciences of the United States of America, 108*(7), 3017–3022. https://doi.org/10.1073/pnas.1015950108.

18. Fox, M. (2017). Poor sleep raises Alzheimer's risk. Retrieved from: https://www.nbcnews.com/health/health-news/poor-sleep-raises-alzheimer-s-risk-n795381.

19. Garcia-Alberca, J. M. (2017). Cognitive-behavioral treatment for depressed patients with Alzheimer's disease: An open trial. *Archives of Gerontology and Geriatrics, 71*, 1–8. https://doi.org/10.1016/j.archger.2017.02.008.

20. Gauthier, S., Cummings, J., Ballard, C., et al. (2010). Management of behavioral problems in Alzheimer's disease. *International Psychogeriatrics, 22*(3), 346–372. https://doi.org/10.1017/S1041610209991505.

21. Gomez-Gallego, M., & Gomez-Amor, J-G. (2012). Determinants of quality of life in Alzheimer's disease: Perspective of patients, informal caregivers, and professional caregivers. *International Psychogeriatrics, 24*(11), 1805–1815. https://doi.org/10.1017/S1041610212001081.

22. Gonfrier, S., Andrieu, S., Renaud, D., et al. (2012). Course of neuropsychiatric symptoms during a 4-year follow-up in the REAL-FR cohort. *The Journal of Nutrition, Health & Aging, 16*(2), 134–137. https://doi.org/10.1007/s12603-011-0147-9.

23. Gooneratne, N. S., & Vitiello, M. V. (2014). Sleep in older adults: Normative changes, sleep disorders, and treatment options. *Clinics in Geriatric Medicine, 30*(3), 591–627. https://doi.org/10.1016/j.cger.2014.04.001.

24. Gradisar, M., & Crowley, S. J. (2013). Delayed sleep phase disorder in youth. *Current Opinion in Psychiatry, 26*(6), 580–585. https://doi.org/10.1097/YCO.0b013e328365aae7.

25. Hoffmann, K., Sobol, N. A., Frederiksen, K. S., et al. (2016). Moderate-to-high intensity physical exercise in patients with Alzheimer's disease: A randomized controlled trial. *Journal of Alzheimer's Disease, 50*(2), 443–453. https://doi.org/10.3233/JAD-150817.

26. Huang, P., Fang, R., Li, B. Y., et al. (2016). Exercise-related changes of networks in aging and mild cognitive impairment brain. *Frontiers in Aging Neuroscience, 8*, 47. https://doi.org/10.3389/fnagi.2016.00047.

27. Jackson, S., Ham, R. J., & Wilkinson, D. (2004). The safety and tolerability of donepezil in patients with Alzheimer's disease. *British Journal of Clinical Pharmacology, 58*(Suppl 1), 1–8. https://doi.org/10.1111/j.1365-2125.2004.02118.x.

28. Jahn, H. (2013). Memory loss in Alzheimer's disease. *Dialogues in Clinical Neuroscience, 15*(4), 445–454.

29. Jia, R. X., Liang, J. H., Xu, Y., et al. (2019). Effects of physical activity and exercise on the cognitive function of patients with Alzheimer's disease: A meta-analysis. *BMC Geriatrics, 19*(1), 181. https://doi.org/10.1186/s12877-019-1175-2.

30. Johnson, D. A., Lane, J., Wang, R., Reid, M., Djonlagic, I., Fitzpatrick, A. L., & Redline, S. (2017). Greater cognitive deficits with sleep-disordered breathing among individuals with genetic susceptibility to Alzheimer's disease: The Multi-Ethnic Study of Atherosclerosis. *Annals of*

the American Thoracic Society. Advance online publication, 14(11), 1697–1705. https://doi.org/10.1513/AnnalsATS.201701-052OC.

31. Kelley, B. J., & Petersen, R. C. (2007). Alzheimer's disease and mild cognitive impairment. *Neurologic Clinics, 25*(3), 577-v. https://doi.org/10.1016/j.ncl.2007.03.008.
32. Khachiyants, N., Trinkle, D., Son, S. J., & Kim, K. Y. (2011). Sundown syndrome in persons with dementia: An update. *Psychiatry Investigation, 8*(4), 275–287. https://doi.org/10.4306/pi.2011.8.4.275.
33. Koivisto, A. M., Hallikainen, I., Valimaki, T., et al. (2016). Early psychosocial intervention does not delay institutionalization in persons with mild Alzheimer's disease and has impact on neither disease progression nor caregivers' well-being: ALSOVA 3-year follow-up. *International Journal of Geriatric Psychiatry, 31*(3), 273–283. https://doi.org/10.1002/gps.4321.
34. Krysta, K., Bratek, A., Zawada, K., & Stepańczak, R. (2017). Cognitive deficits in adults with obstructive sleep apnea compared to children and adolescents. *Journal of Neural Transmission, 124*(Suppl 1), 187–201. https://doi.org/10.1007/s00702-017-1713-0.
35. Lande, R. G., & Gragnani, C. (2010). Nonpharmacologic approaches to the management of insomnia. *The Journal of the American Osteopathic Association, 110*(12), 695–701.
36. Larson, E. B., Wang, L., Bowen, J. D., et al. (2006). Exercise is associated with reduced risk for incident dementia among persons 65 years of age and older. *Annals of Internal Medicine, 144*(2), 73–81. https://doi.org/10.7326/0003-4819-144-2-200601170-00004.
37. Li, D., Thomas, R., Tsai, M. Y., et al. (2016). Vascular biomarkers to predict response to exercise in Alzheimer's disease: The study protocol. *BMJ Open, 6*(12), e011054. https://doi.org/10.1136/bmjopen-2016-011054.
38. Liu, P. Z., & Nusslock, R. (2018). Exercise-mediated neurogenesis in the hippocampus via BDNF. *Frontiers in Neuroscience, 12*, 52. https://doi.org/10.3389/fnins.2018.00052.
39. Millán-Calenti, J. C., Lorenzo-López, L., Alonso-Búa, B., de Labra, C., González-Abraldes, I., & Maseda, A. (2016). Optimal nonpharmacological management of agitation in Alzheimer's disease: Challenges and solutions. *Clinical Interventions in Aging, 11*, 175–184. https://doi.org/10.2147/CIA.S96657.
40. Miller, M. A. (2015). The role of sleep and sleep disorders in the development, diagnosis, and management of neurocognitive disorders. *Frontiers in Neurology, 6*, 224. https://doi.org/10.3389/fneur.2015.00224.
41. Montgomery, P., & Dennis, J. (2004). A systematic review of non-pharmacological therapies for sleep problems in later life. *Sleep Medicine Reviews, 8*(1), 47–62. https://doi.org/10.1016/S1087-0792(03)00023-4.
42. Morgenthaler, T. I., Lee-Chiong, T., Alessi, C., et al. (2007). Practice parameters for the clinical evaluation and treatment of circadian rhythm sleep disorders: An American Academy of Sleep Medicine report. *Sleep, 30*(11), 1445–1459. https://doi.org/10.1093/sleep/30.11.1445.
43. Morris, J. K., Vidoni, E. D., Johnson, D. K., et al. (2017). Aerobic exercise for Alzheimer's disease: A randomized controlled pilot trial. *PLoS ONE, 12*(2), e0170547. https://doi.org/10.1371/journal.pone.0170547.
44. Nordberg, A., & Svensson, A. L. (1998). Cholinesterase inhibitors in the treatment of Alzheimer's disease: A comparison of tolerability and pharmacology. *Drug Safety, 19*(6), 465–480. https://doi.org/10.2165/00002018-199819060-00004.

45. O'Neil, M. E., Freeman, M., Christensen, V., et al. (2011). A systematic evidence reviews of nonpharmacological interventions for behavioral symptoms of dementia. Washington (DC): Department of Veterans Affairs (US). Available at: https://www.ncbi.nlm.nih.gov/books/NBK54971/ (accessed on 29 June 2024).

46. Ohman, H., Savikko, N., Strandberg, T., et al. (2016). Effects of exercise on functional performance and fall rate in subjects with mild or advanced Alzheimer's disease: Secondary analyses of a randomized controlled study. *Dementia and Geriatric Cognitive Disorders, 41*(3–4), 233–241. https://doi.org/10.1159/000445712.

47. Rose, K. M., Fagin, C. M., & Lorenz, R. (2010). Sleep disturbances in dementia: What they are and what to do. *Journal of Gerontological Nursing, 36*(5), 9–14. https://doi.org/10.3928/00989134-20100302-02.

48. Schultz, S. A., Boots, E. A., Almeida, R. P., et al. (2015). Cardiorespiratory fitness attenuates the influence of amyloid on cognition. *Journal of the International Neuropsychological Society, 21*(10), 841–850. https://doi.org/10.1017/S1355617715000843.

49. Sheridan, P. L., & Hausdorff, J. M. (2007). The role of higher-level cognitive function in gait: Executive dysfunction contributes to fall risk in Alzheimer's disease. *Dementia and Geriatric Cognitive Disorders, 24*(2), 125–137. https://doi.org/10.1159/000105126.

50. Siebern, A. T., Suh, S., & Nowakowski, S. (2012). Nonpharmacological treatment of insomnia. *Neurotherapeutics, 9*(4), 717–727. https://doi.org/10.1007/s13311-012-0144-6.

51. Smith, M., Gerdner, L. A., Hall, G. R., et al. (2004). History, development, and future of the progressively lowered stress threshold: A conceptual model for dementia care. *Journal of the American Geriatrics Society, 52*(10), 1755–1760. https://doi.org/10.1111/j.1532-5415.2004.52473.x.

52. Sobol, N. A., Hoffmann, K., Frederiksen, K. S., et al. (2016). Effect of aerobic exercise on physical performance in patients with Alzheimer's disease. *Alzheimer's & Dementia, 12*(12), 1207–1215. https://doi.org/10.1016/j.jalz.2016.05.004.

53. Spalletta, G., Musicco, M., Padovani, A., et al. (2010). Neuropsychiatric symptoms and syndromes in a large cohort of newly diagnosed, untreated patients with Alzheimer's disease. *The American Journal of Geriatric Psychiatry, 18*(11), 1026–1035. https://doi.org/10.1097/JGP.0b013e3181d6b68d.

54. Tarawneh, R., & Holtzman, D. M. (2012). The clinical problem of symptomatic Alzheimer's disease and mild cognitive impairment. *Cold Spring Harbor Perspectives in Medicine, 2*(5), a006148. https://doi.org/10.1101/cshperspect.a006148.

55. Thune-Boyle, I. C., Iliffe, S., Cerga-Pashoja, A., et al. (2012). The effect of exercise on behavioral and psychological symptoms of dementia: Towards a research agenda. *International Psychogeriatrics, 24*(7), 1046–1057. https://doi.org/10.1017/S1041610211002365.

56. Tolppanen, A. M., Solomon, A., Kulmala, J., et al. (2015). Leisure-time physical activity from mid- to late life, body mass index, and risk of dementia. *Alzheimer's & Dementia, 11*(4), 434–443. https://doi.org/10.1016/j.jalz.2014.01.008.

57. Twigg, G. L., Papaioannou, I., Jackson, M., et al. (2010). Obstructive sleep apnea syndrome is associated with deficits in verbal but not visual memory. *American Journal of Respiratory and Critical Care Medicine, 182*(1), 98–103. https://doi.org/10.1164/rccm.200910-1483OC.

58. Urrestarazu, E., & Iriarte, J. (2016). Clinical management of sleep disturbances in Alzheimer's disease: Current and emerging strategies. *Nature and Science of Sleep, 8*, 21–33. https://doi.org/10.2147/NSS.S90675.

59. Valente, S. (2015). Evaluating and managing insomnia: Non-pharmacological treatments. *Journal of Sleep Disorders: Treatment & Care, 4*(2). https://doi.org/10.4172/2325-9639.1000183.

60. Vidoni, E. D., Perales, J., Alshehri, M., et al. (2019). Aerobic exercise sustains performance of instrumental activities of daily living in early-stage Alzheimer's disease. *Journal of Geriatric Physical Therapy, 42*(3), E129–E134. https://doi.org/10.1519/JPT.0000000000000172.

61. Wallace, A., & Bucks, R. S. (2013). Memory and obstructive sleep apnea: A meta-analysis. *Sleep, 36*(2), 203–220. https://doi.org/10.5665/sleep.2372.

62. Yang, S. Y., Shan, C. L., Qing, H., et al. (2015). The effects of aerobic exercise on cognitive function of Alzheimer's disease patients. *CNS & Neurological Disorders Drug Targets, 14*(10), 1292–1297. https://doi.org/10.2174/1871527315666151111123319.

Chapter

8

LIVING WITH AND CARING FOR PATIENTS WITH ALZHEIMER'S DISEASE

Contents

Introduction 270
8.1. Realities of Caring for Someone with Dementia 272
8.2. Everyday Care for a Person With Alzheimer's Disease 275
8.3. Medical Problems and Going to The Doctor 282
8.4. Keeping w Person with Alzheimer's Safe 284
8.5. Adapting Activities for People with Alzheimer's Disease 286
8.6. Caregiver Support and Self-Care 290
8.7. Caring for a Person with Late-Stage Alzheimer's 301
Summary 306
References 307

INTRODUCTION

Care is a complex phenomenon, a cultural experience, and a difficult area in the medical sciences, particularly when it comes to providing care for nursing home patients with Alzheimer's disease (AD) who exhibit behavioral problems and cognitive impairments.

AD currently affects about 27 million people globally, and it's predicted that number will rise by up to 1 million each year. There are 2,500 000 AD patients in Iran.

The creation of an all-encompassing system of care for AD patients is the biggest challenge facing health services today, given the disease's rapid global increase in patients. Because elderly Iranians are accustomed to living with their families, there aren't many nursing homes in the country. Additionally, patients with AD are not housed in special units; instead, they receive care in nursing homes alongside other elderly residents.

Iran's State Welfare Organization is in charge of overseeing its nursing homes. Older patients are increasingly being moved to nursing homes in recent years as a result of shifts in the nuclear family structure and the rise in the number of working women. Additionally, research from other nations to date indicates that the likelihood of institutionalization rises as AD progresses, especially when it comes to the degree of cognitive impairment and aberrant behavior patterns. Increasing the number of nursing homes and raising the standard of care they offer is imperative given the rapidly rising need for institutional care for AD patients in Iranian society as well as the rise in the number of AD patients.

In order to provide AD patients with appropriate care and surroundings, formal caregivers in nursing homes play a crucial role. Many of the difficulties they face on a daily basis have been characterized as emotionally and physically taxing, with significant physical and psychological workloads. These difficulties can have an impact on care, particularly when it comes to individuals who have dementia. Staff burnout has been linked to stressors such as intense involvement with residents. These problems impact resident care quality and the caregivers' capacity to perform their duties. On the other hand, little is known about how caring is experienced culturally. To the best of our knowledge, no research has been done on the treatment of AD patients, especially in Iran. In order to create more effective care programs and education based on our culture for caregivers to reduce their stress in caring for these patients and result in appropriate care for Alzheimer's patients and improve their quality of life, we decided to investigate the experiences of caregivers providing care for patients with AD in Iranian culture in the nursing home.

Orientation and Directional Terms

Term	Definition	Illustration
Advance care planning	Advance care planning is a process that helps people with Alzheimer's disease and other types of dementia share their care preferences with family, care teams, and legal professionals.	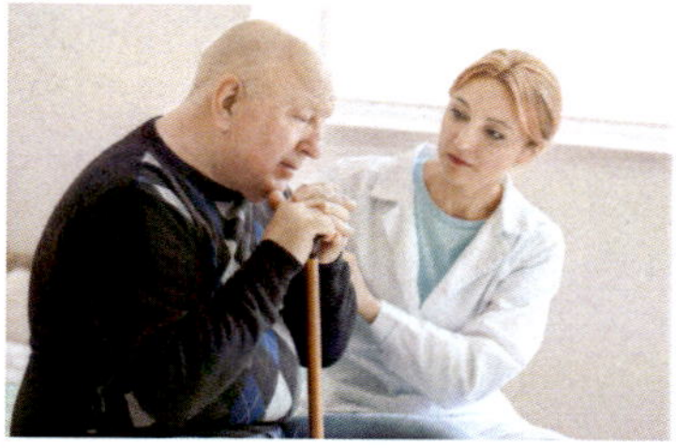
Caregiving	Caregiving is an important job, and caring for a person with Alzheimer's disease comes with unique challenges.	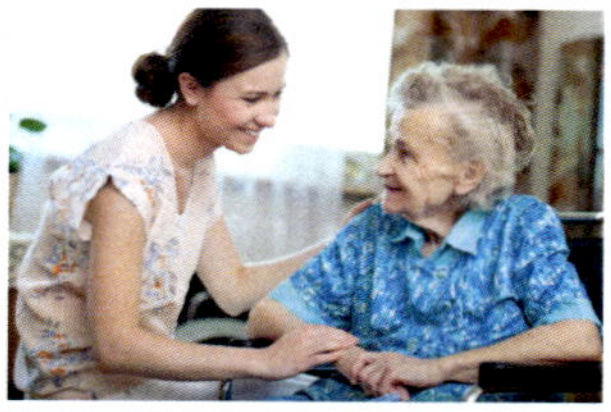
End-of-Life Care	End-of-life care for Alzheimer's disease should support the person's physical, emotional, and relational needs until they die.	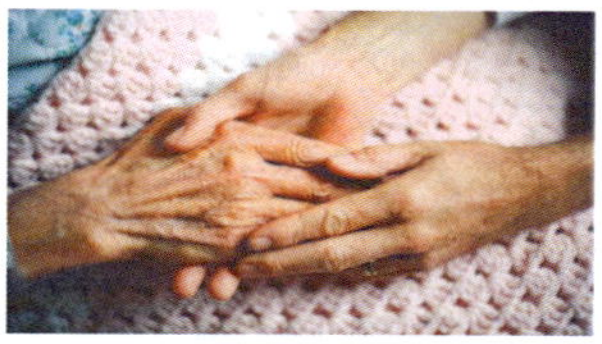
Hospice care	Hospice care is a type of care for people who are terminally ill and focuses on comfort and dignity during the end of life. It can be beneficial for people in the final stages of Alzheimer's disease and their families.	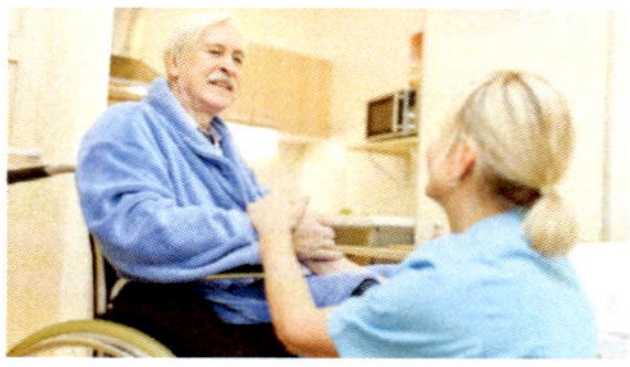
Late Stage Care	The late stage of Alzheimer's disease may last anywhere from several weeks to several years. Intensive, around-the-clock assistance is usually required. Caring for the person with Alzheimer's disease is most successful when the focus is on preserving quality of life and dignity and treating the person with compassion and respect.	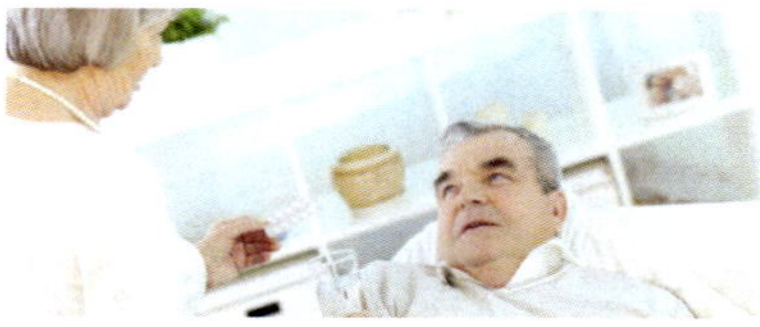
Respite Care	Respite care is a short-term break for caregivers of people with Alzheimer's disease, allowing them time to rest, travel, or spend time with family and friends. The care can last from a few hours to several weeks and can take place at home, in a health care facility, or at an adult day care center.	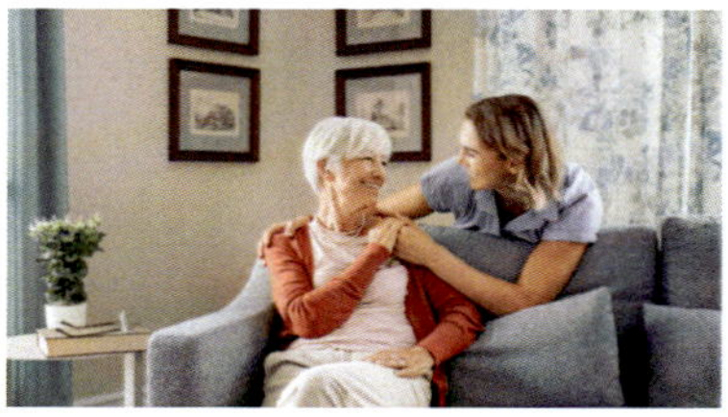

8.1. REALITIES OF CARING FOR SOMEONE WITH DEMENTIA

In the United States, millions of people care for a friend or family member who has Alzheimer's disease or a related dementia. Many families require more than one person to provide care for a loved one who has Alzheimer's. Instead, it's a multi-person role where duties and responsibilities are shared. There might be new difficulties every day, and you might feel helpless.

You can learn more about the realities of providing dementia care in this section. It offers pointers on how to take care of yourself as well as resources for support when caring for others.

8.1.1. Being a Caregiver for Someone with Alzheimer's

Can you recall the moment when you found out about your loved one's diagnosis? While some may not be caught off guard due to the noticeable symptoms of memory loss and cognitive difficulties, the revelation can still be jarring. This leaves many asking themselves: What comes next?

Alzheimer's is a brain disease that impairs the function of a significant number of nerve cells. It's the most prevalent type of dementia, a word used to characterize illnesses that impair a person's memory, reasoning, and good judgment.

Many people do not require full-time caregiving during the early stages of the disease. People with Alzheimer's may require more assistance and struggle to take care of themselves as the disease progresses. A spouse or partner, a member of the family, or a close friend will frequently help with daily tasks, appointments, medication, and other things. Having kind and knowledgeable caregivers is very beneficial at every stage of Alzheimer's.

Giving care can be meaningful and fulfilling, but it can also be difficult. While it's not always feasible, it can be beneficial to have a network or team of caregivers so that the burden of care does not fall solely on one person. Taking care of oneself is crucial for caregivers to maintain their physical and mental well-being. The advice and techniques in this pamphlet are meant to serve as a guide for providing compassionate and efficient dementia care. Since the disease progresses, care methods will also need to adapt.

8.1.2. Helping Friends and Family Understand

It can be challenging to decide when and how to inform friends and family that a loved one has Alzheimer's. You might be concerned about how people will view or handle your loved one. It's acceptable to hold off on telling anyone until you're emotionally ready, or to tell your closest friends and family members only. The people you most trust can assist you and the person with Alzheimer's by being aware of what's going on. The ideas listed below can assist you in getting going.

Family and friends don't understand. Trying to explain it to them is difficult because they believe Alzheimer's to be memory loss only. They are unaware of its complete scope.

8.1.2.1. Tips for Sharing the Diagnosis

It may be hard to share a loved one's Alzheimer's diagnosis with others. Here are a few suggested approaches:

- Realize that family and friends often sense that something is wrong before they are told.
- Be honest with them about the Alzheimer's diagnosis. Explain that Alzheimer's is a brain disease that can have wide-ranging symptoms. Memory loss is a common symptom but it's not the only one. Changes in behavior and communication are also common.
- Share resources (including this guide) to help them understand what you and the person with Alzheimer's are experiencing.
- Give examples of ways they can help, such as visiting, providing meals, or helping with home safety modifications. Let them know you need breaks.

Friends and family may be unsure of how to engage with a person who has Alzheimer's. Give them advice on how to feel more at ease. You can:

- Tell people who visit how much your loved one can understand. For example, if the person is still in the early stage of Alzheimer's, you might say that they can still have a conversation over dinner or play a favorite board game.
- If your loved one has difficulty remembering people, suggest that visitors start a conversation with the person by briefly introducing themselves. For example, "Hello George, I'm John. We used to work together."
- Offer ways to make the conversation easier and more respectful, such as not correcting or arguing with the person with Alzheimer's if they make a mistake or forget something.
- Remind visitors to be patient when the person with Alzheimer's has trouble finding the right words or putting feelings into words.
- 5Suggest activities beyond talking that they can do together, including listening to music or looking through a photo album.

8.1.3. Helping Children Understand

The entire family is impacted by a family member with Alzheimer's, including the children and grandchildren. It's critical to engage with youth and assist them in comprehending the situation (Figure 8.1). For example:

- Answer their questions simply and honestly. You might tell a young child, "Grandma has an illness that makes it hard for her to remember things."
- Reassure them that feelings of sadness and anger are normal.
- Comfort them. Explain that no one caused the disease. Young children may think they did something to hurt their grandparent.

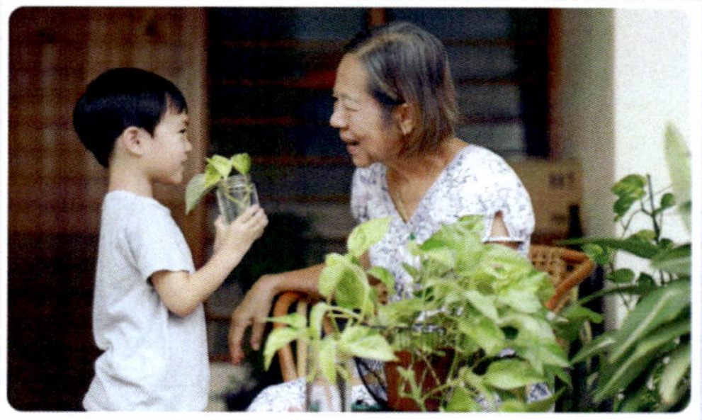

Figure 8.1. *Grandson and grandmother potting plant together.*

Source: https://media.istockphoto.com/id/1530455247/photo/the-grandson-is-helping-his-grandmother-repot-a-house-plant-at-home.jpg?s=1024x1024&w=is&k=20&c=jJm8aJTdsq0Va4uJhmS79evk2cplUetHcsUGMEmIfOI=.

Younger kids might observe your behavior around your Alzheimer's-afflicted loved one. Don't be harsh or use "baby talk" when speaking to your loved one. Youngsters might imitate this behavior after observing it. Make an effort to be aware of the voice you're using and the way you're speaking to them. It's crucial to demonstrate to kids that they can still interact and communicate with the person. There are several things that kids and seniors with Alzheimer's disease can do together.

- Simple arts and crafts
- Playing music or singing
- Looking through photo albums
- Reading stories out loud

It's critical to prioritize the daily needs of your children over your caregiving responsibilities if you and your family live with an Alzheimer's patient. For example:

- Avoid having a young child help take care of or "babysit" the person with Alzheimer's. This may not be safe for the child or that person.
- Make sure the child has time for their own interests and needs, such as playing with friends, school activities, or doing homework.
- Spend quality time with your child so they don't feel that all your attention is on the person with Alzheimer's.

While some kids might not express their emotions verbally, they might act out at home or at school. The behavior of the Alzheimer's patient may embarrass older kids and teenagers. Remind kids that they can talk to you about anything and everything at any time. Social workers and school counselors can also assist kids in learning constructive coping mechanisms for their emotions.

8.1.4. Advance Care Planning

Making future plans is crucial after an Alzheimer's diagnosis, ideally with the patient's assistance while they are still able to contribute to those plans.

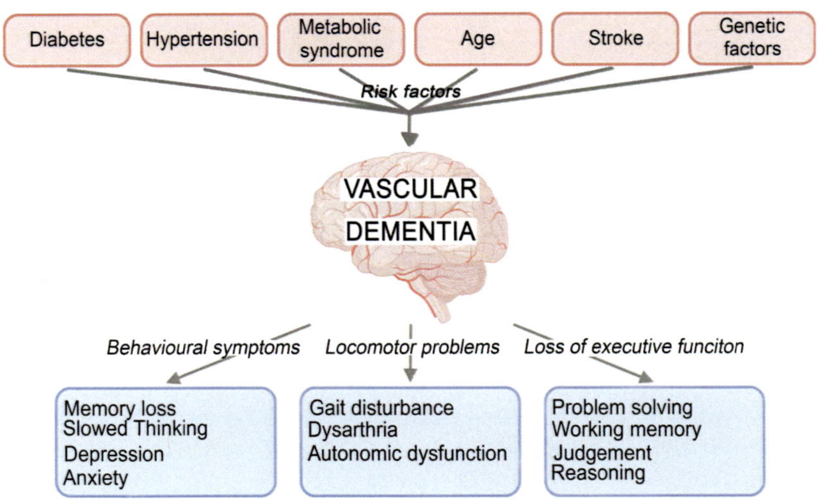

Figure 8.2. *Advance care planning.*

Source: By Mossanen Parsi M, Duval C, Ariëns RAS. – https://www.ncbi.nlm.nih.gov/pmc/articles/PMC8733168/, CC BY 4.0, https://commons.wikimedia.org/w/index.php?curid=147257763.

Advance care planning entails talking about and getting ready to make decisions regarding a person's medical treatment in the event that they become gravely ill or are unable to express their desires. The most crucial aspect of advance care planning is having meaningful conversations with the person who is living with Alzheimer's to find out about their values and preferences.

Official records and legal documents belonging to an elderly person can be kept in one location for easy access when needed. Store these supplies in a location that is both secure and accessible, like a lockbox that is fireproof (Figure 8.2).

8.1.4.1. Prepare and Plan

Having documentation in place can guarantee that the person's preferences are respected when making decisions about their future medical care. Make sure all of their financial, legal, and health information reflects their wishes by carefully reviewing it. Verify that the following documents are current and that you have them.

- **Durable Power of Attorney for Finances:** Provides someone with the power to make legal and financial decisions for the person with Alzheimer's.
- **Durable Power of Attorney for Health Care:** Gives a person — called a health care proxy — the power to make medical decisions for the person with Alzheimer's.
- **Living Will:** Informs doctors how the person with Alzheimer's wants to be treated if they cannot make their own decisions about emergency treatment.
- **Do Not Resuscitate (DNR) Form:** Informs health care staff that the person does not want CPR or other life-support measures to be attempted if their heartbeat and breathing stops.
- **Will:** Provides legal guidance for the distribution of a person's property, belongings, and money after they die.
- **Living Trust:** Informs an individual — called a trustee — about how to distribute the property and money of the person with Alzheimer's while that person is still living but no longer able to manage their own affairs (Drebing et al., 2002; Voutilainen et al., 2006; Carpenter & Thompson, 2008).

8.2. EVERYDAY CARE FOR A PERSON WITH ALZHEIMER'S DISEASE

Alzheimer's affects a person's ability to carry out daily activities like eating, dressing, and taking a shower. They may continue to be largely independent in the early stages of the illness, but eventually they will require more assistance with everyday tasks. The primary objective of a caregiver is to strike a balance between allowing the person to be as independent as possible and offering assistance when required. Finding that balance may involve taking into account what the dementia patient needs to succeed.

This section's subsections provide advice on how to attend to an Alzheimer's patient's needs and make them feel more at ease accepting assistance.

Certain tasks, like taking a shower and putting on clothes, are ones that individuals will probably need assistance with in the past. Your loved one might be ashamed and unwilling to accept assistance. Their inability to take care of themselves could also make them angry. Try to be patient and think of ways to improve the experiences for the two of you (Figure 8.3).

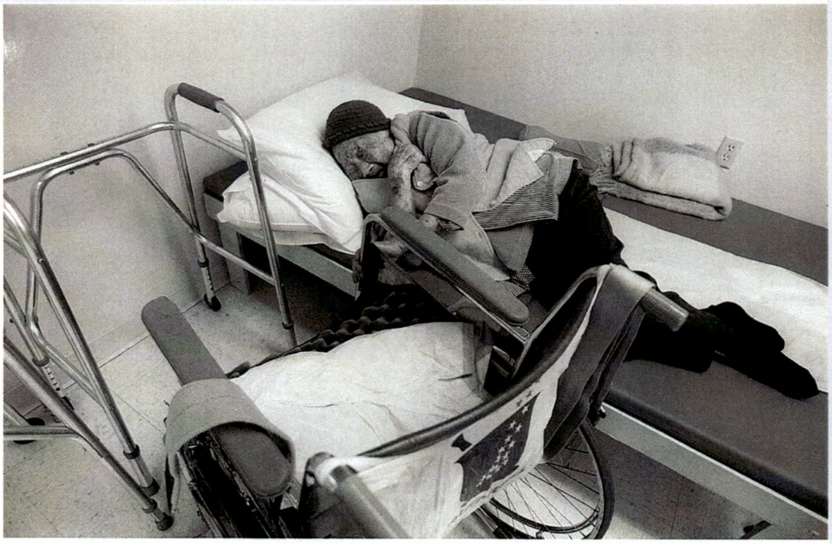

Figure 8.3. *Caring.*

Source: By Nancy Wong – Own work, CC BY-SA 4.0, https://commons.wikimedia.org/w/index.php?curid=81990587.

8.2.1. Bathing

One of the most difficult tasks for caregivers is assisting a person with Alzheimer's disease when taking a bath or shower. A person suffering from this illness may find taking a shower frightening, awkward, or physically uncomfortable. They may also express their discomfort by verbally or physically resisting attempts to assist them in taking a shower.

You can both have a better experience if you plan ahead. To keep your loved one secure and comfortable when taking a bath, use the following advice.

8.2.1.1. Before a Bath or Shower

- Assemble your supplies. Prepare a bath chair, shampoo, towels, soap, and washcloths. Safety bars and a rubber bathmat are additional tools you can use to stop falls. Use of bath oils or anything else that can cause the tub to become slick is not advised. Assemble any extra supplies you may require for yourself, such as gloves.
- Ensure the bathroom is comfortable by keeping the room warm and well lit. Play soft music if it helps to relax the person.
- Make sure the water temperature in the bath or shower is comfortable.

- Be straightforward when taking a bath. "It's time for a bath now," you say. Try offering them an option if they don't react. For instance, inquire, "Would you rather take a shower or a bath now, or in fifteen minutes?"
- Try to schedule bathing at the same time each day

8.2.1.2. During a Bath or Shower

- Allow the person with Alzheimer's to have a role in the bathing process. Even if they are unable to wash their body, they could hold the washcloth, sponge, or shampoo bottle.
- Give the person step-by-step instructions on how to wash their own body if they can. Say things like "wash your stomach," "put your feet in the tub," "sit down," or "take the soap." You can lead the person's hand with your own or model each action.
- If you are bathing the person, use a handheld showerhead. Be gentle and tell the person each step you are going to do before you do it.
- If using a hand-held showerhead, begin by washing hands or feet. These areas are less threatening and can help relax the person before moving to the face, torso, or head.
- Put a towel over the person's shoulders or lap to help them feel less exposed. Then use a sponge or washcloth to clean under the towel.
- Distract the person by talking about something else if they become upset.
- Never leave a person with Alzheimer's alone in the tub or shower.
- If a bath or shower is too upsetting, consider a "wash-up" at the sink. Sometimes washing a person who is sitting in a chair can be a more pleasant experience.

8.2.1.3. After a Bath or Shower

- Using a towel, pat the person's skin dry. Make sure to wipe away any moisture from skin folds and look for rashes. Try applying a moisturizing cream or ointment if you discover a rash. If the rash doesn't seem to be getting better, see a doctor.
- Use petroleum jelly or another protective ointment around the penis, vagina, and rectum if the person struggles with incontinence. If the person with Alzheimer's is capable of doing so, ask them if they would like to take care of this themselves in order to prevent upsetting them.
- Use lotion to keep skin soft and powder and ointments to prevent chafing, as needed.

Although you should be open to a more flexible schedule, try to give the person a bath two or three times per week. On days when a full bath or shower isn't feasible, think about taking a sponge bath to clean the face, hands, feet, underarms, and private areas. Try shampooing the person's hair in the sink with a hose attachment if shampooing is difficult for them.

8.2.2. Dressing

It frequently takes longer for Alzheimer's patients to get dressed. They may find it difficult to decide what to wear, and they may end up buying the incorrect items for the weather. They may also neglect to put on a piece of clothing or wear colors that don't go together. As long as possible, let the person dress themselves. To make dressing easier, try these suggestions:

- Lay out clothes in the order the person should put them on, such as underwear first, then pants, then a shirt, and then a sweater.
- Hand the person one item at a time or give step-by-step dressing instructions.
- Keep only one or two outfits in the closet or dresser at a time to reduce the number of choices.
- Buy three or four sets of the same clothes if the person wants to wear the same clothing every day.
- Buy loose-fitting, comfortable clothing. Short cotton socks and loose cotton underwear are best. Sweatpants and shorts with elastic waistbands are helpful.
- Use fasteners or large zipper pulls for clothing, instead of buttons or buckles. Try slip-on shoes that won't slide off or shoes with hook-and-loop fastener straps instead of shoelaces.

8.2.3. Grooming

People generally feel better when they are happy with their appearance. People with Alzheimer's disease frequently feel more like themselves when grooming assistance is provided. These pointers could be useful.

- **Makeup and Hair**
  - Encourage the person to wear makeup if they have always worn it. If needed, you can offer to apply makeup and face care products.
  - Help them shave as needed if they did this in the past. Use an electric razor for safety. Make sure people with longer facial hair trim it regularly to keep it healthy and make it easier to care for.
  - Take the person to get their hair trimmed and styled. Some barbers or hairstylists may come to your home.
  - Keep the person's nails clean and trimmed. Consider using a nail file if you or your loved one feel uncomfortable using clippers

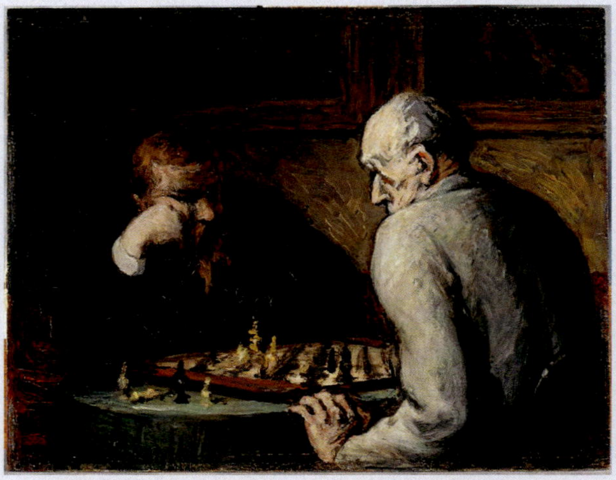

Figure 8.4. *Preventing.*

Source: By https://www.parismuseescollections.paris.fr/fr/musee-de-la-vie-romantique/oeuvres/portrait-du-marechal-de-saxe, Public Domain, https://commons.wikimedia.org/w/index.php?curid=149981C.

- **Brushing and Mouth Care:** Good mouth care helps prevent dental problems such as cavities and gum disease.
    - Assist the individual in brushing their teeth. Proceed cautiously. For instance, take up the toothpaste, unscrew the cap, load the toothbrush with toothpaste, and brush. Don't forget to give the person as much freedom as you can.
    - Try a long-handled, angled, or electric toothbrush if you need to brush the person's teeth for them.
    - If the person bites down on the toothbrush or does not want something in their mouth, sometimes using a child's size toothbrush can be helpful.
    - Use special tools to make flossing easier. Floss holders, floss threaders, oral irrigators, and interdental brushes can be helpful.
    - If the person has dentures, help them keep them clean. Make sure the person uses the denture cleaning material the right way.
    - Ask the person to rinse their mouth with water after each meal and use mouthwash once a day.
    - Take note of dry mouth. It can be difficult to chew, swallow, and speak when you have a dry mouth from certain illnesses or drugs. A dentist can assist in figuring out the cause of dry mouth in the person you are responsible for. In addition, you can advise them to chew sugar-free gum, drink lots of water, abstain from alcohol and caffeine, and use a humidifier at night.
    - Take the individual to the dentist. Seek out a dentist who has experience caring for Alzheimer's patients. To locate a dentist with experience treating Alzheimer's patients, you might need to do some asking around. Make sure you heed the advice of the dentist regarding how frequently to schedule check-ups. Think about mobile dentistry, where patients receive skilled care from professionals in settings that are familiar and comfortable.

8.2.4. Healthy Eating and Mealtimes

A balanced diet is crucial for individuals with Alzheimer's disease, but some may not feel hungry because of medicine, inactivity, or diminished taste and smell perception (Figure 8.5).

To help keep the person nourished, consider the following suggestions:

- Offer healthy foods such as vegetables, fruits, and whole-grain products. Be sure to buy foods that the person likes and can eat.
- Consider taking advantage of meal kit services, or provide foods that are easy to prepare, such as pre-made salads and microwaveable meals.
- If the person is still living alone, call to remind them to eat.
- Offer smaller but more frequent meals, calorie rich snacks, and sweetening food with honey or syrup if you are concerned the person is not eating enough.
- Use a service such as Meals on Wheels, which will deliver meals to the person's home.

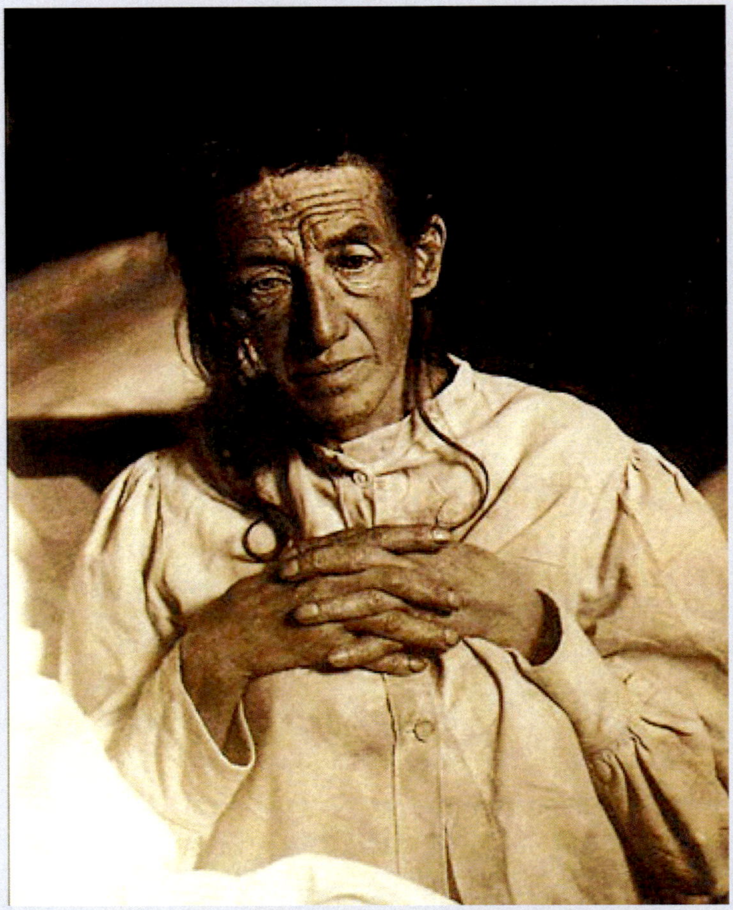

Figure 8.5. *Eating a healthy diet important in Alzheimer's disease.*

Source: https://upload.wikimedia.org/wikipedia/commons/1/1d/Auguste_D_aus_Marktbreit.jpg.

A person with Alzheimer's may find mealtimes challenging, particularly if they have lost some of their independence. To make meals easier, try these suggestions:

- If the person has always eaten meals at specific times, continue to serve meals at those times.
- Serve meals in a consistent, familiar place and way whenever possible.
- Make the eating area quiet. Turn off the TV or radio if they distract the person from eating.
- View mealtimes as opportunities for social interaction. You can set the mood with a warm and happy tone of voice.
- Don't rush and don't push. Be patient and give the person enough time to finish their meal.

Alzheimer's patients may experience difficulty eating over time. To help them eat more easily, consider the following suggestions:

- Offer just one food at a time instead of filling the plate or table with too many options.
- Cut the food into small pieces and make it soft enough to eat, which will help with chewing and swallowing.
- Enable your loved one to feed themselves if they are able. It may require gentle prompting and patience.
- If your loved one is unable to move the food to their own mouth, try putting your hand on their hand while they hold the fork and guide the food to their mouth.
- Consider pureeing food if the person has difficulty swallowing.
- Avoid over-feeding or force-feeding. Keep in mind that in late stages of Alzheimer's, appetite declines.

8.2.5. Exercise and Physical Activity

For an individual with Alzheimer's disease, physical activity maintains the health of their heart, muscles, and joints. Exercise can also enhance sleep quality and mood. Consult their physician prior to beginning a new exercise regimen.

The following advice can be helpful in keeping an Alzheimer's patient engaged:

- Take a walk together each day. Exercise is good for caregivers, too!
- Make sure the person with Alzheimer's has an ID bracelet with your phone number if they walk alone.
- Find exercise videos for older adults online.
- Add music to the exercises if it helps the person with Alzheimer's.
- Make sure your loved one wears comfortable clothes and shoes that fit well and are made for exercise.
- Make sure the person drinks plenty of water or juice during and after exercise.
- Be realistic about how much activity can be done at one time. Several short "mini workouts" may be best.

It's possible that some Alzheimer's patients have trouble moving around. People who struggle with walking might be able to:

- Do simple exercises or yoga while seated in a chair.
- Play games while seated, such as bean bag toss or horseshoe.
- Help with tasks around the home, such as sweeping and dusting.
- Use a stationary bike or pedal exercisers.
- Use soft rubber exercise balls or balloons for stretching or throwing back and forth.
- Use stretching bands, which you can buy in sporting goods stores or online. Be sure to follow the instructions.
- Lift light weights or household items such as soup cans (Drebing et al., 2002; Voutilainen et al., 2006; Carpenter & Thompson, 2008).

8.3. MEDICAL PROBLEMS AND GOING TO THE DOCTOR

As with everyone, an individual with Alzheimer's may eventually develop additional health issues. These issues may lead to increased perplexity and behavioral shifts. It's possible that they are unable to identify the issue. Keep an eye out for symptoms of illness and let the doctor know what you observe.

8.3.1. Common Medical Problems

Among the typical health issues to look out for in individuals with Alzheimer's are:

- Flu, pneumonia, and other respiratory illnesses
- Dehydration
- Constipation
- Diarrhea
- Incontinence
- Urinary tract infection
- Hearing and vision loss

Ensure that the Alzheimer's patient visits a physician on a regular basis. The greatest thing you can do to help prevent or treat medical issues before they worsen is this.

You can take the following actions at home in addition to consulting a doctor to help prevent some common medical issues:

- Make sure the person stays up to date on all recommended vaccinations, including their yearly flu and COVID shots.
- Take note of the amount of liquid the person is consuming. Encourage the person to consume six glasses of liquid or more each day. Try juice, flavored water, broth, milk, decaffeinated coffee, or tea if the person refuses to drink water.
- Urge the person to consume more fiber-rich foods, as these can aid in the relief of constipation and diarrhea. High-fiber foods include whole-grain bread, raisins, prunes, dried apricots, and some dry cereals.
- If possible, ensure the person gets some exercise, such as walking, each day.

8.3.2. Visiting the Doctor

It's critical that the Alzheimer's patient receive ongoing medical attention. To help you prepare for a trip to the doctor, consider the following advice:

- Make an appointment during the person's best time of day and when the doctor's office is less likely to be crowded.
- Let the office staff know before the visit about the person's Alzheimer's. Ask the staff for help to make the visit go as smoothly as possible.
- Share any information with the staff before the visit which might be difficult to discuss in front of the person with Alzheimer's.
- Don't let the Alzheimer's patient know about the appointment until the day of the visit, or even just before it's time to go, if they get anxious when they visit the doctor. Act with positivity and objectivity.
- Pack something they like to eat or drink and any materials or activities the person enjoys.
- Have a friend or family member go with you so that one of you can stay with the person while the other speaks with the doctor.

- Make a quick overview readily available that includes the patient's medical history, primary care physician, and current prescriptions. You might also take into account telehealth, which is a service that allows a patient to see a doctor from home rather than a hospital using video conferencing and other technologies. Rural residents and older adults with limited mobility may find telehealth to be especially beneficial. Inquire about telehealth options with your healthcare provider.

8.3.2.1. Going to the Emergency Room

Both you and the Alzheimer's patient may experience significant stress during an ER visit. Here are a few strategies to handle ER visits:

- Take note of the patient's medications, insurance cards, doctor's contact details, and any advance directives. A living will or other signed document expressing a person's wishes for their care at the end of their life is called an advance directive.
- If you can, ask a friend or family member to go with you or meet you in the ER. They can stay with the person while you complete forms and respond to medical staff's questions.
- Be ready to explain the symptoms and events leading up to the ER visit. You may need to repeat this more than once to different staff members.
- Tell ER staff that the person has Alzheimer's. Explain how best to talk with the person.
- If the person with Alzheimer's must stay overnight in the hospital, try to have a friend or family member stay with them. Talk with the staff about other options for support overnight.

8.3.2.2. Incontinence

A person who is incontinent cannot control their bowels or bladder. Incontinence is a common side effect for most Alzheimer's patients. Although incontinence can occur at any point during the disease, it typically becomes an issue in the later stages. Alzheimer's patients occasionally experience mishaps as a result of their inability to locate the restroom or identify the toilet as one. A person with incontinence may experience embarrassment or shame.

For caregivers, who may need to change clothes, underwear, or bedsheets frequently, incontinence can be especially difficult. A physician can assist in determining the cause of the incontinence. Certain drugs, a urinary tract infection, an enlarged prostate, diabetes, or caffeine consumption can all contribute to incontinence. The incontinence may be treated by the physician in these circumstances. Other situations do not respond to treatment for incontinence.

Here are some tips to cope with incontinence:

- Limit fluids after 6 p.m. if problems happen at night. Give the person fresh fruit before bedtime instead of fluids if they are thirsty.
- Do not give the person caffeinated drinks such as regular coffee or tea.
- Remind the person to go to the bathroom every two to three hours and show them the way.
- Mark the bathroom door with a big sign that reads "Toilet" or "Bathroom."

- Make sure the person wears loose, comfortable clothing that is easy to remove.
- Use a stable toilet seat that is at a good height. A colorful toilet seat may help the person identify the toilet.
- Buy adult disposable briefs or underwear, washable bed protectors, and waterproof mattress covers to make accidents easier to clean up.
- Clean the skin after every leak or accident to avoid irritation and infection. Use a mild soap, rinse, and allow to air dry, if possible. After cleaning, apply moisturizer or petroleum jelly to protect the skin (Drebing et al., 2002; Voutilainen et al., 2006; Carpenter & Thompson, 2008).

8.4. KEEPING A PERSON WITH ALZHEIMER'S SAFE

Making sure the Alzheimer's patient is safe in the car, at home, and while taking medication is crucial. Enhancing safety can not only reduce the risk of accidents but also make an Alzheimer's patient feel more comfortable and enable them to continue living independently for a longer period of time.

8.4.1. Home Safety

0People suffering from Alzheimer's disease will eventually lose their ability to handle household chores. For instance, they might forget how to use the phone in an emergency or to turn off the oven or faucet. Alzheimer's patients may experience changes in their senses of taste, smell, touch, hearing, or vision. There are numerous things you can do as a caregiver to help an Alzheimer's patient feel safer in their home. Here are some tips:

- Mark the edges of steps with brightly colored tape so the person can see the steps as they go up or down stairs.
- Use brightly colored signs or simple pictures to label the bathroom, bedroom, and kitchen.
- Limit the size and number of mirrors in your home and be specific about where you put them. Mirror images may confuse a person with Alzheimer's.
- Set your water heater to 120°F to prevent burns.
- Label hot-water faucets red and cold-water faucets blue or write the words "hot" and "cold" near them.
- Put signs near the oven, toaster, iron, and other things that get hot. The sign could say, "Stop!" or "Don't Touch — Very Hot!" Be sure the sign is not so close that it could catch fire.
- Pad any sharp corners on your furniture or replace or remove furniture with sharp corners.
- Install automatic lights to light up the path to the bathroom when it's dark to help prevent falls.
- Use smoke detectors and natural gas detectors. People with Alzheimer's may not be able to smell smoke or an unlit gas stove.
- Check foods in the refrigerator often. Throw out any that have gone bad.
- Put away or lock up items such as toothpaste, lotions, shampoos, rubbing alcohol, soap, perfume, and laundry detergent pods. They may look and smell like food to a person

with Alzheimer's. Keep the Poison Control number by the phone, on speed dial, or in "favorites" in your phone contacts.

- Learn basic first aid in case the person gets sick or injured. Learn the Heimlich maneuver and CPR, and when to use each.

Examine each room of the house individually to spot any possible concerns and safety hazards. Address any hazards that are present right away, like loose stair railings and dim lighting, before focusing on other strategies to make sure the person will be as safe as possible at home.

- **Paying for Safety Updates:** If the thought of making changes seems too costly, you might be eligible for financial assistance to cover the cost of repairs and safety improvements to an older adult's home. For information on financial aid and discounts, get in touch with your state's housing finance agency, social services division, community development organizations, or the federal government.
- **Preventing Falls:** Seniors are more vulnerable to fractures from falls because their bones deteriorate with age. Because Alzheimer's patients frequently experience changes in depth perception—the capacity to determine how close or far away objects are—they are even more vulnerable to falling. For instance, an individual suffering from Alzheimer's disease might mistakenly perceive a shift in flooring—from carpet to tile, for instance—as a step, leading to falls or stumbles.

8.4.2. Medication Safety

It can be risky to mix certain medications and supplements or take prescriptions incorrectly. Elderly people may take numerous medications and frequently have several medical conditions. Alzheimer's patients frequently require assistance taking their medications. For advice on how to take medications safely, see the section below.

- Be aware of all prescription medications, over-the-counter drugs, vitamins, dietary supplements, and herbal remedies the person takes.
- Keep a list of all medications. Include the time the person should take each medicine, how much they should take, and the reason it was prescribed.
- Set phone alerts or use a chart, calendar, or timer to remind you when it is time for the person to take medicines.
- Use a weekly pill organizer to help keep track of the person's medications.
- If the person lives alone, call to remind them to take their medicine.
- Ask the doctor or pharmacist if the medication is available in liquid form if the patient has difficulty swallowing. In certain situations, crushing pills and combining them with food—like yogurt or applesauce—might help them dissolve more easily. Ask your doctor before attempting this, though, as some medications need to be taken whole in order for them to function properly.
- Speak with the doctor or pharmacist if the patient is having

uncomfortable side effects from a medication. They might be able to recommend an alternative medication or offer you alternative methods of managing side effects. Recall that the patient should never stop taking any medication without first consulting their physician.

8.4.3. Driving Safety

Vigilant drivers think clearly, act fast, and make wise decisions. Driving should be discontinued by someone who has Alzheimer's disease and is unable to perform these tasks. Someone could suffer harm or lose their life if the person with this illness continues to drive after it is no longer safe.

Signs that the person should stop driving include:

- New dents and scratches on the car
- Taking a long time to run a simple errand and not being able to explain why, which may indicate the person got lost
- Two or more traffic tickets, minor accidents, or increased car insurance premiums
- Comments from friends and neighbors about the person's driving
- Speeding or sudden lane changes
- Confusing the brake and gas pedals

Even though they might occasionally be able to drive safely, people with mild memory loss might find it difficult to respond quickly in an emergency situation. The person should cease driving if their reaction time becomes slower. Some individuals with memory loss might be able to drive short distances on neighborhood streets during the day, but they won't be able to drive on a freeway or at night safely. Limit the person's driving durations and distances if this is the case.

When driving becomes unsafe, the person will need to stop driving. Try these tips:

- Explain your concerns to the person.
- Take them to get a driving test or risk screening for older adults at your state's department of motor vehicles.
- Ask the person's doctor to tell the person to stop driving. The doctor can write, "Do not drive" on a prescription pad, and you can show this to the person. If necessary, hide the car keys, disable the car, move it out of sight, or consider selling it.

Learn about community-based services that facilitate the movement of individuals with disabilities. These could be low-cost or free buses, taxis and other private transportation services, or senior citizen carpools. Volunteers from various churches and community organizations transport seniors wherever they desire (Drebing et al., 2002; Voutilainen et al., 2006; Carpenter & Thompson, 2008).

8.5. ADAPTING ACTIVITIES FOR PEOPLE WITH ALZHEIMER'S DISEASE

Alzheimer's patients need to be active and engage in activities they enjoy. But as the illness progresses, they might find it harder to engage in the activities they once found enjoyable. They might struggle to make decisions or get things started. Discover how to modify tasks to make them simpler and more pleasurable. Start with these tips:

- Match the activity with what the person with Alzheimer's can do.
- Choose activities that can be fun for everyone.

- Help the person get started with the activity.
- Decide if they can do the activity alone or need help.
- Watch to see if the person gets frustrated.
- Make sure they feel successful and have fun.
- Let them simply watch if they seem to enjoy that more.

8.5.1. At Home

Try coming up with new daily activities to help keep people with Alzheimer's disease's days lively and interesting. Those who have Alzheimer's disease may find the following everyday activities enjoyable:

- **Cooking and Baking**: Gather materials, measure ingredients, mix and pour, or tell someone else how to prepare a recipe.
- **Exercise**: Take a walk together, use a stationary bike, use stretching bands, throw a soft ball or balloon back and forth, lift weights or household items such as soup cans, or follow along with exercise videos or programs for older adults.
- **Music and Dancing**: Play music, talk about the music and the artist, ask what the person with Alzheimer's was doing when the song was popular, sing or dance to well-known songs, or attend a concert or musical program in the community.
- **Pets**: Feed, groom, walk, or sit and hold a pet.
- **Gardening**: Take care of indoor or outdoor plants, plant flowers and vegetables, water the plants when needed, or talk about how much the plants are growing.
- **Household Chores**: Wash dishes, set the table, prepare food, sweep the floor, dust, sort mail and clip coupons, sort socks and fold laundry, or sort recycling materials or other items.
- **Visiting with Children**: Play a simple board game, read stories or books, visit family members who have small children, walk in the park or near schools, or go to school events. If you don't have children to visit, talk about fond memories from childhood.

8.5.2. Going Out

People with Alzheimer's may continue to enjoy the same kinds of trips they used to enjoy in the early stages of the disease. As long as you feel comfortable, keep going outside. Schedule activities for when the person is most productive. Make sure you don't spend too much time away from home so the Alzheimer's patient doesn't become overly fatigued. Your loved one might like to visit the following locations:

- Favorite restaurant
- Zoo or aquarium
- Park or nature trail
- Shopping mall
- Swimming pool (during a slow time of day at the pool)
- Museum, theater, or art exhibits for short trips

A senior center could be enjoyable for the Alzheimer's patient as well. Because it offers an activity for the person with Alzheimer's and a break for the caregiver, this kind of "going out" could also be categorized as respite care.

8.5.3. Eating Out

While dining out can be a pleasant change, there are drawbacks as well. The following advice can be helpful when dining out with an Alzheimer's patient:

- Choose a restaurant that the person likes, is quiet, and has quick service and understanding staff.
- Visit restaurants during "off hours" when they're less likely to be crowded.
- Consider going to the restaurant earlier in the day so the person is not too tired. Bring supplies such as utensils, a towel, and wipes that the person uses at home.
- At the restaurant, ask for a table near the bathroom.
- Help the person choose their meal, if needed. Read parts of the menu or show the person a picture of the food. Suggest food you know the person likes.
- Ask the server to fill glasses half full or leave the drinks for you to serve.
- Order some finger food or appetizers before the main meal to hold the attention of the person with Alzheimer's.

8.5.4. Traveling

It can be difficult to take an Alzheimer's patient on a trip because the condition can make the patient more anxious and confused. You might find the following advice useful.

- Before you leave, talk with the person's doctor about medicines to calm someone who gets upset while traveling.
- Think about the person's unique needs and preferences when choosing transportation, such as a plane, train, or car. Go with the option that provides the most comfort and least anxiety.
- Pack an extra set of clothing and items they enjoy looking at or holding in a carry-on bag.
- Talk to the person about travel plans in advance, but not too far ahead if traveling makes them feel anxious.
- Do not plan too many activities, and plan rest periods.
- During the trip, follow a routine like the one you use at home. Try to have the person eat, rest, and go to bed at the same time as usual.
- Be prepared to cut your visit short if necessary.
- In case the person with Alzheimer's gets lost, make sure they wear or have something with them that tells who they are, such as an ID bracelet.

8.5.5. Managing Finances

Having trouble handling money could be among the earliest obvious symptoms of dementia. A family member or close friend can offer support while honoring the person's independence by doing the following:

- **Watching for Signs of Money Problems:** A stack of unopened bills or difficulty paying for a purchase could be signs of financial difficulties. Have a discussion with the Alzheimer's patient about the resources that are available to assist with their costs. Restricting credit card use and giving the person small amounts of cash to keep on hand could aid in money management.

- **Setting Up Automated Bill Payments:** Make plans for automatic withdrawals from a bank account to cover their rent, utilities, and other costs. The timely and accurate payment of bills can be guaranteed by automated payments. Make sure all of the transactions are correct by reviewing the automated payments.
- **Protecting Against Scams or Fraud:** Put the person's number on the National Do Not Call Registry to reduce the likelihood of telemarketing schemes. If the person has a bank, credit card company, national credit bureau, or other credit monitoring service, think about enrolling them in fraud alerts. Get in touch with your local police department if you believe the person is a potential victim of fraud.

8.5.6. Spiritual Activities

Someone with Alzheimer's disease may feel more socially connected and able to recall happy memories if they are a part of a religious community. These suggestions should be useful:

- Involve the person in spiritual activities that they have known well. These might include worship services, religious or other readings, sacred music, prayer, meditation, and holiday rituals.
- Tell people in the preferred faith community about the person's Alzheimer's. Encourage them to talk with the person and show they still care.
- Find worship services or readings online if the person is more comfortable at home.

8.5.7. Holidays

The additional demands that holidays place on their time and energy can cause anxiety for those who care for those who have Alzheimer's. Here are some ideas to help make the holidays simpler:

- Understand that things will be different and be realistic about what you can do.
- Incorporate the holiday traditions of the person with Alzheimer's.
- Create a quiet space in case the individual with Alzheimer's needs a break. Have their favorite activities or calming music in that space.
- Ask friends and family to visit. Limit the number of visitors at any one time.
- Avoid crowds, changes in routine, and strange places that may make the person with Alzheimer's feel confused or nervous.
- Remember to enjoy yourself. Find time for the holiday activities you like to do. Ask a friend or family member to spend time with the person while you're out.

8.5.8. Visitors

People who are suffering from Alzheimer's value visitors. Even though they don't always recall the visitor's identity, they frequently appreciate their company. Remind visitors to:

- Be calm and speak in a normal tone. Don't use a loud voice or talk to the person as if they were a child.

- Consider bringing along some kind of activity to share with the person, such as a well-known book or photo album.
- Respect the person's personal space and don't get too close.
- Make eye contact and call the person by name to get their attention.
- Try not to take it personally if the person doesn't recognize them, is unkind, or gets angry.
- Avoid asking, "Don't you remember?" or correcting or arguing with the person if they say something wrong or unusual.
- Respond to the feelings that the person expresses. If the person seems confused, try to distract them by talking about something different instead of arguing (Drebing et al., 2002; Voutilainen et al., 2006; Carpenter & Thompson, 2008).

8.6. CAREGIVER SUPPORT AND SELF-CARE

One of the most crucial things you can do as a caregiver is to look after yourself. This could be enlisting the aid of friends and family, scheduling fun activities, using adult day care facilities, or receiving assistance from a nearby home health care provider. You may experience some relief if you follow these steps. It might also prevent you from getting sick or depressed. The following are some self-care strategies:

- Ask for help when you need it.
- Join a caregiver support group.
- Take breaks each day.
- Spend time with friends.
- Keep up with your hobbies and interests.
- Eat healthy foods.
- Exercise as often as you can.
- See your doctor on a regular basis.
- Keep your health, legal, and financial information up to date (Drebing et al., 2002; Voutilainen et al., 2006; Carpenter & Thompson, 2008).

8.6.1. Getting Help from Friends and Family

It's acceptable to request assistance and set aside time for oneself. Still, a lot of caregivers find it difficult to ask for help. It's possible that you think you should be able to handle everything on your own, that leaving the person with someone else is wrong, or that if you asked for help, none of your friends or family would be willing to lend a hand. Recalling that you are not alone and that it is acceptable to ask for assistance is crucial. Try utilizing some of these suggestions if you find it difficult to ask for help:

- Ask people to help out in specific ways, like making a meal, visiting the person, or taking the person out for a short time.

- Join a support group in person or online to share advice and understanding with other caregivers.
- Get help from home health care or adult day care services when you need it.
- Use national and local resources to find out how to pay for professional help or get respite care services.

Everyone occasionally requires assistance. Understand that an individual with Alzheimer's disease frequently requires more care than one person can give them alone. Think about "Plan B"—what you would do if you needed more help and your loved one's care requirements increased.

8.6.2. Your Emotional Health

It requires a lot of time and work to care for someone who has Alzheimer's. When the person you are taking care of loses their identity, becomes irate with you, or hurts your feelings, your job as a caregiver may become even more difficult. You might have intense feelings of discouragement, sadness, loneliness, frustration, confusion, or anger at times. These emotions are typical.

The following are some self-talk suggestions that may make you feel better:

- I'm doing the best I can.
- What I'm doing would be hard for anyone.
- I'm not perfect, and that's okay.
- I can't control everything that happens.
- Sometimes, I just need to do what works for right now.
- Even when I do everything I can think of, the person with Alzheimer's will still have problem behaviors because of the illness.
- I will enjoy the moments when we can be together in peace.
- I will seek help from professionals if caregiving becomes too much for me.

Attending a church, temple, or mosque can be a helpful coping mechanism for caregivers who are overwhelmed by the demands of their daily lives. For some, finding balance and tranquility comes from just believing that there are greater forces at play in the universe.

8.6.2.1. More Tips for Self-Care

- Understand that you may feel sad and hopeless about what's happening to the person you care for.
- Remember the reasons behind your decision to care for the person suffering from Alzheimer's. Consider whether you made this decision out of loyalty, love, a sense of moral or religious obligation, or a desire to support your family.
- Let yourself feel day-to-day "uplifts." These might include good feelings about the person you care for, support from other caring people, or time to spend on your own interests and hobbies.
- Experiment with relaxation techniques such as meditation, tai chi, or yoga. Download a smartphone app with guided meditations or relaxing music. Many of these apps are free (Figure 8.6).
- Find a connection to something "higher than yourself." This may be a belief in a higher power or religious faith or believing that something good comes from every life experience.

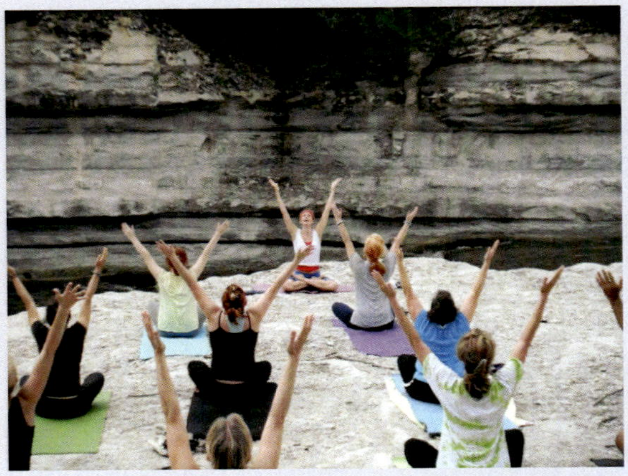

Figure 8.6. *Yoga.*

Source: https://upload.wikimedia.org/wikipedia/commons/6/65/Yoga4Love_Freedom_Gratitude.jpg.

8.6.3. Finding Help with At-Home Caregiving

When a person has Alzheimer's disease in its early stages, some caregivers require assistance. When the patient is nearing the end of their illness, other caregivers search for assistance. Asking for assistance when you need it is acceptable.

There is presently no known cure for Alzheimer's, despite the fact that some people can slow the progression of the disease and treat its symptoms with medications. This implies that as Alzheimer's progresses, symptoms like disorientation and memory loss will worsen and the patient will require more care.

It's a common misconception that asking for assistance indicates weakness or indifference, but this is untrue. Seeking assistance is a sign of strength. It indicates that you are aware of your boundaries and when to get help.

Many caregivers believe that creating a network of local support is essential to getting assistance. A caregiver support group, community and nonprofit organizations, family, friends, and religious groups can all be a part of your support network.

The services listed below can assist you in providing at-home care for a person with Alzheimer's, along with information on how to find out if they are available in your area.

8.6.3.1. Home Care Services

Home care services, which should not be confused with home health care services, provide you with an assistant to help you take care of an Alzheimer's patient at home. These assistants offer the person companionship and/or personal care. They help with everyday tasks like getting dressed and bathing. They can also offer light housekeeping, transportation, and errand assistance. Aides are typically not medical professionals, and they do not offer expert medical care. A home care aide may visit for a few hours or remain overnight and for the entire day.

- What to Know About Costs:
  - Home care services generally charge by the hour. Some services charge a flat rate for staying overnight.
  - Medicare and private health insurance may cover some home care costs, though nonmedical care is generally not covered. Check with your health care provider.
  - Long-term care insurance may cover personal care and housekeeping services.
- How to Find These Services:
  - Ask the person's doctor or another health care professional, family, and friends to recommend home care services in your area.
  - Use an online tool such as the

Home Care/ Hospice Agency Locator tool from the National Association for Home Care & Hospice.

8.6.3.2. Home Health Care Services

These are usually doctor-ordered, part-time medical services for a particular condition. A person recovering from surgery, an accident, or an illness may benefit from in-home nursing care. Also included in home health care may be speech, occupational, or physical therapy. The provider could come and go in a few hours or all day.

- What to Know About Costs
  - Home health services charge by the hour.
  - Medicare has limited coverage of home health service costs.
  - he services must be short-term and provided by agencies certified by Medicare. Medicaid also provides coverage for home health service costs, but these benefits vary by state.
  - Most private health insurance plans do not cover these costs.

You must pay all costs not covered by Medicare, Medicaid, or insurance.

- How to Find These Services
  - Ask the person's doctor or another health care professional for a list of agencies that serve your area.
  - Use the Home Health Compare tool.
  - Search the Eldercare Locator.

8.6.3.3. Meal Services

Meal services provide wholesome, nourishing meals to a person's home either every day or once a week. Many of these services can accommodate dietary restrictions and provide options for special diets. But the delivery personnel don't help with feeding the person or preparing meals at home.

- What to Know About Costs
  - In some cases, a person must qualify for the service based on certain guidelines. These can include age, mobility, and economic need.
  - Medicare does not generally cover meal delivery services, although under certain circumstances, it will provide this benefit for a short time. Medicaid may pay for some meal delivery services if the person is eligible.
  - Some meal delivery services do not require payment. Others charge a fee or accept donations.
- How to Find These Services
  - Use the Eldercare Locator.
  - Call Meals on Wheels America.
  - Some local governments provide low- or no-cost meals to older adults. Call or check their websites for details.
  - Your health care provider or local senior center may also be able to recommend a service.
  - There are many subscription services that deliver ready-to-eat meals and meal kits. These can be arranged online and generally involve a regular weekly or monthly charge.

8.6.3.4. Adult Day Care Services

Adult day care facilities can give caregivers at home a much-needed break. These programs offer senior citizens in a nearby facility a secure atmosphere staffed by trained personnel. In addition to meals, exercise, personal care, and basic medical services, adult day care centers may provide social activities. Some will arrange for transportation; contractors or facility employees may pick up the individual, drive them to day care, and then drop them off at home.

- What to Know About Costs
  - Adult day care tends to be less expensive than in-home or nursing home care.
  - Charges can be hourly or by the day.
  - Medicare will not pay for adult day care, but Medicaid and other government programs may provide coverage.
  - Most private health insurance plans don't cover the costs of adult day care. Some long-term care insurance plans pay a portion of the costs.

You must pay all costs not covered by a government program or insurance.

- How to Find These Services
  - Call the National Adult Day Services Association.
  - Use the Eldercare Locator.

8.6.3.5. Respite Care

An older adult receiving respite care can stay at home, in a healthcare facility, or at an adult day care center for a brief period of time. A few hours to several weeks may pass during the course of the care. With the help of these services, regular caregivers can take a break and go on a trip, relax, or see friends and family.

- What to Know About Costs
  - Respite services charge by the hour or by the number of days or weeks that services are provided.
  - For a person receiving hospice care, Medicare will cover most of the cost for up to five consecutive days of respite care in a hospital or skilled nursing facility. Medicaid also may provide payment assistance.
  - Most private health insurance plans do not cover these costs.
  - Some long-term care insurance plans may help pay for respite care.

You must pay all costs not covered by insurance or government programs.

- How to Find These Services
  - Visit the ARCH National Respite Locator.
  - Use the Eldercare Locator.

8.6.3.6. Geriatric Care Managers

Often a licensed nurse or social worker with expertise in geriatrics—the medical care of the elderly—a geriatric care manager is also known as an aging life care expert. In order to determine needs, create a care plan, and locate community resources, geriatric care managers collaborate with elderly individuals and their families. When a caregiver is located far away, they can be extremely useful.

- What to Know About Costs
  - The cost of an initial evaluation varies and may be expensive.
  - Geriatric care managers charge by the hour.
  - Medicare and Medicaid do not pay for this service.
  - Most private health insurance plans don't cover these costs. Long-term care insurance may pay for some of the costs; check the plan to see if it includes coverage.
  - Most people must pay for some or all of this service themselves.
- How to Find Them
  - Call the Aging Life Care Association.

8.6.3.7. Hospice Services

A person who is nearing the end of their life and is no longer receiving treatment to cure their serious illness can receive care from hospice services. Hospice services aim to provide the dying individual with the utmost comfort and pain relief, either in their residence or at a hospice facility. They assist the family by giving care for the dying. If a patient wants to resume receiving life-prolonging treatments, they are free to discontinue hospice services at any time.

- What to Know About Costs
  - Medicare, Medicaid, the Veterans Health Administration, or private insurance plans may cover all hospice costs.
  - If you receive hospice services in an assisted living facility or nursing home, you may need to pay for room and board. You must pay all costs not covered by insurance.
  - Some nonprofit organizations and hospice providers help cover hospice costs on a sliding scale for low-income patients.
  - Once you've chosen to receive hospice services, any medicines intended to treat Alzheimer's will not be covered.
- How to Find These Services
  - Call the National Association for Home Care & Hospice.
  - Call the Hospice Foundation of America.
  - Call the National Hospice and Palliative Care Organization (Drebing et al., 2002; Voutilainen et al., 2006; Carpenter & Thompson, 2008).

8.6.4. Choosing a Long-Term Care Facility

You might eventually be unable to provide the Alzheimer's patient with at-home care. You'll have to find that person a new place to live when that occurs. Although this choice may make you feel bad or angry, as the illness progresses, it might be the only or best way to give your loved one the best care possible. Keep in mind that a lot of caregivers get to this stage. You might feel more at ease if the individual is placed in a care facility.

It can be difficult to choose the best location even after you've determined that the person needs to move. Finding out about long-term care facilities, scheduling visits, and making the appropriate inquiries are all part of the process.

8.6.4.1. Different Types of Long-term Care Facilities

Facilities for long-term care are not one size fits all. Group homes, nursing homes, and assisted living facilities are examples of facility-based long-term care services.

While some facilities only provide lodging and housekeeping, many more also offer medical and personal care services. Numerous establishments provide specialized programs for those suffering from dementia, including Alzheimer's. Find out what kinds of places your family member will feel most at ease by learning about the various kinds of places.

- **Assisted Living Facilities:** In assisted living facilities, there are apartments or rooms. They are intended for those who don't require 24-hour care but might require some assistance with everyday duties. Certain assisted living communities have dedicated Alzheimer's units staffed by caregivers who monitor and assist those suffering from dementia. The cost of the room or apartment is your responsibility, and any additional costs for any special care might apply. A bigger company that provides care at different levels also owns some assisted living facilities. For instance, independent living and skilled nursing care are also provided in continuing care retirement communities.
- **Group Homes:** People who are unable to care for themselves can live in a group home. The house is home to multiple individuals receiving care. There is always at least one caregiver on the property. The staff prepares meals, assists with personal hygiene and medication administration, and attends to other needs of the residents. Even though these homes might not be regulated or inspected, they might nevertheless offer top-notch care.
- **Nursing Homes:** Individuals who are unable to care for themselves and may require continuous medical attention are placed in nursing homes. There are specialized Alzheimer's care units in some nursing homes. These units, which are frequently located in different parts of the building, are staffed by staff members who have received specialized training in dementia care. Certain apartments are designed to give the impression that the occupant is in their own home. They offer meals, medical attention, and special activities. State governments oversee and inspect nursing homes.

8.6.4.2. Visiting Facilities

Select a few locations to visit once you've determined what kind of long-term care facility best suits the needs of your loved one. Find out what locations people in your religious community, social workers, friends, and family recommend. Ask medical professionals about the best nursing homes they believe to offer quality care. To arrange a visit or to find out more, give the facilities a call. To fully grasp how the facility operates and handles its residents, visit at various times of the day and have a meeting with its leaders.

- Ask Yourself
  - How does the staff care for the residents?
  - Is the staff friendly?
  - Does the place feel comfortable?
  - How do the people who live there look? Are they clean and well cared for?
  - Are mealtimes comfortable for people living there?
  - Is the facility well-maintained? Does it look and smell clean?
  - Do staff members speak to residents with patience and respect?
- Ask the Staff
  - What activities are planned for residents?
  - How many staff members are at the facility? And how many of them are trained to provide medical care if needed?
  - How many residents in the facility have Alzheimer's?
  - Does the facility have a special unit for people with Alzheimer's? If so, what kinds of services does it provide? Are the costs for this unit different than the rest of the facility?
  - Is there a doctor who checks on residents on a regular basis? How often?
  - What is a typical day like for the person with Alzheimer's?
  - Is there a safe place for the person to go outside?
  - What is included in the fee? What services or options would cost extra?
  - How would my loved one get to medical appointments?

Speak to other caregivers who have a family member residing in the facility. Ask them about their impressions of the location. Inquire about the entire cost of the care. Since every facility is unique, you should ascertain whether any expenses will be covered by Medicare, Medicaid, or long-term care insurance.

If you're asked to sign a contract, ensure you understand what you are agreeing to.

8.6.4.3. Making Moving Day Easier

For the person with Alzheimer's disease and their carers, moving them into an assisted living community, group home, or nursing home is a significant adjustment. You might experience a wide range of feelings, such as relief, guilt, or even a sense of loss and sadness. You are allowed to feel all of these things. You might be able to plan for and cope with this significant change with the assistance of a social worker or a private service provider. It's critical to have assistance during this challenging phase.

Here are some things that may help:

- Know that the moving day can be very stressful.
- Talk to a social worker about your feelings about moving the person into a new place. Find out how to help the person with Alzheimer's adjust.
- Get to know the staff before the person moves into a facility.

- Talk with the staff about ways to make the change to the assisted living facility or nursing home go smoothly.
- Don't argue with the person with Alzheimer's about why they need to be there.

8.6.4.4. Be an Advocate

Check in with the person to see how they are doing after they have moved into their new residence. You probably know the person best as the caregiver. Seek indications that they might require additional care, be taking excessive or insufficient amounts of medication, or not be receiving the necessary attention. Establish a rapport with the employees so that you can collaborate as care partners.

8.6.4.5. Private Financing Options for Long-Term Care

There are a number of private payment options for long-term care in addition to government programs and personal funds. These include annuities, trusts, reverse mortgages, long-term care insurance, and certain life insurance policies. The optimal course of action for an individual is contingent upon various factors, such as their age, health, financial situation, and propensity to require medical attention (Drebing et al., 2002; Voutilainen et al., 2006; Carpenter & Thompson, 2008).

8.6.5. Paying for Care

The way that individuals pay for long-term care, whether it is received at home, in a hospital, assisted living community, or nursing home, is determined by their financial circumstances and the services they require. Some people think that their long-term care needs will be covered by their current health or disability insurance, but the majority of these policies have little to no long-term care benefits. People frequently have to rely on a range of funding sources, such as private financing options, government programs, and personal funds.

8.6.5.1. Personal Funds (Out-of-Pocket Expenses)

At first, personal care and other services, like transportation, might be given without charge by family and friends. However, when a person's needs grow, they might require paid services.

In addition, a large number of senior citizens pay for their own meals, adult day care programs, and other community-based services rendered by nonprofit organizations and local governments. These programs enable them to stay in their houses.

In assisted living facilities and continuing care retirement communities, professional care is almost always paid for out of pocket; however, in certain states, Medicaid may reimburse some costs for individuals who meet certain health and financial requirements.

8.6.5.2. Government Programs

Government health care benefits may be available to older adults. Caregivers can support older adults by helping them apply for aid when necessary and by learning more about potential financial resources.

Assistance with health care-related expenses is offered by a number of federal and state programs. The benefits and qualifying standards of these programs are subject to change over time, and some benefits are state-specific. The most up-to-date information can be obtained by directly contacting each program.

- **Medicare:** People 65 years of age and older, as well as those under 65 with certain disabilities and serious medical conditions, can receive some financial assistance for medical costs through this federal government health insurance program. Hospital stays, physician visits, some home health care, hospice care, and immunizations are among the preventive services that are covered. Long-term care or assisted living are not covered by the program. Part A (hospital insurance), Part B (medical insurance), and Part D (drug coverage) are the components of Medicare. A different way to get Part A and Part B coverage is through Medicare Advantage.

- **Medicaid:** Medicaid is a state-federal program designed for low-income individuals. For those who fit the eligibility criteria and have a low income, this program pays for certain long-term care options as well as medical expenses. States differ in terms of covered services and eligibility.
- **Program of All-Inclusive Care for the Elderly (PACE):** PACE, a program that combines Medicare and Medicaid, is available in some states and offers services and care to individuals who might otherwise require it in a nursing home. PACE provides long-term care, social services, and medical cost coverage. For an individual with Alzheimer's, it might cover all or part of their long-term care expenses. For the majority of qualifying individuals, PACE allows them to stay in their homes rather than entering long-term care facilities. A group of medical specialists provides participants with coordinated care.

You must ascertain whether the individual in need of care is eligible for PACE and whether a PACE program exists in your area. A monthly fee might apply. Only a few states and specific areas within those states offer PACE.

- **Social Security Administration Programs:** People with disabilities can receive financial aid through the Social Security Disability Insurance (SSDI) and Supplemental Security Income (SSI) programs. SSDI is for individuals who meet the Social Security Administration's definition of disability and are under 65. In order to be eligible, you have to demonstrate that:
  - You worked in a job covered by Social Security.
  - You are unable to work because of your medical condition.
  - Your medical condition will last at least a year or is expected to result in death.

An SSDI application's processing period may last three to five months. To help people with some serious medical conditions, like early-onset Alzheimer's and other forms of dementia, receive disability benefits more quickly, Social Security offers what are known as "compassionate allowances."

Another program that pays monthly benefits to disabled adults 65 years of age and older is called SSI. Your resources and income must be below certain thresholds in order to be eligible.

- **State Health Insurance Assistance Program (SHIP):** One-on-one counseling and assistance with Medicaid, Medicare, and Medicare supplemental insurance (Medigap) is provided by SHIP, a nationwide program available in every state.

Navigating eligibility, coverage, appeals, out-of-pocket expenses, and your family's particular needs can be made easier with SHIP's assistance.

- **Department of Veterans Affairs:** For certain veterans, the US Department of Veterans Affairs (VA) pays for long-term care in a facility or at home. Find out from the VA or contact the closest VA medical facility if your loved one qualifies for benefits for veterans. A waiting list for VA nursing homes might exist.
- **National Council on Aging (NCOA):** BenefitsCheckUp is a free service offered by the private National Council on Aging. This service can assist you in locating state and federal assistance programs for senior citizens. You can view a list of potential benefit programs to look into after giving some basic information about the person in need of care. Prescription medication, utilities, housing, meal programs, and legal services can all be paid for with the assistance of these programs. Using this service does not require you to give your name, address, or Social Security number.

8.6.5.3. Can I Get Paid to Take Care of My Family Member with Alzheimer's?

Family caregivers give up a lot to take care of ailing, elderly, or disabled family members. Some even left their jobs to provide full-time care for the individual. Giving care involves a lot of expenses, such as paying for bills, purchasing necessities for the home, and covering travel costs. Caregivers may face a heavy financial burden as a result of these expenses.

Family caregivers are eligible for financial assistance from many states; however, each state has its own set of regulations, qualifications, and funding sources. Medicaid is the most popular form of assistance, providing a range of state-based programs to qualified individuals based on their income or disability. Medicaid personal care services, adult foster care, and home and community-based services are some of these programs. To find out more, get in touch with your state's Medicaid office. Home care is typically covered by long-term care insurance. Different policies apply to who can provide that care, though. Sometimes the only payment for long-term care is for a professional service. In other situations, the policy will cover the cost of having a family member give care. To find out the specifics of your policy, get in touch with your long-term care insurance provider.

8.6.6. Tips for Finding and Hiring In-Home Care Services

There are excellent care services and bad care services. Request testimonials from customers of the providers' services. Look up any complaints that have been made about a service, if you can. You can get in touch with the local Better Business Bureau or inquire with the county, city, or state organizations that oversee health care.

Get as much information as you can about the services, costs, terms, and limitations of a care provider before signing an agreement (Drebing et al., 2002; Voutilainen et al., 2006; Carpenter & Thompson, 2008).

8.7. CARING FOR A PERSON WITH LATE-STAGE ALZHEIMER'S

Caretakers may face new difficulties as the disease progresses. At this point, the Alzheimer's patient might not be able to move or speak, and they might need 24-hour care. Caregiving suggestions are provided in this section to assist during this time (Figure 8.7).

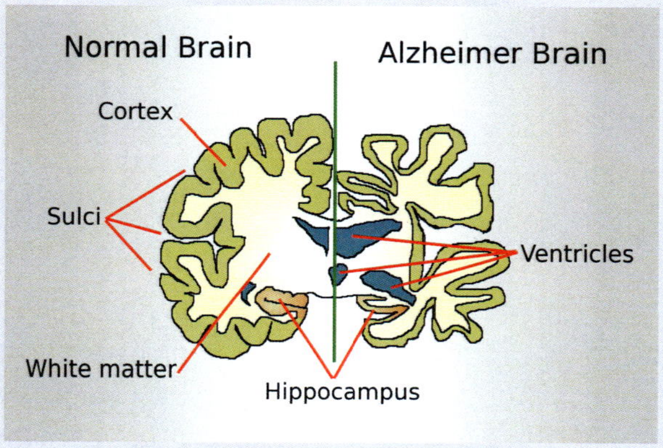

Figure 8.7. *Care in the last stages of Alzheimer's.*

Source: https://en.wikipedia.org/wiki/File:Brain-ALZH.png.

Daily caregiving may become even more difficult as a person enters the later stages of Alzheimer's. This section offers coping mechanisms for the changes that occur in late-stage Alzheimer's disease.

8.7.1. When the Person with Alzheimer's Can't Move

Ask your doctor, the hospice or palliative care team, or other caregivers for a referral or information on resources if the person with Alzheimer's is unable to move around independently. You can learn safe movement techniques for the individual, like shifting their position in bed or a chair, from a physical or occupational therapist, home health aide, or nurse.

Additionally, a physical therapist can demonstrate range-of-motion exercises for you to use on the patient. You move and bend the person's arms or legs one at a time, multiple times a day, while performing these exercises. Stiffness in the arms, hands, and legs is avoided through movement. Additionally, it guards against bedsores, which are open sores that can appear from prolonged standing.

- How to Make Someone with Late-Stage Alzheimer's More Comfortable
  - Invest in pressure sore-preventing wedge-shaped seat cushions and special mattresses. These can be purchased online, at a pharmacy, or from a medical supply company. Find out how to use them optimally from the home health aide, nurse, or physical therapist.
  - Move the person to a different position at least every two hours.
  - Use a lap board to rest the person's arms and support the upper body when they are sitting up.
  - Give the person something to hold, such as a washcloth, while being moved. The person will be less likely to grab onto you or the furniture. If they are weak on one side, stand on the weak side to help the person change positions.
- To Avoid Hurting Yourself When Moving Someone with Alzheimer's
  - When moving or lifting someone, be aware of your limitations and avoid overextending yourself. Additionally, pay attention

to how you hold your body. Make sure you have any extra supports in place before moving the person, such as a back brace.

- Bend at the knees and then straighten up by using your thigh muscles, not your back.
- Keep your back straight, and don't bend at the waist.
- Hold the person as close to you as possible to avoid reaching away from your body.
- Place one foot in front of the other, or space your feet comfortably apart for a wide base of support.
- Take small steps to move the person from one seat to another. Don't twist your body (Drebing et al., 2002; Voutilainen et al., 2006; Carpenter & Thompson, 2008).

8.7.2. How to Make Sure the Person Eats Well

Alzheimer's patients frequently lose interest in food. This could begin in the early phases of the illness and get worse with time. By cooking food according to the guidelines on page 25 and utilizing the following advice, you can assist the person with late-stage Alzheimer's in eating healthily:

- Give the person small amounts of food at a time.
- Describe to them the food they are eating.
- Sit to the side of the person while helping them eat because sitting in front may be intimidating.
- Encourage eating by switching between a bite of the meal and a bite of something sweet.
- Make sure the person has swallowed before introducing more food. Sometimes food can be pocketed in the cheeks.
- Serve the patient high-calorie, healthful foods and beverages, like protein shakes or meals made with good fats. Consult the patient's physician about taking a dietary supplement if they are still not receiving enough calories.
- Ask the doctor whether the person would benefit from a multivitamin — a tablet, capsule, powder, liquid, or injection that adds vitamins, minerals, and other important nutrients to a person's diet.

It can be very taxing to assist an Alzheimer's patient with eating. You can find this task a little easier if you plan your meals in advance and prepare the food. But keep in mind that persons suffering from Alzheimer's disease might feel more like eating at other times and not eat much during certain periods. When the food is ready to be served, the person might not be hungry, no matter how carefully you prepare.

8.7.3. What to Do About Swallowing Problems

The likelihood of choking increases when a person has Alzheimer's disease because they may find it difficult to chew and swallow food. Food particles may end up in the person's lungs if they choke on a food bite. Pneumonia may result from this, and pneumonia can be fatal.

The following suggestions may help with swallowing:

- When preparing liquid meals and beverages, think about adding a thickener like maltodextrin, xanthan gum, or corn starch. Liquids that are thicker pass down the throat more gradually, reducing the possibility of the fluid entering the lungs. Most pharmacies sell thickening agents, both generic and brand-name.

- Cut food into small pieces and make sure the food is soft enough for the person to eat.
- Grind or blend food to make it easier to eat.
- Offer soft foods, such as yogurt, applesauce, mashed avocado, sweet potatoes, and bananas.
- Don't use a straw, which may cause more swallowing problems. Instead, have the person drink small sips from a cup.
- Offer drinks of different temperatures — warm, cold, and room temperature — to see which might be easiest for the person to drink.
- Don't hurry the person. Give them time to chew and swallow each mouthful before taking another bite.
- Encourage the person to feed themselves as much as possible during meals. If the person needs support, try using overhand, underhand, or direct hand feeding approaches.
- Don't feed a person who is drowsy or lying down. They should be in an upright, seated position during the meal and for at least 20 minutes after the meal.
- Say "swallow" to remind the person to swallow.

Speak with the patient's physician or the home health care team if you believe the person with Alzheimer's may have difficulty swallowing. Physicians can assess a patient's ability to swallow and offer expert guidance on how to lower the risk of choking.

8.7.4. Body Jerking

Myoclonus, which is characterized by abrupt muscle spasms or jerks in the arms, legs, or entire body, can occur in some Alzheimer's patients. Although it may appear like a seizure, the person is not unconscious. Inform the physician immediately if you observe any myoclonus symptoms. To help with symptom relief, the doctor may recommend one or more medications.

8.7.5. Skin Problems

People frequently get sores or other skin problems if they stop walking or remain still for an extended period of time. Skin issues can cause great discomfort to a person nearing the end of their life. Creams and ointments that act as barriers can keep someone's skin hydrated and clean. In addition to protecting the skin, massaging the area with an unscented lotion can ease discomfort and provide comfort. You can also try these tips:

- Apply a balm or petroleum jelly to the lips.
- Gently dab an eye cream or gel around the eyes.
- Try placing a damp cloth over the person's closed eyes.

- If the inside of the mouth seems dry, giving ice chips (if the person is conscious) or wiping the inside of the person's mouth with a damp cloth, cotton ball, or specially treated swab might help.

Constant pressure from sitting or lying down can cause painful bedsores, also known as pressure ulcers, on delicate skin. The skin becomes discolored or darker when a bedsore initially appears. Keep a close eye out for these discolored areas, particularly on the back of the head, heels, hips, and lower back. Consult the patient's physician for advice if you notice any sores or redness. Making an early appointment with a physician can help avert more severe skin damage. To help prevent skin or pressure sores, you can:

- Move the person at least every two hours if they are sitting up.
- Move the person at least every hour if they are lying down.
- Put foam, gel, air, or a water pad on top of the mattress. The pad should be comfortable and fit snugly around the person's body.

28.7.6. Foot Care

The Alzheimer's patient must take good care of their feet. If they are unable to, you will have to assist them. Here's what to do:

- Soak the person's feet in warm water; wash the feet with a mild soap; and check for cuts, corns, and calluses.
- Put lotion on the feet so that the skin doesn't become dry and cracked.
- Cut or file their toenails.
- Talk to a foot care doctor, call a podiatrist if the person has diabetes or sores on the feet (Drebing et al., 2002; Voutilainen et al., 2006; Carpenter & Thompson, 2008).

A Closer Look

End-of-Life Care

Planning for the end of a person's life and knowing what to expect can make this time easier for everyone. Often, hospice and palliative care programs can help coordinate care, get referrals, and provide additional resources.

Both palliative care and hospice care are intended to improve the quality of life for the patient and their family. Palliative care is specialized medical care for people living with a serious illness, including Alzheimer's that provides relief from the symptoms and stress of the illness. This type of care can be helpful at any stage of illness. Hospice care is designed to relieve symptoms, such as pain and discomfort, at the end of life. Palliative or hospice care teams may be able to help identify when someone with dementia is in the last days or weeks of life.

In the final stages of Alzheimer's, a person may not be able to tell you that they are in pain. Instead, people with Alzheimer's may express pain with groans or sighs and may grimace when touched. They may become upset or aggressive and may sit in unusual positions to guard the part of their body that hurts. If you think the person with Alzheimer's is in pain, talk with the health care team about pain medication and other forms of pain management.

You may find it hard to provide emotional or spiritual comfort at this stage of the disease. However, even in the advanced stages of dementia, a person may benefit from such connections. Try telling the person a story or showing those photos. Being touched or massaged can also be soothing. Listening to music, white noise, or sounds from nature seems to relax some people and lessen agitation. Just being present can be calming to the person.

Caring for people with Alzheimer's or another form of dementia at the end of life can be physically and emotionally demanding.

When a person with Alzheimer's dies, their caregivers can experience a range of emotions. These may include sadness, loss of purpose, guilt, and relief. It is important to realize such feelings are normal.

Hospice care experts can provide support to family caregivers near the end of life as well as help with their grief (Drebing et al., 2002; Voutilainen et al., 2006; Carpenter & Thompson, 2008).

SUMMARY

- Care is a multidimensional phenomenon, a cultural experience and a challenging domain in medical sciences, especially when it involves care for patients in nursing homes who have Alzheimer's disease (AD) with cognitive deficits and behavioral disturbances.
- Alzheimer's is a brain disorder that causes large numbers of nerve cells to not work properly. It's the most common form of dementia, a term used to describe conditions that cause people to lose their ability to remember, think, and use good judgment.
- Advance care planning involves discussing and preparing for decisions about the person's medical care if they become seriously ill or unable to communicate their wishes. Having meaningful conversations with the person living with Alzheimer's to learn about their values and preferences is the most important part of advance care planning.
- The ability to perform daily tasks, such as bathing, dressing, and eating, changes when a person has Alzheimer's. During the earlier stages of the disease, they may remain relatively independent, but there will come a point when they need more help with daily activities. For a caregiver, the main goal is to find the balance of letting the person be as independent as possible while providing support when needed.
- Physical activity helps keep the muscles, joints, and heart of someone with Alzheimer's in good shape. Exercise can also improve mood and sleep. Check with their doctor before starting a new fitness routine.
- Meal services deliver healthy, nutritious meals to a person's home on a daily or weekly basis. Many of these services offer options for special diets and can handle dietary restrictions. However, the delivery staff do not assist with making meals at home or feeding the person.
- Adult day care services can provide a much needed break for caregivers at home. These programs provide a safe environment for older adults with trained staff in a nearby facility. An adult day care center may offer social activities, exercise, meals, personal care, and basic health care services.
- Respite services provide short-term care for an older adult at home, in a health care facility, or at an adult day care center. The care may last anywhere from a few hours to several weeks at a time. These services provide regular caregivers with a break to rest, travel, or spend time with other family and friends.
- A geriatric care manager, also called an aging life care expert, is usually a licensed nurse or social worker who specializes in geriatrics, which is health care for older adults. Geriatric care managers work with older adults and their families to identify needs, make a care plan, and find services in the community. They can be especially helpful when a caregiver lives far away.
- Hospice services provide care for a person who is near the end of life and no longer receiving treatment to cure their serious illness. Hospice services keep the person who is dying as comfortable and pain-free as possible in the person's home or a hospice facility.

They also support the family by providing end-of-life care. A person can stop hospice services at any time if they wish to receive life-prolonging treatments again.

- The last stages of Alzheimer's can bring different challenges for caregivers. In this stage, the person with Alzheimer's may not be able to move or talk and may require around-the-clock care.

REFERENCES

1. Ayalon, L., & Huyck, M. H. (2001). Latino caregivers of relatives with Alzheimer's disease. *Clinical Gerontologist, 24*(3, 4), 93–106.
2. Bakhtiari, S., Mohammadzadeh, S., & Moshtagh, Z. (2009). Obstacles in nurse-elderly patient relationship from the patients' point of view. *Iranian Journal of Nursing and Midwifery Research, 14*(2), 77–82.
3. Carpenter, J., & Thompson, S. A. (2008). CNAs' experiences in the nursing home: "It's in my soul." *Journal of Gerontological Nursing, 34*(9), 25–32.
4. Chang, E. M., Hancock, K. M., Johnson, A., Daly, J., & Jackson, D. (2005). Role stress in nurses: Review of related factors and strategies for moving forward. *Nursing & Health Sciences, 7*(1), 57–65.
5. De Geest, G. (2003). The relation between the perceived role of family and the behavior of the person with dementia. *American Journal of Alzheimer's Disease and Other Dementias, 18*(3), 181–187.
6. Drebing, C., McCarty, E. F., & Lombardo, N. B. (2002). Professional caregivers for patients with dementia: Predictors of job and career commitment. *American Journal of Alzheimer's Disease and Other Dementias, 17*(6), 357–366.
7. Fallahi Khoshknab, M., & Mazaheri, K. (2009). *Living with Alzheimer*. Tehran: Resanehaie Takhasosi.
8. Fjelltun, A. M., Henriksen, N., Norberg, A., Gilje, F., & Normann, H. K. (2009). Functional levels and nurse workload of elderly awaiting nursing home placement and nursing home residents: A comparative study. *Scandinavian Journal of Caring Sciences, 23*(4), 736–747.
9. Kane, M. N. (2002). Awareness of ageism, motivation, and countertransference in the care of elders with Alzheimer's disease. *American Journal of Alzheimer's Disease and Other Dementias, 17*(2), 101–109.
10. Lancioni, G. E., Singh, N. N., O'Reilly, M. F., Sigafoos, J., Pangrazio, M. T., Megna, M., et al. (2009). Persons with moderate Alzheimer's disease improve activities and mood via instruction technology. *American Journal of Alzheimer's Disease and Other Dementias, 24*(3), 246–257.
11. Lynn-McHale, D. J., & Deatrick, J. A. (2000). Trust between family and health care provider. *Journal of Family Nursing, 6*(3), 210–230.
12. McGoldrick, M., Giordano, J., & Garcia-Preto, N. (2005). *Ethnicity and Family Therapy*. New York: Guilford Press.
13. Morgan, D. G., Semchuk, K. M., Stewart, N. J., & D'Arcy, C. (2002). Job strain among staff of rural nursing homes: A comparison of nurses, aides, and activity workers. *Journal of Nursing Administration, 32*(3), 152–161.

14. Norbergh, K. G., Helin, Y., Dahl, A., Hellzén, O., & Asplund, K. (2006). Nurses' attitudes towards people with dementia: The semantic differential technique. *Nursing Ethics, 13*(3), 264–274.

15. Polit, D. F., Beck, C. T., & Hungler, B. P. (2001). *Essentials of Nursing Research* (5th ed.). Philadelphia: Lippincott.

16. Sanders, S., Ott, C. H., Kelber, S. T., & Noonan, P. (2008). The experience of high levels of grief in caregivers of persons with Alzheimer's disease and related dementia. *Death Studies, 32*(6), 495–523.

17. Schermer, M. (2003). In search of 'the good life' for demented elderly. *Medicine, Health Care and Philosophy, 6*(1), 35–44.

18. Smith, G. E., Kokmen, E., & O'Brien, P. C. (2000). Risk factors for nursing home placement in a population-based dementia cohort. *Journal of the American Geriatrics Society, 48*(5), 519–525.

19. Stolley, J. M., Reed, D., & Buckwalter, K. C. (2002). Caregiving appraisal and interventions based on the progressively lowered stress threshold model. *American Journal of Alzheimer's Disease and Other Dementias, 17*(2), 110–120.

20. Voutilainen, P., Backman, K., Isola, A., & Laukkala, H. (2006). Family members' perceptions of the quality of long-term care. *Clinical Nursing Research, 15*(2), 135–149.

21. Yaffe, K., Fox, P., Newcomer, R., Sands, L., Lindquist, K., Dane, K., et al. (2002). Patient and caregiver characteristics and nursing home placement in patients with dementia. *JAMA, 287*(16), 2090–2097.

22. Ying, L., Kunaviktikul, W., & Tonmukayakul, O. (2007). Nursing competency and organizational climate as perceived by staff nurses in a Chinese university hospital. *Nursing & Health Sciences, 9*, 221–227.

23. Zimmerman, S., Williams, C. S., Reed, P. S., Boustani, M., Preisser, J. S., Heck, E., & Sloane, P. D. (2005). Attitudes, stress, and satisfaction of staff who care for residents with dementia. *The Gerontologist, 45*, 96–105.

Chapter 9

EPIDEMIOLOGIC AND BIOLOGIC MARKERS FOR ALZHEIMER'S DISEASE

Contents

Introduction 309
9.1. Epidemiology of Alzheimer's Disease 311
9.2. Blood-Based Biomarkers for Alzheimer's Disease 312
9.3. Alzheimer's Disease Biomarker Profiling in a Memory Clinic Cohort Without Common Comorbidities 322
Summary 342
References 342

INTRODUCTION

Epidemiologic studies have provided valuable insights into the risk factors associated with Alzheimer's disease (AD). Age remains the strongest risk factor, with prevalence increasing dramatically in individuals over 65. Gender also plays a role, with women having a higher likelihood of developing AD compared to men. Genetics significantly influence susceptibility, with mutations in genes like APP, PSEN1, and PSEN2 contributing to familial forms of the disease. Additionally, the presence of the APOE ε4 allele increases the risk of developing AD, although not everyone with this allele will develop the condition. Biologically, AD is characterized by the accumulation of amyloid-beta plaques and tau tangles in the brain, leading to neuronal damage and cognitive decline. Biomarkers such as amyloid-beta and tau proteins in cerebrospinal fluid or detected through imaging techniques like positron emission tomography (PET) can aid in the early detection and monitoring of AD progression. Understanding both epidemiologic and biologic markers is crucial for advancing diagnostic methods and developing targeted interventions for this debilitating neurodegenerative disease.

Orientation and Directional Terms

Term	Definition	Illustration
Hypertension	Hypertension (high blood pressure) is when the pressure in your blood vessels is too high (140/90 mmHg or higher). It is common but can be serious if not treated. People with high blood pressure may not feel symptoms. The only way to know is to get your blood pressure checked.	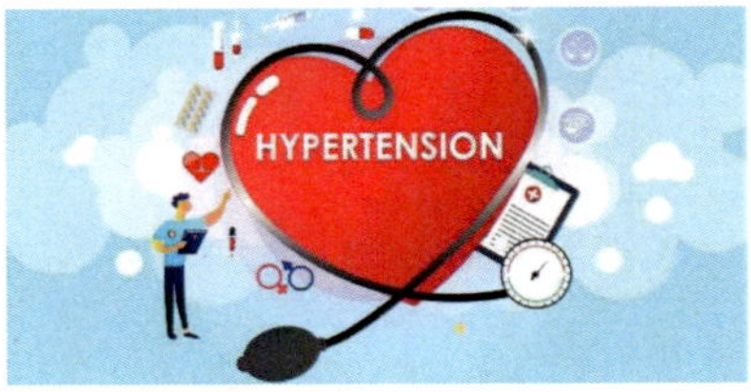
Positron Emission Tomography	Positron emission tomography (PET) is a type of nuclear medicine procedure that measures the metabolic activity of the cells of body tissues.	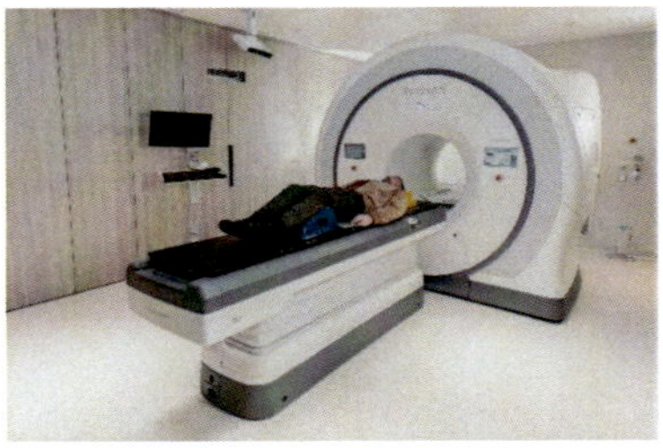
Apolipoprotein E4	APOE4 is the strongest risk factor gene for Alzheimer's disease, although inheriting APOE4 does not mean a person will definitely develop the disease. The study suggests that dementia may be caused by lipid imbalances in brain cells.	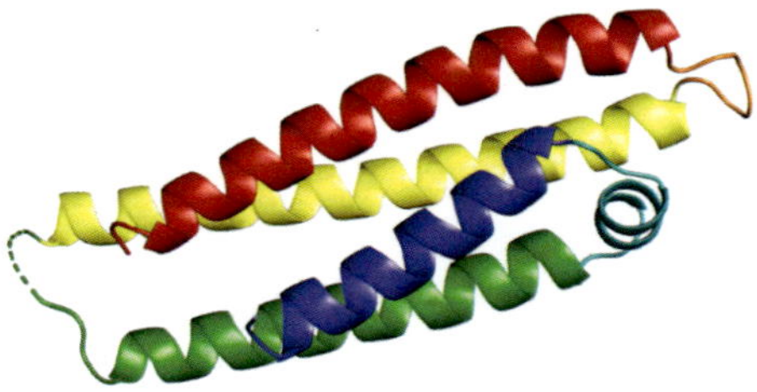
Vascular Endothelial Growth Factor (VEGF)	Vascular endothelial growth factor (VEGF) represents a growth factor with important pro-angiogenic activity, having a mitogenic and an anti-apoptotic effect on endothelial cells, increasing the vascular permeability, promoting cell migration, etc.	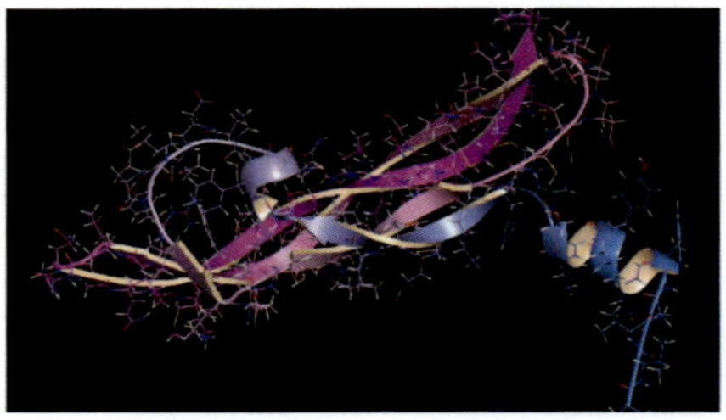
Medial Temporal Lobe (MTL)	The medial temporal lobe (MTL) is a brain region that is known to mediate functions of episodic memory and learning. It is an area with extensive bi-directional connections to the rest of the brain, and thus often thought to integrate complex sets of information from multiple sensory modalities.	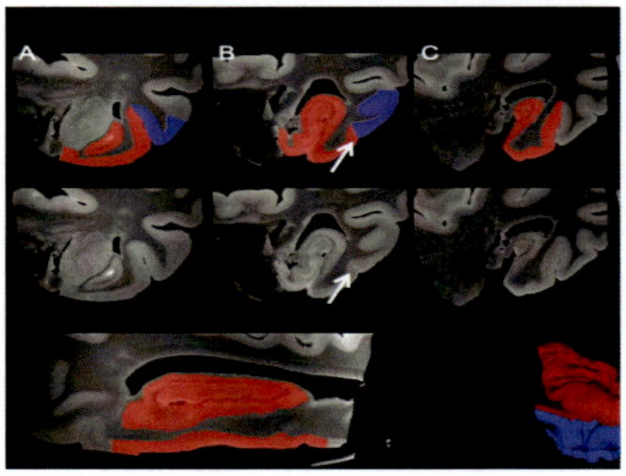

9.1. EPIDEMIOLOGY OF ALZHEIMER'S DISEASE

Alzheimer's disease is a neuropsychological condition marked by progressive neuronal degeneration leading to mental impairment and dementia. The illness is characterized by mild cognitive impairment symptoms that progress to total memory loss, mental confusion, poor decision-making, and increased dependency. Even the most ordinary activities in their lives are forgotten by disease-affected patients. As the illness worsens, performing any kind of task gets harder. Apathy and social disengagement are additional behavioral symptoms that Alzheimer's patients experience. They also experience bipolar mood swings and depression. There are various classifications for Alzheimer's disease, including late-onset and early-onset, severe, moderate, and mild, as well as inflammatory, non-inflammatory, and cortical responses. The development of beta-amyloid protein plaques in the brain and the formation of neurofibrillary tangles of a protein called "tau," which is essential to the brain's normal function, are the hallmarks of Alzheimer's disease. Cell death ultimately follows from these alterations that cause a loss of cell-to-cell communication. The Hippocampus area of the brain is the primary target of Alzheimer's disease (Hansson, 2021; Scheltens et al., 2021).

9.1.1. Incidence and Distribution

Approximately 47 million people worldwide suffered from dementia in 2016. 70% of dementia cases are caused by Alzheimer's disease, making it the most prevalent dementia cause. Few patients with Alzheimer's have early onset in their 40s or 50s, and the majority of patients have late onset, occurring at 65 years of age or later. The geographic distribution of Alzheimer's disease exhibits a slight skew. The highest rates of Alzheimer's are found in North America and western Europe, with Western-Pacific, China, and Latin America following. Except for the fact that Alzheimer's disease is more common in Latin America than in western European nations, the incidence rates also paint a similar picture. Approximately 5.7 million Americans suffer from Alzheimer's disease. It ranks as the sixth most common cause of death in the US, and between 2000 and 2015, the number of deaths increased by 123%.

9.1.2. Epidemiological Factors

Alzheimer's is believed to be the culmination of several different types of risk factors:

- Genetic Risk Factors

The majority of early-onset Alzheimer's cases show mutations in three different genes: APP, PSEN1, and PSEN2. Particularly in non-Hispanic White people, a mutation in the Apolipoprotein E4 (ApoE4) gene is primarily linked to late-onset Alzheimer's. In people of different ethnicities, the relationship between ApoE4 and Alzheimer's disease was not always direct. Though no conclusive evidence has been found, there may be a correlation between Alzheimer's and numerous other genes.

- Non-Genetic Factors

An important risk factor for Alzheimer's is age. Actually, the primary cause of Alzheimer's disease is aging. Because they typically live longer than men, women are more likely than men to develop Alzheimer's disease. In certain studies, it has been discovered that hypertension and Alzheimer's disease coexist. It is generally accepted that elevated blood pressure may compromise the blood-brain barrier's integrity, which could allow hazardous substrates to enter the brain and cause neuronal damage and cognitive decline. Alzheimer's disease also has cerebrovascular disease as a risk factor. Vasculopathy and ischemic infarcts in the brain are very dangerous. These have been linked to a higher risk of Alzheimer's. The mechanism is still unknown, though.

Diabetes type 2 doubles the risk of Alzheimer's disease. Although the exact cause is unknown, inflammation in the brain as a result of glucose hypometabolism is thought to be the cause. Moreover, there is a strong correlation between elevated plasma lipid levels and a higher risk of Alzheimer's. This risk is further supported by a genetic connection involving lipid metabolism-related gene mutations.

An individual's body weight may also pose a risk. Both a high and a low body weight are thought to increase the likelihood of Alzheimer's later in life. Alzheimer's disease can be influenced by physical activity. It is commonly known that physical activity can improve cognitive and logical thinking abilities by upregulating a number of neurotransmitters in the brain. Therefore, engaging in physical activity may lower the chance that the illness will manifest and worsen. Studies have connected memory loss symptoms to metabolic syndrome. Conversely, past records suggest that a traumatic brain injury can raise the risk of developing Alzheimer's and other dementias.

The disease may also arise as a result of one's diet. The Mediterranean-DASH Intervention for Neurodegenerative Delay (MIND) diet is advised for patients with Alzheimer's disease in order to slow down the disease's progression and significantly reduce the risk of Alzheimer's disease. This includes, among other things, eating berries, nuts, beans, wine, whole grain carbohydrates, and green leafy vegetables. Conversely, the diet suggests staying away from processed foods, dairy products, and sweets. Alzheimer's disease risk may also rise as a result of pollution exposure. Particulate matter is a major cause of Alzheimer's disease, including magnetite and nickel. When combined with other risk factors, air pollution increases the risk of Alzheimer's disease even though its role as a direct causative agent has not been established. Although most people agree that smoking is unhealthy and should be avoided, there is conflicting evidence regarding the relationship between smoking and the onset of Alzheimer's disease. Last but not least, behavioral and observational research show that people who engage in activities like reading, playing games, and learning new things have a considerable protective advantage against dementia (Hansson, 2021; Scheltens et al., 2021).

9.2. BLOOD-BASED BIOMARKERS FOR ALZHEIMER'S DISEASE

In clinical trials, biomarkers that accurately reflect the pathology of Alzheimer's disease during life are a crucial component of the inclusion criteria. In clinical practice, they are also crucial for diagnosis, especially with the advent of disease-modifying treatments. The traditional pathophysiological indicators of Alzheimer's disease, such as tau, amyloid β [Aβ], and neurodegeneration, can presently be identified through CSF or imaging methods; in clinical trials, amyloid-PET and tau-PET scans are the gold standards for determining amyloid and tau pathology. Nevertheless, these techniques are highly costly, invasive, or both. Finding affordable biomarkers that can be measured serially and that are easier to obtain in a less invasive way is therefore critically important from a medical standpoint. Blood-based biomarkers are probably going to meet this need. Alzheimer's disease and other dementias are starting to have blood-based biomarkers. The utilization of blood markers of neurodegeneration, such as neurofilament light chain [NfL], as well as the core pathological biomarkers, such as Aβ and phosphorylated tau [pTau], has great potential, according to the results obtained from well-defined cohorts. These findings demonstrate that these plasma biomarkers are aberrant in synchrony with CSF biomarker values in individuals with Alzheimer's disease. As a result, these biomarkers may prove to be effective tools for early and accurate diagnosis, prognosis, or tracking the course of the disease and the effects of treatment in both clinical practice and research trials. The discovery of blood markers is a significant development in the field since it may offer a less invasive and more affordable means of diagnosing patients with cognitive issues.

The state of the art in the rapidly developing and highly dynamic field of blood-based biomarkers for Alzheimer's disease is presented here. Researchers offer a thorough summary of current developments with an emphasis on three biomarkers—amyloid, pTau, and NfL—that are most likely to be used in clinical settings. The study presented here also talks about the new and developing biomarker for astrocytes called glial fibrillary acidic protein (GFAP). Finally, they outline a clinical implementation roadmap for blood-based biomarkers, outlining the specific steps required to enable their use in trials and clinical care as well as the advancements made thus far.

9.2.1. Blood-Based Biomarkers in Sporadic Alzheimer's Disease

9.2.1.1. $A\beta_{1-42}$ and $A\beta_{1-40}$

Alzheimer's disease is primarily characterized by Aβ pathology, and abnormalities in CSF and PET biomarkers for Aβ pathology appear decades before symptoms of dementia manifest. A 2016 meta-analysis revealed no differences in the plasma concentrations of $A\beta_{1-42}$ and $A\beta_{1-40}$ between Alzheimer's patients and controls. But more encouraging results have recently been obtained thanks to the development of extremely sensitive assays and technologies. There are currently numerous dependable techniques for the accurate and robust quantification of plasma $A\beta_{1-42}$ and $A\beta_{1-40}$, each with pros and cons related to practicality and cost. Automated ultrasensitive immunoassays (like the single molecule array; panel 1) and mass spectrometry assays can measure the peptides' full-length ($A\beta_{1-42}$ and $A\beta_{1-40}$) or N-terminally truncated ($A\beta_{x-42}$ and $A\beta_{x-40}$) forms. In order to identify Aβ pathology, a plasma test based on the mass spectrometry analysis of Aβ has been approved under the Clinical Laboratory Improvement Amendments (CLIA). Alternative techniques can identify the amyloid oligomerization or structural alterations unique to Alzheimer's disease in these plasma peptides.

Several cohorts spanning the whole spectrum of Alzheimer's disease have validated the clinical utility of these assays for measuring plasma Aβ. The assays have also been compared to baseline and longitudinal changes in cognitive performance and cognitive decline, as well as established biomarkers of Alzheimer's disease (CSF $A\beta_{1-42}$ and Aβ-PET). Accuracy ranged from 82 to 97% for mass spectrometry assays and from 62 to 79% for immunoassays when identifying abnormal amyloid CSF or PET status in individuals across the clinical Alzheimer's disease continuum using the ratio of plasma $A\beta_{1-42}$ to $A\beta_{1-40}$, or Aβ42/40. Classification performance improved after adjusting for APOE ε4 allele carriership, with dementia patients performing better than those with mild cognitive impairment. Significantly, compared to those without cerebral Aβ pathology, there was a drop in plasma $A\beta_{42/40}$ of less than 20% in those with this pathology. On amyloid PET scans, however, people with pathological findings of Alzheimer's disease showed a roughly 50%

decrease in CSF Aβ42/40 compared to those without this pathology. This difference could be explained by a number of factors, such as liver metabolic rates, binding to peripheral blood proteins (which are present in plasma at 200-fold higher concentrations than in CSF), and the production of plasma Aβ from peripheral sources. Consistent with CSF or PET amyloid data, low plasma Aβ42/40 or the presence of misfolded $A\beta_{1-42}$ are linked to cognitive decline and the risk of Alzheimer's disease progression in individuals who are cognitively normal, subjectively cognitively declining, or have mild cognitive impairment. There is currently no research on the diagnostic utility of plasma Aβ42/40 to distinguish Alzheimer's disease from other types of dementias.

9.2.1.2. pTau Forms

Alzheimer's disease is also characterized by tangles that contain full-length or truncated forms of hyperphosphorylated tau, which is another important pathological marker. Thus far, research utilizing ultrasensitive technologies to measure plasma total tau has revealed excessive overlap between clinical groups and low diagnostic value. This discovery stands in sharp contrast to the outcomes of the examination of tau's post-translationally altered forms. Over 70 posttranslational modification sites, including over 40 phosphorylation sites and multiple truncated forms, have been identified in tau. There are distinct pTau forms that can be found in plasma and CSF. Similar to Aβ, a variety of techniques are available to detect amyloid or tau pathology with high accuracy (80–98%), including mass spectrometry and immune-based approaches. Those with clinically diagnosed Alzheimer's disease have significantly higher (more than two-fold) concentrations of plasma tau phosphorylated at different sites (pTau181, pTau217, or pTau231) than do controls or individuals with dementias other than Alzheimer's disease. Since the first report revealed a correlation between tauPET and plasma pTau181 concentrations in Alzheimer's disease patients, plasma pTau181 has gained popularity as a biomarker. Subsequent independent studies' findings strongly imply that plasma pTau181 reflects neuropathology unique to Alzheimer's disease, as pTau181 is elevated in Alzheimer's patients relative to those with dementias other than Alzheimer's disease, such as other tauopathies. Based on a prospective cohort study involving individuals with and without cognitive impairment, changes in plasma pTau181 at baseline and over time were linked to widespread tau aggregation six years later. Moreover, pTau181 correlated with elevated tau-PET, especially in brain regions impacted by Alzheimer's disease pathology, and distinguished individuals with amyloid pathology across various clinical stages. Moreover, higher plasma concentrations of pTau181 were linked to gray matter atrophy. The observation of these correlations solely in individuals with Aβ pathology supports the specificity of pTau181 for neuropathological alterations linked to Alzheimer's disease. In addition to being able to distinguish between patients with mild cognitive impairment who developed Alzheimer's disease and those who did not, pTau181 performed better as a plasma biomarker than Aβ42/40. Comparable outcomes have been noted in people without dementia, where a high pTau181 level is linked to an increased risk of developing Alzheimer's disease.

There are more pTau markers that appear promising. When employing mass spectrometry techniques, CSF pTau217 demonstrated more variations between Alzheimer's disease and controls than pTau181. The results of a sizable, multicenter cohort study demonstrated that plasma pTau217 can accurately (96%) distinguish Alzheimer's disease from non-Alzheimer's disease dementias, matching the performance of recognized CSF or tau-PET biomarkers. Additionally, plasma pTau217 accurately detected tau-PET positive cases. The specificity of plasma pTau for Alzheimer's disease tau pathology is highlighted by the correlation between plasma pTau217 concentrations and the density of cortical tau pathology in Alzheimer's disease, but not in other tauopathies like FTD-tau, based on neuropathological ratings of cerebral tau-tangle pathology. Consistent with findings indicating that plasma pTau217 becomes abnormal prior to tau-PET, the study also demonstrated that plasma pTau217 begins to increase approximately 20 years prior to the onset of mild cognitive impairment in autosomal dominant Alzheimer's disease. This discovery raises the possibility that the biological mechanisms generating the tau-PET signal may not be the same as the source of plasma pTau alterations. Studies that conducted direct comparisons between pTau217 and pTau181 using mass spectrometry and immunochemical platforms revealed that both modalities—tau-PET negativity, Aβ-PET negativity, and autopsy-confirmed Alzheimer's disease versus frontotemporal lobar degeneration—perform well in terms of discriminating. Nevertheless, pTau217 demonstrated superiority in identifying Aβ-PET positivity, especially when employing mass spectrometry methodologies. Additionally, pTau217 demonstrated a stronger correlation with tau-PET and marginally improved accuracy in differentiating Alzheimer's disease from other dementias.

A study compared plasma pTau231 with plasma pTau181, analyzing plasma pTau231 in multiple cohorts, including a neuropathological cohort of people with dementias other than Alzheimer's disease. pTau231 distinguished dementias other than Alzheimer's disease from dementias not caused by Alzheimer's disease with a performance comparable to pTau181. However, pTau231 began to alter in earlier stages of the pathology of Alzheimer's disease based on both tau Braak and Aβ-PET, indicating that pTau231 might be particularly useful as an early pathological marker of Alzheimer's disease even before symptoms appear. However, the superiority of pTau231 over pTau181 or pTau217 for predicting tau-PET or amyloid was not replicated in another study involving a community-based population. 57 Future research ought to focus on the significance of various pTau forms, namely whether the variations are actually biological or merely a result of the technology employed.

As pTau forms have the ability to identify pathology related to Alzheimer's disease throughout the clinical continuum, they may be employed as diagnostic markers unique to Alzheimer's disease. A critical next step is evaluation in the early stages of Alzheimer's disease and in people without cognitive impairment. The best model for predicting Alzheimer's disease, according to a recent study in a cohort of people with mild cognitive impairment or subjective cognitive decline, was a combination of plasma pTau217 or pTau181, the APOE genotype, and three quick cognitive tests measuring executive function and memory. Given the simplicity of blood testing in comparison to CSF analysis or PET scans, the combination of these tests and biomarkers may make it easier to recruit participants for Alzheimer's disease trials. This model was not influenced by the plasma NfL concentration or plasma Aβ42/40 measured using immunoassays. Another study, however, found that for the purpose of detecting Aβ-PET positivity in participants without dementia, plasma Aβ42/40 measured by mass spectrometry performed better than both plasma pTau181 concentration and plasma Aβ42/40 measured by single molecule array. To ascertain the test's specificities and the best environment in which to use them, more research is required. Furthermore, in contrast to plasma Aβ42/40, the concentration of plasma pTau increases gradually as the disease progresses, indicating that pTau may be a valuable marker for disease stage. This characteristic could be helpful in clinical trials of medication candidates meant to slow the course of disease. The primary constraint on the studies conducted thus far is that they have mostly been carried out by a small number of groups in specialized centers with retrospective cohorts. The inclusion of more diverse populations and prospective validation are two essential next steps in the research process.

Besides phosphorylated sites, the differential truncation patterns observed in circulating tau fragments could themselves capture important aspects of Alzheimer's disease-related neurodegeneration and cognitive decline. The N-terminal fragment of tau (NT1) in plasma is increased in individuals with Alzheimer's disease compared with cognitively unimpaired controls and predicts cognitive decline and neurodegeneration among cognitively unimpaired elderly individuals.

9.2.1.3. Neurofilament Light Chain

NfL is a primary neurofilament protein in the central nervous system, along with α-internexin. It functions as an axonal scaffolding protein. Neurofilaments are critical for the CNS's synaptic organization and function in addition to axon growth and stability. NfL has become a potent candidate for a cross-disease neurodegeneration biomarker. This biomarker is measurable in CSF and blood, and it was the first neurospecific biomarker for which an ultrasensitive assay was developed and clinical value was demonstrated in numerous publications. There is a good to excellent correlation (r values of 0·70–0·97) between CSF and blood concentrations of NfL in neuroinflammatory and neurodegenerative diseases. The conditions with the highest concentrations of NfL include atypical parkinsonian disorders, amyotrophic lateral sclerosis, frontotemporal, vascular, and HIV-associated dementias. After CSF total tau [tTau], CSF NfL exhibits the second-highest fold-change among fluid biomarkers associated with Alzheimer's disease in sporadic cases of the disease. A higher overlap across groups than in familial Alzheimer's disease is observed between elevated concentrations of NfL in CSF and plasma and longitudinal neurodegeneration as assessed by MRI, as well as amyloid-PET and tau-PET positivity. The results are more difficult to interpret when NfL concentrations rise with age. Regardless of the underlying cause, NfL is utilized as a general biomarker of neuroaxonal injury or degeneration in clinical research and practice. In patients exhibiting psychiatric symptoms, it can serve as an indicator of a neurodegenerative process. In order to learn more about the underlying cause of the neurodegeneration, the biomarker may be used as a first diagnostic test. If the test is positive, it may lead to further examinations using more focused biomarkers. In clinical trials of disease-modifying therapies, NfL may also be used as a biomarker of disease severity. It may also be used, as it is in multiple sclerosis, to optimize and track the effects of treatment in clinical settings.

9.2.1.4. Glial Fibrillary Acidic Protein

One important component of the cytoskeleton of astrocytes is GFAP. Reactive astrocytosis has been suggested as a possible cause or consequence of the pathological alterations associated with Alzheimer's disease. Both GFAP expression and protein concentrations were higher in the vicinity of dense Aβ plaques and increased with tau accumulation in a neuropathology study involving a population-based cohort. Although GFAP has not been studied as much as Aβ, tau, and NfL, ultrasensitive immunoassays have produced encouraging results regarding GFAP's utility as a fluid biomarker. GFAP concentrations in plasma or serum are higher in people who fall somewhere along the clinical Alzheimer's disease spectrum. When examining the full clinical spectrum, from cognitively unimpaired to Alzheimer's disease,

GFAP concentrations can distinguish abnormal Aβ-PET status with approximately 81% accuracy; when considering individuals without dementia, the accuracy ranges from 76% to 80%. When the Aβ-PET burden increased, plasma GFAP concentrations rose linearly; however, this linear relationship vanished at high Aβ-PET burdens. Moreover, correlations with the diagnosis of a syndrome, performance on neuropsychological tests, and measurements of MRI atrophy indicated that elevations in plasma or serum GFAP were also associated with clinical disease severity. Alzheimer's disease development was predicted by plasma GFAP in patients with mild cognitive impairment. Moreover, higher serum GFAP concentrations were linked to steeper rates of cognitive decline and an increased risk of dementia in people without cognitive impairment.

It is noteworthy that plasma Aβ42/40 has no bearing on the predictive value of plasma or serum GFAP. Given that astrocyte activation is not exclusive to the pathophysiology of Alzheimer's disease, GFAP may also serve as a viable biomarker for other forms of dementia. In fact, some research discovered that subtypes of frontotemporal dementia had higher serum or plasma GFAP concentrations. In addition, concentrations in Lewy body dementia were higher than in Parkinson's disease patients and controls.

Thus, serum or plasma GFAP could be used for prognosis as well as diagnosis (in diagnostic panels). To clarify these possible therapeutic uses for various forms of dementia and neurodegenerative illnesses, more research is necessary. Given the prognostic significance of GFAP and its early and gradual increases in conjunction with amyloid pathology, plasma GFAP may also be used in trials to support inclusion of patients in the early stages of Alzheimer's disease, enrichment, and treatment response monitoring.

9.2.2. Blood-Based Biomarkers in Genetically Determined Alzheimer's Disease

A rare form of Alzheimer's disease is caused by a monogenetic mutation in the APP, PSEN1, PSEN2, or APP gene, or by an APP gene multiplication, which is also present in Down syndrome because of the trisomy of chromosome 21. One benefit of researching genetically determined Alzheimer's disease is that, because the disease typically manifests at a young age (40–60 years), general aging has less of an impact on biomarker concentrations. Furthermore, the age of onset is consistent with each mutation. This has greatly advanced our conceptual understanding of the progression of changes in Alzheimer's disease and made it possible to study biomarkers throughout the course of the illness. 5,81 Numerous large and small cohort studies—but not GFAP—have examined plasma Aβ, pTau, and NfL in genetically determined Alzheimer's disease since the advent of high-sensitivity assays.

9.2.2.1. Increased Plasma $A\beta_{1-42}$

In contrast to Alzheimer's disease that occurs randomly, people with Down syndrome, including children, and carriers of autosomal dominant Alzheimer's disease mutations have higher plasma concentrations of Aβ1–42 and Aβ42/40, respectively, and these levels do not correlate with CSF counterparts. Increased levels of Aβ1–42 in blood are likely the result of overproduction of Aβ1–42 due to APP processing mutations in individuals with genetic Alzheimer's disease. It is still unclear how plasma Aβ1–42 concentrations in genetic Alzheimer's disease vary over time. Depending on the type of mutation, a mass spectrometry analysis revealed a relative decrease in plasma Aβ42/40 towards the onset of dementia and an increase in Aβ42/40 in symptomatic individuals. The blood levels of Aβ1–42 and Aβ42/40 in individuals with Down syndrome first increased, but they then decreased closer to the onset of symptoms, and then increased again. Applying these findings to elderly people (e.g., 75–80 years old) with intermittent Alzheimer's disease should be done with caution. Overall, these findings indicate that, in patients with genetic Alzheimer's disease, plasma Aβ concentrations are elevated and vary throughout life based on genetic variation and the stage of the disease; the underlying mechanisms for these relationships remain unclear.

9.2.2.2. Increased Plasma pTau and NfL

The dynamics of pTau and NfL biomarkers in people with genetically determined Alzheimer's disease are in line with observations made in people with sporadic Alzheimer's disease and offer information on when these biomarkers change. In terms of pTau forms, 16–24 years prior to the onset of symptoms in autosomal dominant Alzheimer's disease, plasma concentrations of pTau181 and pTau217 start to rise, which corresponds with the beginning of amyloid accumulation in the brain as determined by Aβ-PET and CSF Aβ.

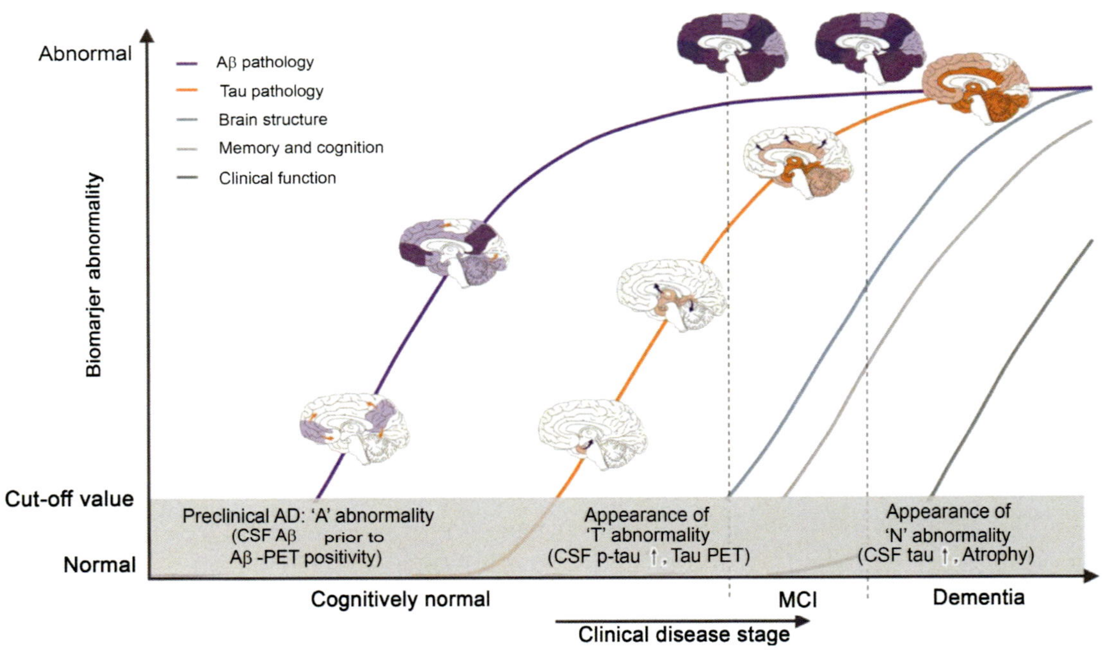

Figure 9.1. *Biomarkers and changes in spatiotemporal pattern of Aβ and NFT deposit during disease cascade. Abnormality in CSF Aβ42 and Aβ-PET ('A' abnormality) are biomarkers in pre-clinical stage, followed by abnormality in CSF p-tau or tau-PET and 'N' abnormality (increased CSF T-tau and hippocampal atrophy).*

Source: Mankhong S, Kim S, Lee S, Kwak HB, Park DH, Joa KL, & Kang JH, (2022). Development of Alzheimer's disease biomarkers: From CSF- to blood-based biomarkers. Biomedicines, 10(4), 850. https://doi.org/10.3390/biomedicines10040850.

After symptoms appear, plasma pTau concentrations seem to stabilize and may even slightly decline, much like the CSF biomarkers of Alzheimer's disease. Additionally, blood NfL concentrations rise early: in the Dominantly Inherited Alzheimer 'sNetwork cohort study, they do so approximately 16 years before symptoms appear, and in the Colombian kindred study, they do so 22 years before symptoms appear. But only three years prior to the onset of symptoms, plasma NfL was able to differentiate between mutation carriers and unaffected family controls. As in the case of intermittent Alzheimer's disease, symptomatic individuals showed a persistent rise in NfL concentrations. Additionally, plasma NfL started to rise in Down syndrome patients more than 20 years before dementia symptoms appeared. Additionally, increases in NfL predicted future cognitive decline, and baseline and longitudinal NfL concentrations correlated well with other neurodegenerative signs and clinical diagnosis. The potential use of plasma pTau181, pTau217, and NfL for diagnostic, prognostic, and disease monitoring purposes very early in the disease course is supported by these findings in genetically determined Alzheimer's disease.

9.2.3. Factors Associated with Heterogeneity

To properly interpret the results, it is crucial to comprehend the factors influencing the concentrations of blood-based biomarkers of amyloid and tau pathology and neurodegeneration as they get closer to clinical use (Figure 9.1). Particular importance is given to this data in the creation of reference ranges. The analysis of blood markers and factors influencing them in various population-based and community-based cohorts is essential, as initial blood biomarker studies are conducted in well-characterized populations. This is particularly significant from the perspective of primary care, where blood-based biomarkers are more appropriate than intrusive and expensive CSF and neuroimaging markers. Patients receiving primary care, however, exhibit the greatest heterogeneity with regard to comorbidities and neurodegenerative illnesses.

Blood biomarkers can be clinically interpreted differently depending on factors like age, sex, comorbidities, medication, lifestyle factors, and genetic variation. The majority of research findings indicate that while Aβ42/40 decreases with age, blood concentrations of NfL, GFAP, pTau181, pTau217, and total tau rise with age. Changes in the turnover of the biomarkers and an increased prevalence of neuropathology at older ages could explain this finding. Therefore, it is crucial to stratify by in-vivo assessments of amyloid and tau pathology and investigate age-related associations of these blood biomarkers (Aβ, pTau) among cognitively unimpaired individuals who do not have pathology. Studying the age-related characteristics of non-specific neurodegeneration markers (NfL, GFAP) is more challenging. Variations have been observed in the biomarker concentrations according to gender. While some studies have found no differences in total tau concentrations between the sexes, one study found higher concentrations for women. Studies have not found any differences in NfL concentration (measured in serum or plasma) or Aβ42/40 by sex.

Higher body-mass index (BMI) individuals, especially those who fall into the overweight or obese categories, have lower plasma NfL concentrations. 100 Lower concentrations of plasma pTau181, pTau217, and NfL were linked to higher BMI in an ethnically diverse population study, but not tTau or Aβ42/Aβ40. While there is a correlation between obesity and brain atrophy, this finding is mostly explained by the increased blood volume that comes with weight gain. Before going into clinical use, more research on how BMI affects other blood-based indicators of Alzheimer's disease is required. Blood biomarker concentrations have also been demonstrated to be impacted by cardiovascular comorbidities. According to one study, people with diabetes, ischemic heart disease, and hypertension had lower plasma Aβ concentrations. Replication in bigger cohorts and with the investigation of additional biomarkers is nevertheless required. Because of decreased clearance, renal disease can also have an impact on blood biomarker concentrations.

It is necessary to investigate blood-based biomarkers in various communities to comprehend how racial, ethnic, and geographic variations impact Aβ-PET and CSF biomarker values for Alzheimer's disease. Blood biomarker studies in a variety of populations revealed that sex, race, or ethnicity had no effect on biomarker concentrations. However, in an autopsy study, non-Hispanic Black individuals' plasma pTau181 and pTau217 were better than non-Hispanic White individuals' (0·65–0·75) at identifying the presence of Alzheimer's disease neuropathology changes (area under the curve: 0·94–0·96). Notably, it's critical to avoid overinterpreting the data and to take variations in blood biomarker concentrations into account in relation to other variables. As previously noted, concentrations of blood-based biomarkers linked to Alzheimer's disease can be impacted by BMI and renal disease. Compared to White people, Black and Hispanic women and men have a higher age-adjusted prevalence of obesity, which is also more prevalent in rural than in urban areas. This also applies to kidney disease that is chronic. Therefore, rather than just saying that there are racial or ethnic differences in the biomarker itself without providing any additional context, it is crucial to take into account racial and ethnic differences in the frequency of comorbidities and other factors (Hansson, 2021; Scheltens et al., 2021).

9.2.4. The Road Towards Clinical Implementation

When introducing novel fluid biomarkers into clinical practice, a number of issues must be methodically taken care of. The Geneva roadmap outlines a biomarker development framework that is divided into five phases. Phase 1 exploratory studies must be followed by phase 2 clinical assay development and biomarker validation. Phase 3 should involve studying biomarker use in retrospective and longitudinal cohorts. Phase 4 should involve evaluating biomarkers in prospective validation studies conducted in real-world settings. Phase 5, the final stage, is devoted to clinical implementation. In order to accommodate technical analytical elements for blood-based biomarkers, we have modified this roadmap (Figure 9.2). For Aβ, pTau, and NfL, the majority of the implementation roadmap's phases 1 and 2 have been completed. Phases 1 and 2 of GFAP and phase 3 of all biomarkers are still under development. It is still necessary to address phases 4 and 5 for every biomarker.

Assay requirements for phases 1–3 of the roadmap can be met by using fully validated laboratory-developed tests or assays intended solely for research use (panel 2). In-vitro diagnostic assays that are scalable and robust and have been approved by the certifying bodies are required for the use of diagnostic assays in clinical care (phases 4 and 5 of the roadmap). Developing standardized operating procedures for processing and storage—preferably ones that can handle the analysis of multiple biomarkers—is another important requirement before integrating biomarkers into clinical trials or other settings. As part of the Global Biomarker Standardization Consortium, the effects of various preanalytical factors are being meticulously mapped. No matter what technology is used, studies conducted by the Consortium have demonstrated that processing blood after it has been collected or centrifuged too soon has a negative impact on Aβ concentrations when it is stored at room temperature. Nevertheless, by keeping the samples cold, this reduction can be lessened. No such effect was seen for GFAP, NfL, or pTau. Repeated freezing and thawing also had no effect. A standard operating procedure for blood-based biomarker collection was developed as a result of the study's findings.

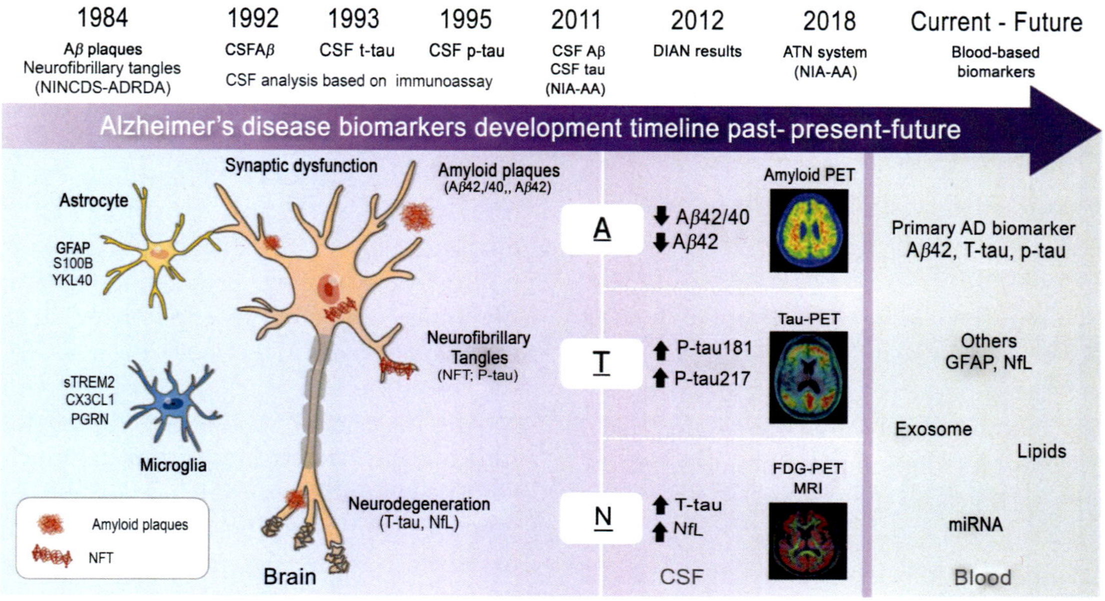

Figure 9.2. *Roadmap for the five phases in the development of blood-based biomarkers for the diagnosis of Alzheimer´s disease.*

Source: Mankhong S, Kim S, Lee S, Kwak H-B, Park D-H, Joa K-L, Kang J-H, (2022). Development of Alzheimer's disease biomarkers: From CSF- to blood-based biomarkers. Biomedicines, 10(4), 850. https://doi.org/10.3390/biomedicines10040850.

The development of diagnostic decision tools, such as algorithms that take into account data gathered from the biomarkers during their evaluation in diagnostic panels, is another aspect of phase 3 of the roadmap, which pertains to combined analyzes for multiple biomarkers and validates biomarkers in retrospective samples. It's critical to determine whether within-individual rates of change yield more information than absolute values, given that blood-based biomarkers enable serially repeated measurements. In contrast to absolute values, which may be more helpful during the symptomatic phase, the rate of change in serum NfL concentration can, for example, distinguish mutation carriers—that is, people with presymptomatic familial AD—from non-mutation carriers earlier. Phase 4 should define the criteria for using biofluid-based biomarkers appropriately for each patient, including when and how to use them. Using biomarkers at the prodromal and presymptomatic stages of a disease presents a particularly difficult task. There have been reports of personalized dementia risk prediction for mild cognitive impairment based on MRI and CSF biomarkers. Such customized models might be created for blood-based biomarkers as well, given that the predictive value of plasma pTau181 is comparable to that of CSF pTau181. The dissemination of biomarker results to patients and potential users (i.e., clinicians) will be crucial in phase 5 of the implementation roadmap. People still place a high value on information even in the absence of curative treatments. For instance, they need information to better manage symptoms, understand the cause of their complaints, plan for advanced care, and make future decisions. Within the next three to five years, blood-based biomarkers may be used in specialized memory clinics. It is possible that within the next 5 to 10 years, the diagnostic process will begin in primary care settings. Population screening is a long-term goal that is frequently carried out in a primary care setting.

Amyloid PET and CSF biomarkers are expensive and hard to come by, which limits the current state of Alzheimer's disease biomarker research. Thus, widespread testing for Alzheimer's disease may be made possible by blood-based biomarkers. However, the results of upcoming blood-based biomarker research will not be the only factor influencing implementation; treatment options and the structure of the local healthcare system may also play a role. For example, approval in other regions of the world is still pending for aducanumab, an antiamyloid drug that was approved by the US Food and Drug Administration on June 7, 2021. Furthermore, the only methods that are currently advised for measuring amyloid status are CSF and PET. Nonetheless, blood-based biomarkers may already be used by certain specialized healthcare providers to choose the right patients. Blood-based biomarkers will likely enter clinics more quickly as a result of aducanumab's anticipated approval in other regions of the world as well as the anticipated approval of other comparable medication candidates that are currently undergoing testing.

9.2.4.1. Implementation in Clinical Trials

The development of new blood-based biomarkers for Alzheimer's disease will probably enhance the planning and execution of clinical trials assessing treatment-modifying interventions. The inclusion of individuals in clinical trials who are in the early stages of preclinical Alzheimer's disease will depend on biological markers due to the disease's protracted preclinical stage. Blood-based biomarkers may be employed as treatment efficacy and target engagement indicators, as well as inclusion criteria (enrichment and stratification). In order to identify patients who are eligible for treatments like aducanumab, an antiamyloid medication, blood-based biomarkers that identify the presence of pathological features of Alzheimer's disease, such as tau tangles and amyloid plaques, are crucial. As an illustration, pTau concentrations in plasma are used as an inclusion criterion in innovative drug trials intended to treat Alzheimer's disease (Teunissen CE, unpublished observation). Furthermore, it will be crucial to identify biomarkers that indicate the existence of additional mechanisms (like neuroinflammation) in order to decide whether to prescribe additional treatments or combinations of treatments. Blood-based biomarkers may prove beneficial in observing biological efficacy (such as the analysis of tau and amyloid aggregate clearance by plasma Aβ and pTau), treatment outcomes, adverse events (like abnormalities in imaging related to amyloid), and the safety of increasing the dosage interval. In this case, blood-based biomarkers are preferable over CSF and imaging biomarkers because they are non-invasive, less expensive, and less taxing on patients and healthcare systems (e.g., in terms of tracer cost and scanning time). On the other hand, the visibility of accumulated damage and spatial resolution are benefits of imaging (Hansson, 2021; Scheltens et al., 2021).

9.3. ALZHEIMER'S DISEASE BIOMARKER PROFILING IN A MEMORY CLINIC COHORT WITHOUT COMMON COMORBIDITIES

When it comes to its clinical symptoms, rate of progression, neuropathological profiles, and biomarkers, Alzheimer's disease (AD) is a heterogeneous disorder. Numerous factors, such as age at onset, comorbidities, lifestyle factors, and the apolipoprotein E (APOE) genotype and other risk genes, account for this heterogeneity. With the goal of achieving more harmonized cohort studies, the National Institute on Aging-Alzheimer's Association research framework proposed a biological definition of Alzheimer's disease based on biomarkers of tau, β-amyloid, and neurodegeneration. A thorough understanding of the heterogeneity of Alzheimer's disease is necessary for the development of effective, individualized treatments. Studies of additional cerebrospinal fluid (CSF) biomarkers offer information on co-existing, inducing, and/or interacting mechanisms in Alzheimer's disease, complementing the findings of β-amyloid and tau markers. Thus, the discovery of more fluid biomarkers may contribute to the development of a toolkit for patient group stratification for mechanism-targeted therapeutic strategies.

In one study discussed below, 13 biomarkers representing various mechanisms pertinent to brain health were included in addition to the core CSF pathology markers for Alzheimer's disease. Synaptosomal-associated protein 25 kDa (SNAP-25), synaptotagmin 1 (SYT-1), and neurogranin (NG) are three examples of these biomarkers that are synaptic proteins. Presynaptic neurotransmitter release is associated with both SNAP-25 and SYT-1, while the postsynaptic protein NG is involved in the calcium signaling pathway through calmodulin. Elevated CSF concentrations of these proteins, which have been linked to preclinical and clinical stages of Alzheimer's disease4, suggest loss or dysfunction of synapses. Within the central and peripheral nervous systems lies the neurofilament light chain (NFL), a subunit of the neurofilament protein. It has been suggested that this compound serves as a general biomarker of axonal injury, and its concentration in CSF rises in Alzheimer's disease and other neurodegenerative disorders. The study also included markers of inflammatory processes that have been shown to be altered in Alzheimer's disease: calprotectin (S100A8/A9), an inflammatory mediator produced by glial cells and implicated in Aβ pathology; astrocytic IL-15, which contributes to tissue damage in both neurodegeneration and acute brain injury; and the heterodimeric interleukin-12/23p40 (IL-12/IL-23p40), which is produced, e.g., by microglia, and influences pro-inflammatory pathways in the brain. Additionally evaluated were the antioxidants thioredoxin-1 (TRX-1) and thioredoxin-80 (TRX-80), which are cleaved forms of TRX-1. It has been discovered that both types offer protection against Aβ-induced toxicity, while Alzheimer's disease brains and CSF exhibit reduced levels of TRX-80. Regarding whether brain TRX-1 levels are impacted, the data are not always consistent.

It has been demonstrated that insulin resistance raises the risk of Alzheimer's disease. since it has been suggested that elevated CSF levels of ectonucleotide pyrophosphatase/phosphodiesterase 2 (ENPP-2) in Alzheimer's disease represent abnormal brain glucose homeostasis, we measured this enzyme, also referred to as autotaxin. The bioactive lipid lysophosphatidic acid, which is produced by ENPP-2, has a variety of actions in the central nervous system and numerous other tissues. Although VEGF is primarily recognized for its role in angiogenesis, it also affects neurogenesis and neuronal regeneration in addition to helping to regulate the vasculature of the brain. Upregulation of VEGF in Alzheimer's disease may be an attempt to make up for abnormal vasculature. One of the initial processes in the renin–angiotensin system (RAS) is the conversion of AGT to Angiotensin I by renin. Astrocytes are the primary producers of AGT in the brain. It has been demonstrated that an upregulated RAS causes CSF AGT to be elevated in Alzheimer's disease. Below are the findings of a case study of research published in Brain Communications by Daniilidou et al. (2023).

9.3.1. GEDOC Memory Clinic Subcohort

A portion of the broader GEDOC study, which focuses on Alzheimer's disease (AD) and related dementias, is known as the GEDOC memory clinic subcohort. Patients who have been evaluated or are currently being evaluated at memory clinics are specifically included in this subcohort. These clinics focus on diagnosing dementia, evaluating cognitive function, and offering complete care to patients with memory and cognitive issues.

These are the demographic details listed in Table 9.1. A detailed description of the memory clinic's clinical evaluation can be found elsewhere. In summary, it includes a full medical history review, a physical and neurological examination, the Mini-Mental State Examination (MMSE), extensive neuropsychological testing, routine blood tests, brain imaging (MRI or CT), and CSF sampling to measure biomarkers for Alzheimer's disease (Aβ42, t-tau, and p-tau). By consensus in multidisciplinary meetings of the clinic staff, diagnoses were made, on average, within two months of the start of the assessment period using all available clinical data, including CSF biomarker data, in an unblinded manner. The consensus criteria for mild cognitive impairment, which call for the presence of both subjective and objective cognitive impairments affecting one or more cognitive domains but not dementia or impairment to activities of daily living, were used to diagnose mild cognitive impairment. A test result that is 1.5 standard deviations (SD) below the expected range for the given age and educational background was considered objective cognitive impairment. The Diagnostic and Statistical Manual of Mental Disorders criteria were used to diagnose dementia, and the National Institute of Neurological and Communicative Disorders and Stroke–Alzheimer's Disease and Related Disorders were used to diagnose the etiology of Alzheimer's disease. Subjective cognitive decline was the term used to describe patients who did not fit the diagnostic criteria for dementia or mild cognitive impairment. The exclusion criteria for this research included having diabetes, hypertension, high cholesterol, stroke, or another neurodegenerative condition.

Table 9.1. Summary of the CSF Study Population Characteristics

Demographics	**SCD (*n* = 30)**	**MCI (*n* = 30)**	**AD (*n* = 30)**	***P*-value**
Age, years	62.4 (4.38)	65.6 (7.48)	68.2 (7.86)	0.005
Female	60%	50%	50%	0.668
APOE e4 carriera	31%	71%	76%	0.077
Cognition				
MMSE scoreb	28.1 (2.0)	27.7 (2.1)	23.2 (5.6)	<0.0001
Core AD CSF biomarkers				
Aβ42, pg/mL	988.5 (217.6)	569.2 (60.7)	555.3 (128.7)	<0.0001
t-tau, pg/mL	251.1 (95.1)	464.3 (219.8)	551.3 (215.1)	<0.0001
p-tau, pg/mL	61.4 (27.9)	68.4 (23.3)	74.0 (21.4)	0.108

p-tau/Aβ42	0.06 (0.03)	0.12 (0.05)	0.14 (0.05)	<0.0001
Chronic conditions				
Cardiovascularc	3.3%	6.7%	0%	0.355
Autoimmuned	3.3%	6.7%	6.7%	0.809
Osteoarthritis	13.3%	13.3%	6.7%	0.638

Data are shown as unadjusted mean (SD), unless otherwise stated. *P*-values were calculated by ANCOVA, adjusting for age for continuous variables or by χ^2 for categorical data.

[a]*APOE* e4 carrier data were available for 13 SCD, 17 MCI and 17 AD participants.

[b]MMSE score was available for 29 SCD, 29 MCI and 26 AD participants.

[c]Coronary heart disease in one SCD and two MCI participants.

[d]Autoimmune conditions found in the cohort included psoriasis in one SCD and two MCI participants, Crohn's disease and ulcerative colitis in two AD participants, respectively.

Source: Daniilidou M, Eroli F, Alanko V, Goikolea J, Latorre-Leal M, Rodriguez-Rodriguez P, Griffiths WJ, Wang Y, Pacciarini M, Brinkmalm A, Zetterberg H, Blennow K, Rosenberg A, Bogdanovic N, Winblad B, Kivipelto M, Ibghi D, Cedazo-Minguez A, Maioli S, & Matton A, (2023). Alzheimer's disease biomarker profiling in a memory clinic cohort without common comorbidities. Brain Commun., 5(5), fcad228. doi: 10.1093/braincomms/fcad228. PMID: 37680670; PMCID: PMC10481253.

9.3.2. Human Brain Tissue

Samples of human hippocampi from six patients with Alzheimer's disease and six healthy individuals. The Consortium to Establish a Registry for Alzheimer's disease states that every participant with the disease satisfied the requirements for having Alzheimer's disease. There were no recognized neurological or psychiatric conditions in the non-demented control subjects. At the time of their deaths, none of the donors had been taking medication for diabetes, hypercholesterolemia, or hypertension (Daniilidou et al., 2023).

9.3.3. CSF Sampling

Using a 25-gage needle, lumbar punctures were performed between the L3/L4 and L4/L5 intervertebral spaces to obtain CSF samples. Using a commercially available enzyme-linked immunosorbent assay, samples were collected in polypropylene tubes, centrifuged within two hours, and evaluated for Aβ42, t-tau, and p-tau 181 concentrations. Extra sample aliquots were kept in storage at -80°C until they were examined in more detail.

9.3.4. CSF Biomarker Measurements

- **AGT, ENPP-2, TRX-1, TRX-80, NG and NFL:** The CSF protein levels of AGT, ENPP-2, and TRX-1 were measured using the following commercially available ELISAs: ENPP-2, TRX-1. All ELISAs were carried out using samples that were diluted 1:200 for AGT, 1:40 for ENPP-2, and 1:2 for TRX-1 following the manufacturer's instructions.

ELISA was used to determine NG and NFL, as previously mentioned. TRX-80 was measured using an internal ELISA. Samples underwent duplicate testing, with the average being taken into account for statistical analysis. For all of the ELISAs, the computed intra- and inter-assay coefficients of variation (CV percent) were less than 6 and less than 15%, respectively. Samples that had duplicate CVs greater than 15% had to be remeasured or were not included in the analysis. A microplate reader was used to measure absorbance. GraphPad Prism 9 software was used to compute concentrations by interpolating from the standard curves using a 4PL curve fit.

- **IL-12/IL-23p40, IL-15, VEGF and Calprotectin:** They measured VEGF, calprotectin, IL-15, IL-12/IL-23p40, and VEGF using the highly sensitive Mesoscale Discovery immunoassays. The preconfigured V-PLEX Human Cytokine Panel 1 was used to select IL-12/IL-23p40, IL-15, and VEGF. The R-Plex Human calprotectin antibody set was used to analyze calprotectin in accordance with the manufacturer's instructions. For IL-12/IL-23p40 and IL-15, a two-fold dilution was used; however, VEGF and calprotectin samples were run without dilution. Each array was scanned using an MSD QuickPlex 120, and Discovery Workbench 4.0 was used to retrieve concentration data. Samples with an intra-assay CV of less than 20% and above the lowest limit of detection were taken into consideration for analysis. The inter-assay CV for every analyte was less than 20%.
- **SNAP-25, SYT-1 and 27-OH:** We measured SYT-1 and SNAP-25 using a previously defined protocol. After sterol esters were alkaline hydrolyzed, 27-OH was examined using liquid chromatography–mass spectrometry with charge-tagging methodology, also known as "Enzyme-Assisted Derivatization for Sterol Analysis," as previously mentioned.

9.3.5. Immunofluorescence Staining

The brain tissue sections were deparaffinized and the antigen was extracted according to the previously mentioned procedures. Sections were blocked in 0.1 percent Triton X-100 (Sigma-Aldrich), 2% normal goat serum, and 1% bovine serum albumin (Sigma-Aldrich) in phosphate-buffered saline (PBS) for one hour at room temperature following washing with PBS. After that, sections were incubated for an additional night at +4°C with primary antibodies diluted in blocking buffer. Following a 1-hour incubation period at room temperature with secondary antibodies and DAPI (2-(4-Amidinophenyl)-1H-indole-6-carboxamidine), they were washed for 3 minutes in 0 percent Triton X-100 in PBS. 1000 mouse anti-phospho-tau (Thr212, Ser214) (MN1060), 1000 rabbit anti-TRX-1 (MA532569), 1000 rabbit anti-AGT (MA529010), 1000 Alexa Fluor fluorescently conjugated secondary goat anti-rabbit and anti-mouse antibodies (Thermo Fisher Scientific), and 1000 DAPI (1351303; Bio-Rad, USA) dilutions and antibodies were employed. Sections were treated for 5 minutes in PBS to quench the lipofuscin's autofluorescence, and then they were incubated with 0.1 percent w/w Sudan Black B in 70% ethanol. Sections were cleaned with Triton X-100 in PBS 2 × 10min and 10min with PBS before mounting.

9.3.6. Image Biomarkers: PiB PET, FDG PET, and MRI

A much deeper understanding of the intricately intertwined pathophysiological mechanisms underlying AD has been made possible by advancements in imaging technologies. PET allows for the visualization of the two primary proteins involved in the pathological process: Tau and Aβ. Moreover, the precise nature of the local effects of neurodegeneration can also be determined: brain network disruption, regional tissue atrophy, and abnormalities in brain glucose metabolism can all be evaluated using structural magnetic resonance imaging (MRI), functional MRI, and PET, respectively. Therefore, meticulously obtaining information from imaging the spatiotemporal dynamics of AD pathophysiology ought to provide additional understanding of the biology and evaluation of the disease's progression in actual patients.

9.3.6.1. Amyloid-PET

Using radiopharmaceuticals like PIB or 18F-florbetapir, which have a high specificity and sensitivity for binding to amyloid plaques, this technique allows one to see aggregated forms of Aβ but not the more pathogenic oligomeric soluble forms. Notably, there is general agreement that the AD brain experiences a notable elevation in Aβ accumulation. Large regions in the medial and lateral association cortex are particularly vulnerable to Aβ deposition, even in people without dementia, according to research on brain Aβ mapping. Notably, Aβ deposition in the medial parietal cortex appears to be the initial step in the development of AD. In fact, it appears that Aβ deposition occurs in the striatum and medial temporal lobe (MTL) in patients with autosomal-dominant Alzheimer's disease (ADAD) up to 20 years prior to the onset of the disease, and that Aβ deposition starts in the medial parietal and frontal cortex in patients with AD on an aging background. It is noteworthy that while Aβ accumulation occurs all over the association cortex, there is very little correlation between it and symptoms. The amyloid-PET technique appears to be the only one where more or less reliable cut-points for AD are emerging. A thorough analysis comparing various techniques for establishing cut-points has revealed that a universal centiloid value of 19 for amyloid-PET appears to be a well-established cut-point in AD.

9.3.6.2. Tau-PET

Given that Tau-PET ligands are relatively new, not many longitudinal studies about Tau accumulation have been done. Nevertheless, a second generation of Tau tracers (such as 18F-RO-948) was created after the first generation, whose main issue was off-target binding. At the moment, several studies are providing more insight into the spatiotemporal dynamics of Tau accumulation. The MTL may be the starting point for Tau pathology, even though its exact timing and location are unknown. Patients with AD have shown markedly elevated levels of Tau tracer retention in the MTL, inferior lateral temporal, posterior cingulate, and lateral parietal regions. Second-generation Tau tracers have made it possible to confirm that AD patients show increased tracer signals in the prefrontal cortex, posterior cingulate, lateral parietal and occipital lobes, and medial temporal areas. Nevertheless, there are still very few clinical and experimental validations of Tau tracers, and it is unknown how much hyperphosphorylated Tau is present in the brain below the detectable threshold. These are a few of the causes behind the lack of a trustworthy Tau-PET cut-point for AD diagnosis.

9.3.6.3. FDG-PET

Using FDG, a glucose analog, PET can be used to map brain glucose metabolism. This allows for the characterization of metabolic activity, which is often linked to the loss of neuronal and/or synaptic function in AD. However, it could also reflect changes in glial cell function, which is essential for understanding AD neuropathology. Hypometabolism differs in location among AD syndromes, providing an opportunity to discern the specific phenotype: it begins in the MTL before the onset of the disease, spreading to the lateral parietal cortex in ADAD; it is related to Tau deposition in early-onset Alzheimer's disease; and it is prominent in the MTL and medial parietal lobe in late-onset Alzheimer's disease. In contrast, hypometabolism does not follow a distinct pattern in normal aging. As the disease progresses, characteristic brain hypometabolism appears in the temporoparietal and posterior cingulate cortices. However, the specific grade and location of hypometabolism necessary to establish a reliable threshold value for AD patients has not yet been determined.

9.3.6.4. Structural MRI

Structural MRI allows for precise, noninvasive measurement of brain tissue volumes based on an internal signal. This allows for the accurate localization of pathophysiological features such as white matter damage, gray matter loss, or regional brain atrophy. The primary results obtained from brain volumetric measurement techniques have revealed gray matter atrophy of MTL structures occurring in both AD and MCI. It appears that the left MTL atrophy is the most reliable biomarker for conversion from MCI to AD. A more nebulous cortical loss in AD and a decrease in the gray matter volumes of the hippocampal and parahippocampal regions are additional factors that predict the transition from MCI to AD. Furthermore, degradation of some major tracts in AD has been detected by diffusion imaging techniques, which use the anisotropic nature of microscopic water diffusion in the human brain to identify white matter tracts. The cingulum, which links MTL structures to the rest of the brain, is primarily disrupted during the phases that separate normal aging from Alzheimer's disease. There has also been evidence of damage to the uncinate fasciculus, a region involved in memory and emotional processing. However, the quantity of data needed to establish a trustworthy threshold value for cortical thinning is currently lacking, and it is unknown how many brain cells or white matter tracts must be lost to identify and characterize atrophy in AD (Daniilidou et al., 2023).

9.3.6.5. Functional MRI

Functional MRI (fMRI) measures MRI signals reflecting tissue perfusion in the brain, identifying synchronous signal fluctuations among different brain regions to determine connectivity within brain networks. Disruption of these signals indicates changes in network connectivity and can be studied to understand alterations in brain connectivity. Loss of functional connectivity in critical regions of the default-mode network (DMN) has been observed before gray matter loss in Alzheimer's disease (AD). Changes in DMN connectivity signals detected by fMRI may serve as a potential biomarker for AD, as disruptions in other brain networks are characteristic of different types of dementia. Disconnection in the hippocampus and medial prefrontal cortex also aligns with AD neuropathology. However, the lack of established cut-points for fMRI signal alterations hinders the use of fMRI as a diagnostic tool for distinguishing individuals with AD.

9.3.7. CSF Study Population Characteristics

Table 9.1 presents the clinical and demographic characteristics of the CSF cohort, categorized by diagnosis. In summary, participants with Alzheimer's disease were considerably older than those with subjective cognitive decline and mild cognitive impairment (P = 0.005), but there was no difference in the distribution of sexes between the three diagnostic groups (P = 0.68). Furthermore, following age adjustment, the MMSE score for those with Alzheimer's disease was lower than that of the other two groups ($P < 0.0001$). When comparing individuals with Alzheimer's disease to those with subjective cognitive decline and mild cognitive impairment, CSF Aβ42 levels were significantly lower and t-tau levels were higher ($P < 0.0001$ for both comparisons). However, after age correction, p-tau levels did not change ($P = 0.108$). Patients with Alzheimer's disease tended to be more likely to be APOE e4 carriers ($P = 0.077$). Between the groups, there were no variations in the prevalence of other recognized chronic conditions.

9.3.8. CSF Levels of the Biomarkers Stratified by Diagnostic Groups and -Amyloid Pathology Status

They first investigated the CSF levels of each individual biomarker, stratified by diagnosis, as illustrated in Figure 9.3 A–K. The age difference between the groups may have had a confounding effect, so all analyzes were conducted after age adjustment.

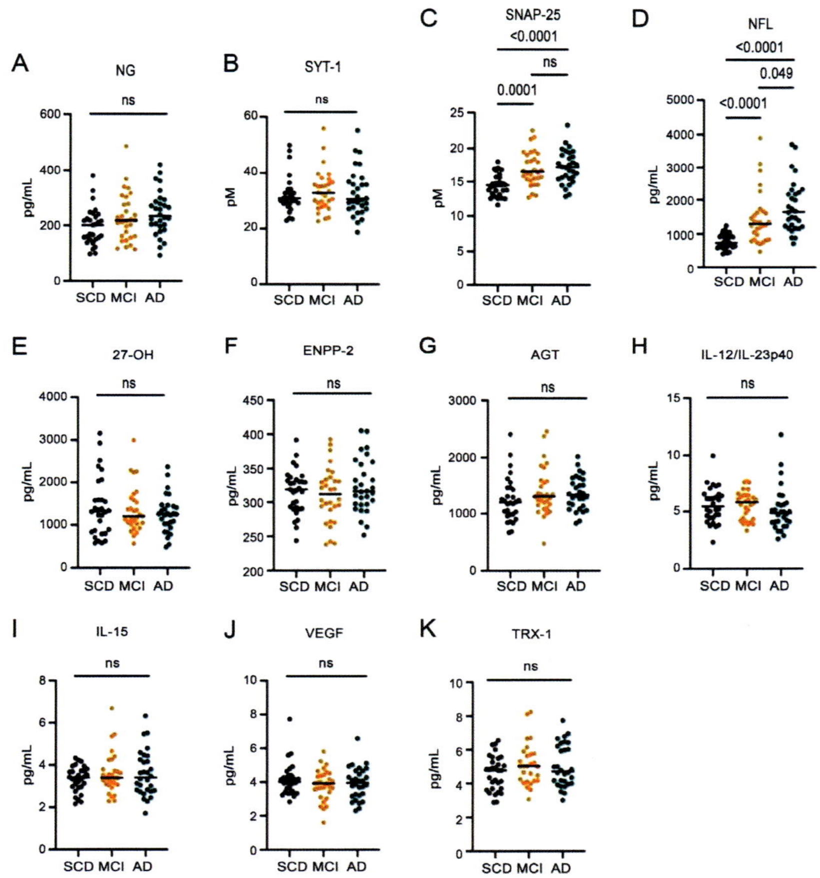

Figure 9.3. *Scatter plots depicting biomarker levels across clinical groups (A–K). Biomarker concentrations are on the y-axis. The median is shown as a horizontal line. P-values were calculated by ANCOVA, adjusting for age.*

Source: *Daniilidou M, Eroli F, Alanko V, Goikolea J, Latorre-Leal M, Rodriguez-Rodriguez P, Griffiths WJ, Wang Y, Pacciarini M, Brinkmalm A, Zetterberg H, Blennow K, Rosenberg A, Bogdanovic N, Winblad B, Kivipelto M, Ibghi D, Cedazo-Minguez A, Maioli S, Matton A.*

There were notable differences in SNAP-25 and NFL between the three diagnostic groups. To be more precise, SNAP-25 was higher in mild cognitive impairment and Alzheimer's disease compared to subjective cognitive decline (P = 0.0001 and P < 0.0001, respectively; Figure 9.3C). NFL was greater in participants with Alzheimer's disease than in those with mild cognitive impairment or subjective cognitive decline (P = 0.049 and P < 0.0001), as well as in mild cognitive impairment compared to subjective cognitive decline (P < 0.0001; Figure 9.3D). For the remaining biomarkers, there were no additional group-level differences that could be found.

TRX-80 and calprotectin were not present in enough CSF samples for further analysis. Out of 90 individuals, 34 had detectable calprotectin and 31 had detectable TRX-80. There were no differences in detection rates among diagnostic groups for either biomarker (P = 0.231 for calprotectin, P = 0.640 for TRX-80) or in levels among individuals with quantifiable data (P = 0.466 for calprotectin, P = 0.546 for TRX-80). When comparing biomarker levels by amyloid pathology status (A− for CSF Ab42 levels >550 pg/mL, A+ for CSF Ab42 levels <550 pg/mL), several markers were higher in A+ participants compared to A− participants; NG (P = 0.021), SNAP-25 (P < 0.0001), NFL (P < 0.0001), 27-OH (P = 0.027), IL-15 (P < 0.001), and TRX-1 (P = 0.041).

9.3.9. CSF Biomarker Correlations to Age, Sex and One Another

The associations between each marker and age, sex, and other markers—as well as with the known biomarkers for Alzheimer's disease (Aβ42, t-tau, and p-tau)," were then investigated. P = 0.037 and P = 0.048 showed that women had higher levels of NG and IL-12/IL-23p40 than men did. Figure 9.4 displays correlation maps showing relationships to age and among markers.

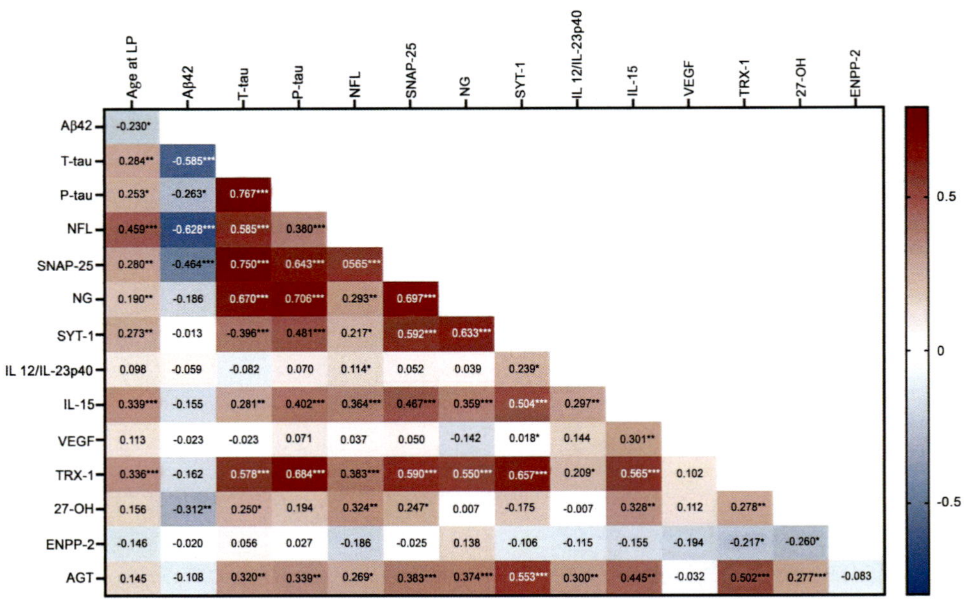

Figure 9.4. *Correlation matrix of the analyzed biomarkers.*

Source: Daniilidou M, Eroli F, Alanko V, Goikolea J, Latorre-Leal M, Rodriguez-Rodriguez P, Griffiths WJ, Wang Y, Pacciarini M, Brinkmalm A, Zetterberg H, Blennow K, Rosenberg A, Bogdanovic N, Winblad B, Kivipelto M, Ibghi D, Cedazo-Minguez A, Maioli S, Matton A.

SNAP-25, NFL, SYT-1, IL-15, TRX-1, Aβ42, t-tau, and p-tau all correlated with age, according to our data. T-tau, p-tau, NFL, SNAP-25, and 27-OH levels all showed a negative correlation with Aβ42 levels. An increase in NFL, synaptic markers, IL-15, TRX-1, and AGT was linked to higher t-tau and p-tau levels. Moreover, a positive correlation was observed between 27-OH and t-tau. Correlation map: After the core biomarkers for Alzheimer's disease and synaptic biomarkers, the most significant correlations were found with IL-15, TRX-1, and AGT. IL-12/IL-23p40, NFL, synaptic markers, 27-OH, and each other were all correlated with all three. In addition, TRX-1 and ENPP-2 had a negative correlation with IL-15 and a positive correlation with VEGF.

9.3.10. Associations Between Mechanistic Biomarkers and Key Elements of Alzheimer's Disease Pathogenesis

The relationship between Alzheimer's disease pathology, synaptic dysfunction, neurodegeneration, and cognition was further investigated, as were the potential associations between the biomarkers of cholesterol dysmetabolism (27-OH), vascular function (AGT, VEGF), inflammation (IL-12/IL-23p40, IL-15), oxidative stress (TRX-1), and glucose homeostasis (ENPP-2). In order to achieve this, we ran independent linear regression models using the p-tau/Aβ42, SNAP-25, NFL, and MMSE scores as outcome variables and the regressors being each of the various biological mechanism biomarkers. Age, sex, and diagnosis were taken into account for all models. Since it has been demonstrated to be more effective at determining β-amyloid pathology than individual markers, the p-tau/Aβ42 ratio was chosen as a specific marker for Alzheimer's disease. They selected SNAP-25 as a synaptic dysfunction outcome measure because it was the only synaptic marker that varied between the clinical groups in our material and because research has shown that it has the best discriminatory power to separate patients with Alzheimer's disease from those without the disease when compared to other synaptic biomarkers.

A summary of the analysis' findings can be found in Table 9.2. IL-15, TRX-1, and AGT exhibited the strongest correlations, which is consistent with our correlation analysis results. In particular, IL-15 and TRX-1 were positively correlated with the p-tau/Aβ42 ratio (β = 0.300, P = 0.0001 and β = 0.451, P = 0.0001, respectively), SNAP-25 (β = 0.507, P = 0.0001 and β = 0.593, P = 0.0001, respectively), and NFL (β = 0.371, P = 0.0001 and β = 0.310, P = 0.0001, respectively). NFL (β = 0.160, P = 0.047) and SNAP-25 (β = 0.354, $P < 0.0001$) were linked to AGT. Additionally, it was found that 27-OH and IL-12/IL-23p40 were linked to NFL (β = 0.223, P = 0.007 and β = 0.260, P = 0.001). NFL and ENPP-2 showed a negative correlation (β = -0.162, P = 0.047). The MMSE score (β = 0.259, P = 0.015) was only correlated with IL-15. With regard to VEGF, no correlations were found. The outcomes remained unchanged when osteoarthritis, autoimmune diseases, or cardiovascular disease were added to each model independently.

Table 9.2. Linear Regression Models

	p-tau/Aβ42 β (P-value)	SNAP-25 β (P-value)	NFL β (P-value)	MMSE β (P-value)
Single Biomarkers				
AGT	0.103 (0.202)	0.354 (<0.001)	0.160 (0.047)	0.104 (0.301)
27-OH	0.150 (0.067)	0.168 (0.092)	0.223 (0.007)	0.172 (0.090)
IL-12/IL-23p40	0.074 (0.369)	0.134 (0.173)	0.260 (0.001)	−0.003 (0.977)
IL-15	0.300 (<0.001)	0.507 (<0.0001)	0.371 (<0.0001)	0.259 (0.015)
TRX-1	0.451 (<0.0001)	0.593 (<0.0001)	0.310 (<0.001)	0.094 (0.391)
VEGF	0.128 (0.117)	0.116 (0.240)	0.067 (0.419)	0.043 (0.673)
ENPP-2	0.018 (0.829)	−0.024 (0.809)	−0.162 (0.047)	−0.148 (0.136)
Composites				
Vascular/ metabolic	0.143 (0.080)	0.298 (0.002)	0.115 (0.164)	0.047 (0.641)
Inflammatory	0.237 (0.004)	0.374 (<0.001)	0.412 (<0.0001)	0.141 (0.180)
Survival	0.357 (<0.0001)	0.448 (<0.0001)	0.249 (0.003)	0.092 (0.390)

Source: Daniilidou M, Eroli F, Alanko V, Goikolea J, Latorre-Leal M, Rodriguez-Rodriguez P, Griffiths WJ, Wang Y, Pacciarini M, Brinkmalm A, Zetterberg H, Blennow K, Rosenberg A, Bogdanovic N, Winblad B, Kivipelto M, Ibghi D, Cedazo-Minguez A, Maioli S, Matton A.

The data from independent linear regression models that used each individual biomarker or composite score as a regressor and p-tau/Aβ42, SNAP-25, NFL, or MMSE as the outcome measure. Standardized β coefficients (P-values) are displayed for the data, adjusted for age, sex, and diagnosis.

9.3.11. Stratification of Biomarkers Into Composite Scores

They then sought to determine whether it would be possible to gather more data and improve our comprehension of the contributing mechanisms to Alzheimer's disease by classifying the various biomarkers into biological pathways. Consequently, they arranged them according to their correlation with particular biological processes, giving rise to three theoretical variables, denoted by composite scores: vascular/metabolic, inflammatory, and survival. Z-scores for AGT, 27-OH, and ENPP-2 were averaged to calculate the vascular/metabolic composite. Z-scores for IL-12/23p40, IL-15, and TRX-1 and VEGF were averaged to calculate the inflammatory composite. Figure 9.5 illustrates how the composite scores were distributed among the clinical groups. Not a single composite showed any discernible variation between the clinical groups. The survival component score was higher in subjects with amyloid pathology when the patients were categorized as amyloid positive versus negative.

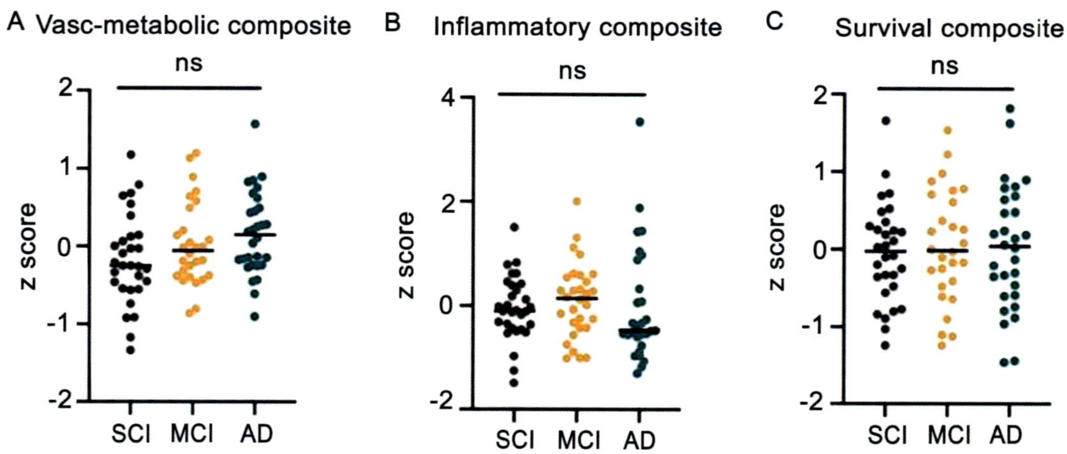

Figure 9.5. *Scatter plots of CSF biomarker composite scores in SCD, MCI and AD.*

Source: Daniilidou M, Eroli F, Alanko V, Goikolea J, Latorre-Leal M, Rodriguez-Rodriguez P, Griffiths WJ, Wang Y, Pacciarini M, Brinkmalm A, Zetterberg H, Blennow K, Rosenberg A, Bogdanovic N, Winblad B, Kivipelto M, Ibghi D, Cedazo-Minguez A, Maioli S, Matton A.

The association between each composite score and the pathology of Alzheimer's disease (p-tau/Aβ42), synaptic dysfunction (SNAP-25), neurodegeneration (NFL), and cognition (MMSE) was then investigated using linear regression models that controlled for age, sex, and diagnosis (Table 9.2). For vascular/metabolic, inflammatory, and survival composite, the SNAP-25 composite scores were as follows: $\beta = 0.298$, $P = 0.002$, $\beta = 0.374$, $P < 0.0001$, and $\beta = 0.448$, $P < 0.0001$, respectively. Additionally, p-tau/Aβ42 ($\beta = 0.237$, $P = 0.004$ and $\beta = 0.357$, $P < 0.0001$) and NFL ($\beta = 0.412$, $P < 0.0001$ and $\beta = 0.249$, $P = 0.003$) were linked to inflammatory and survival composites. They were all unrelated to cognition. The outcomes remained unchanged when additional chronic medical conditions were added one at a time to each model.

9.3.12. Patient Clustering by Biological Mechanisms

They conducted a two-step clustering analysis on the entire data set ($n = 86$; four samples were excluded owing to missing data) in order to evaluate the various biomarker profiles within the cohort. The seven comparatively unknown biomarkers linked to pathways that confer an elevated risk of Alzheimer's disease served as the foundation for this data-driven, unbiased clustering. There were two clusters found (Figure 9.6A), with TRX-1, AGT, and IL-15 acting as the main drivers of this stratification. When compared to Cluster 2, the individuals assigned to Cluster 1 showed parallel increases in CSF TRX-1 ($P \ll 0.0001$), AGT ($P \ll 0.0001$), IL-15 ($P \ll 0.0001$), 27-OH ($P = 0.004$), and IL-12/IL-23p40 ($P = 0.002$), as shown in Figure 9.6A and Table 9.3. Of the cohort population, 37% belonged to Cluster 1 ($n = 32$), which included 30% of the groups with subjective cognitive decline, 42% to those with mild cognitive impairment, and 40% of those with Alzheimer's disease (Figure 9.6B). Individuals in Cluster 1 were older ($P < 0.0001$), had higher levels of NFL and SNAP-25 ($P < 0.0001$ and $P = 0.011$, respectively), and had a tendency toward an increased p-tau/Aβ42 ratio (P = 0.080; Table 9.3) in comparison to Cluster 2. Between the two clusters, there were no variations in the levels of VEGF (P = 0.434) and ENPP-2 (P = 0.224). Furthermore, the clinical group distributions in both clusters were comparable (P = 0.590, Pearson's $\chi 2$).

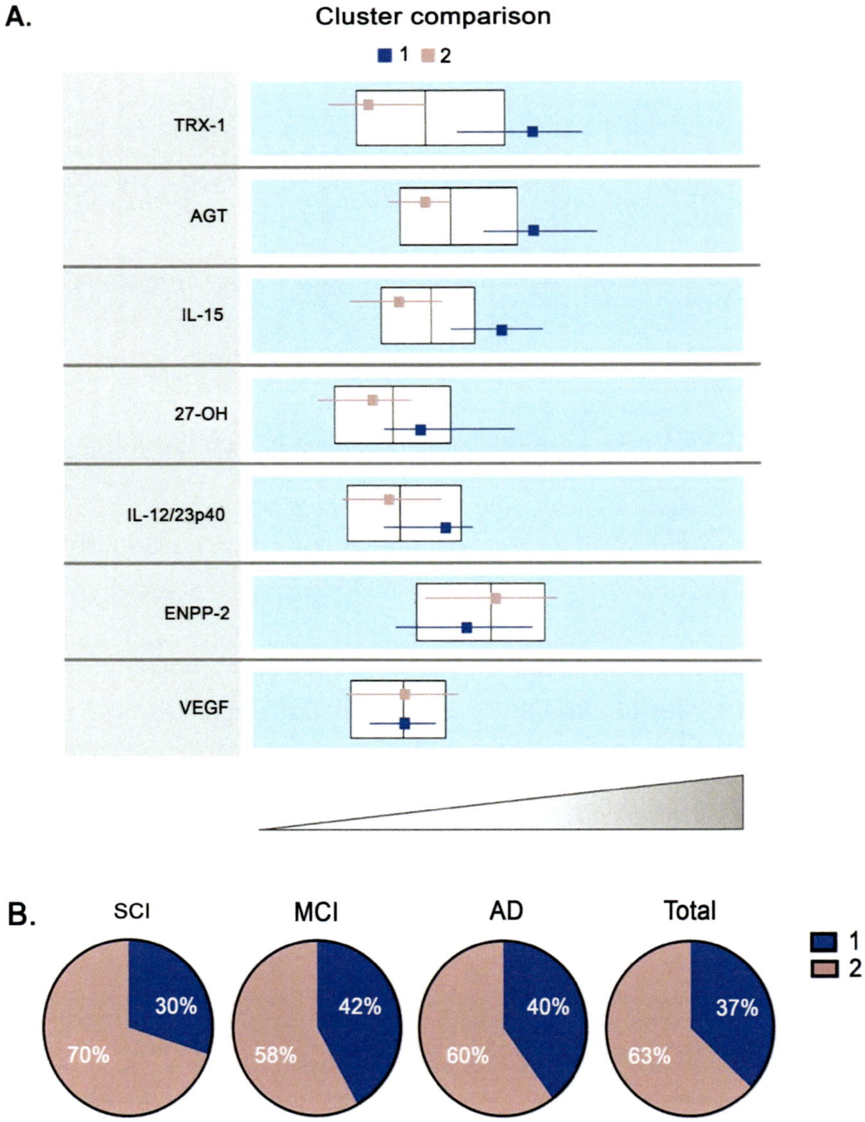

Figure 9.6. *Multivariate clustering of patients.*

Source: Daniilidou M, Eroli F, Alanko V, Goikolea J, Latorre-Leal M, Rodriguez-Rodriguez P, Griffiths WJ, Wang Y, Pacciarini M, Brinkmalm A, Zetterberg H, Blennow K, Rosenberg A, Bogdanovic N, Winblad B, Kivipelto M, Ibghi D, Cedazo-Minguez A, Maioli S, Matton A.

Table 9.3. Demographic, Cognition and Biomarker Comparisons Between Clusters

	Cluster 1 (*n* = 32)	Cluster 2 (*n* = 54)	*P*-value
Age	68.4 (7.1)	63.2 (5.9)	<0.0001
Female, %	62.5%	46.3%	0.146
MMSE	27.4 (2.5)	25.8 (4.9)	0.016
p-tau/Aβ42	0.12 (0.06)	0.10 (0.05)	0.080
SNAP-25, pM	17.5 (2.3)	15.3 (2.0)	<0.0001
NFL, pg/mL	1654.8 (848.8)	1123.5 (551.8)	0.011
TRX-1, ng/mL	5.9 (0.9)	4.3 (0.8)	<0.0001
AGT, ng/mL	1646.1 (373.4)	1148.7 (234.3)	<0.0001
IL-15, pg/mL	4.1 (0.8)	3.1 (0.6)	<0.0001
27-OH, pg/mL	1565.5 (0.630.6)	1196.2 (486.1)	0.004
IL-12/IL-23p40, pg/mL	6.0 (1.7)	5.1 (1.4)	0.002
ENPP-2, ng/mL	310.1 (40.4)	323.3 (34.8)	0.224
VEGF, pg/mL	3.9 (0.6)	4.0 (1.1)	0.434

Source: Daniilidou M, Eroli F, Alanko V, Goikolea J, Latorre-Leal M, Rodriguez-Rodriguez P, Griffiths WJ, Wang Y, Pacciarini M, Brinkmalm A, Zetterberg H, Blennow K, Rosenberg A, Bogdanovic N, Winblad B, Kivipelto M, Ibghi D, Cedazo-Minguez A, Maioli S, Matton A.

Despite individuals in Cluster 1 showing increased CSF levels of synaptic biomarkers (suggesting higher neurodegeneration), their overall cognitive performance in MMSE was found higher than in Cluster 2 ($P = 0.016$; Table 9.3).

9.3.13. Immunofluorescence Staining of TRX-1 and AGT in the Human Brain

They investigated the distribution and levels of TRX-1 and AGT in hippocampal sections from Alzheimer's disease and age-matched, non-demented subjects (controls), as they were two of the CSF markers with the strongest associations to neurodegenerative markers and, at the same time, relatively little research in human brain tissue. Co-staining the sections for p-tau was necessary because it was one of the markers in the CSF where correlations to AGT and TRX-1 were discovered. Both Alzheimer's disease and control cases showed a nuclear and cytoplasmic distribution of TRX-1 (Figure 9.7A). There were no differences in the two groups' levels of TRX-1 immunofluorescence that we could see. P-tau was primarily found in the cytoplasm in Alzheimer's disease brains, whereas it seemed to be mostly localized in the nuclei in control brains. In both groups, TRX-1 co-localized with p-tau to a comparable degree (Figure 9.7A and B). In comparison to control samples, immunofluorescence labeling for AGT was more prominent in Alzheimer's disease samples (Figure 9.7C). There was a noticeable co-staining between AGT and p-tau in the sections on Alzheimer's disease (P = 0.004; Figure 9.7C and D).

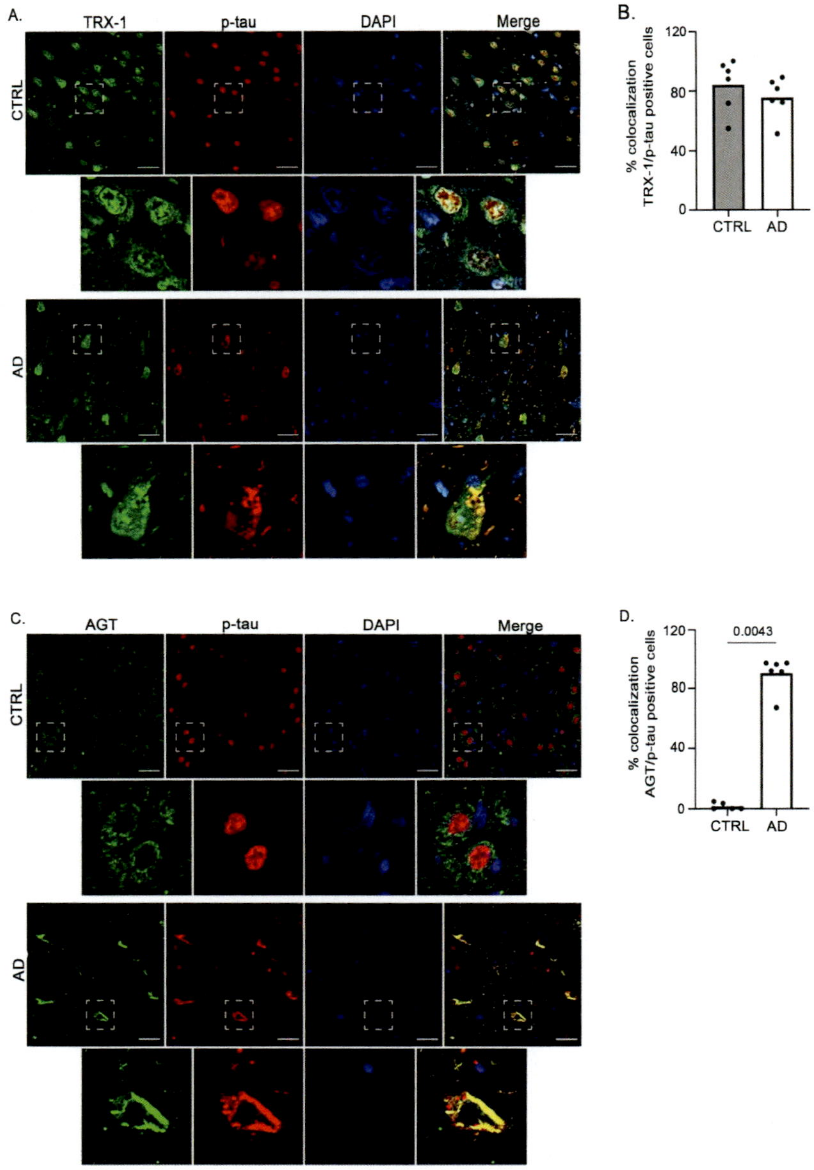

Figure 9.7. *Immunofluorescence co-staining of p-tau with thioredoxin-1 (TRX-1) or angiotensinogen (AGT) in human hippocampal sections.*

Source: Daniilidou M, Eroli F, Alanko V, Goikolea J, Latorre-Leal M, Rodriguez-Rodriguez P, Griffiths WJ, Wang Y, Pacciarini M, Brinkmalm A, Zetterberg H, Blennow K, Rosenberg A, Bogdanovic N, Winblad B, Kivipelto M, Ibghi D, Cedazo-Minguez A, Maioli S, Matton A.

9.3.14. CSF Biomarkers as Evidence of the Pathological Process

An early-stage biological marker of AD should ideally identify a key aspect of the disease's pathology with high accuracy. The intracellular build-up of abnormally hyperphosphorylated tau protein and the extracellular deposits of Aβ peptide are the main pathological characteristics of AD. The CSF is an ideal source of pathophysiological markers because it has direct contact with the brain's extracellular space and typically reflects pathological changes in the brain. Currently, β-amyloid peptide (Aβ42), total Tau (Tau), and the isoforms of phosphorylated Tau (P-Tau181 and P-Tau231) are the primary biological biomarkers used in AD diagnosis. Studies have looked into the relationships between AD-type neuropathologic alterations in the brain and antemortem CSF biomarker levels (Tau, P-Tau, and Aβ proteins). These clinico-pathological data demonstrated that P-tau represents tangle pathology and total Tau represents the degree of neuronal degeneration in the CSF.

Additionally, it has been shown that the numbers of Aβ plaques at post-mortem examination are inversely correlated with antemortem Aβ42. Furthermore, positron-emission tomography research reveals an inverse relationship between CSF Aβ42 levels and the total retention of the amyloid tracer Pittsburgh compound B (PiB). The amount of amyloid plaques and hyperphosphorylated Tau in cortical brain biopsies are associated with low CSF Aβ42 and high CSF levels of Tau markers, respectively. This finding was recently confirmed by a study that examined relationships between AD pathology in cortical brain biopsy and AD biomarkers in a series of 182 patients. Additionally, a sample of patients from a memory clinic showed a 94% concordance between CSF markers and neuropathological diagnosis (Daniilidou et al., 2023).

9.3.15. Sensitivity and Specificity of CSF Biomarkers for Alzheimer's Disease

Numerous studies have repeatedly shown that, in comparison to healthy controls, AD patients have lower levels of CSF Aβ42 and higher levels of CSF Tau and P-tau. Each of these biomarkers distinguishes AD patients from age-matched controls with 80–90% sensitivity and specificity, according to data from these studies. Compared to age-matched normal subjects, AD patients have CSF Aβ42 levels that are approximately 50% lower. The proposed explanations for the decline in CSF Aβ42 levels in AD patients include the aggregation of Aβ protein in amyloid plaques and the ensuing decrease in its availability in the CSF. However, it should be mentioned that other illnesses like Lewy body dementia, vascular dementia, and cerebral amyloid angiopathy can also cause a decrease in CSF Aβ42 levels. Therefore, while a lower level of Aβ42 is indicative of AD, it is insufficient to establish the etiology of the disease. Tau is thought to be a non-specific neuronal lesion marker linked to numerous biological processes. Total Tau CSF levels in AD patients are roughly three times higher than in age-matched controls. In addition to head trauma, stroke, and Creutzfeldt-Jakob disease, isolated elevated total Tau protein levels have also been linked to other acute neurodegenerative diseases and brain lesions. Conversely, the most specific biomarker of AD is P-Tau protein (subtypes P-Tau181 and P-Tau231), which is normal in non-AD diseases including those where Tau protein levels may be elevated, like stroke and Creutzfeldt-Jakob disease.

Total Tau, P-Tau, and Aβ42 are the three primary AD CSF markers. It is well known that the combination analysis of two or more of these markers yields the best accuracy in the differential diagnosis between AD patients and controls. When compared to any of the markers alone, the association between Aβ42 and Tau or P-Tau improves the sensitivity and specificity of AD diagnosis. A study that included neuropathological confirmation of the diagnosis proved the value of the combined approach of CSF biomarkers, showing that the ratio P-Tau/Aβ42 has a sensitivity of 91.6% and a specificity of 85.7% for AD diagnosis. A number of ratios have been proposed to take into account the combined analysis of biomarkers. These include the AD-CSF-Index, the ratios Tau/Aβ42 and P-Tau/Aβ42, and the Innotest Amyloid-Tau Index (IATI), which is defined by the ratio Aβ42/(240+1.18 x Tau). Although it has been suggested that an IATI score of less than 1 is suggestive of AD, this cut-off does not appear to be specific given the high prevalence (31%) of control subjects with this profile who do not have cognitive impairment (Daniilidou et al., 2023).

9.3.16. CSF Biomarkers in the Prodromal Stage (Pre-Dementia) of Alzheimer's Disease

Decades before the disease's clinical manifestation, the pathophysiological process of AD begins, with a progressive loss of synapses, axons, and neurons that occurs before the first cognitive symptoms—episodic memory impairment, in most cases—appear. Thus, there is a clinical phase prior to the dementia that characterizes the severe stage of the disease, during which the patients exhibit memory impairment to a degree that falls between that of age-matched normal controls and those who meet the clinical criteria for AD. This symptomatic predementia phase, also known as mild cognitive impairment (MCI), is distinguished by the preservation of autonomy. Extensive cohort studies conducted over the past 10 years have consistently demonstrated that an AD biomarker profile can accurately (up to 95% sensitivity) differentiate MCI patients who will progress to AD from healthy controls, as well as from MCI patients who will maintain cognitive stability during treatment. These long-term studies demonstrated that, in contrast to "MCI-stable" patients, "MCI-converters" have a normal biomarker profile and low Aβ42 levels linked to high levels of CSF total Tau and P-Tau. When combined, these findings provide credence to the usefulness of CSF markers in diagnosing AD incipients among patients experiencing mild cognitive impairment. These individuals may be referred to as "prodromal AD" if they exhibit an AD signature at CSF analysis, an objective memory deficit, and preserved autonomy.

Along with predementia stages of AD, abnormalities on CSF measures can eventually be seen in subjects who do not exhibit cognitive complaints; this is consistent with current understanding of the pathophysiology of AD. As per this theory, a protracted pathophysiological process comes before the onset of clinical symptoms in AD. The data from clinical trials, it should be noted, do not support the notion that asymptomatic individuals with any particular AD biomarker progress from normal cognition to AD. In light of this, the term "preclinical AD" is currently limited to research purposes and cannot be used to suggest clinical practices (Daniilidou et al., 2023).

9.3.17. The Prognostic Value of CSF Biomarkers

Whether CSF biomarkers are associated with clinical and imaging indicators of AD severity was the subject of several studies. According to data from a longitudinal study, during a one-year follow-up, low Aβ42, elevated Tau levels, and high Tau/Aβ42 are predictive of a faster rate of cognitive decline. Individuals who exhibit significant changes in CSF biomarkers, such as a reduction in Aβ42 and an increase in total Tau and P-Tau, seem to have an adverse course, characterized by a more severe cognitive decline, a poor response to anticholinesterase treatment, and a higher mortality rate. Additionally, subgroups of AD patients with unique clinical and neuropsychological profiles that may be linked to more severe cognitive impairment may be identified using CSF markers. Increased levels of Tau markers (total Tau and P-Tau) have also been linked to a significant positive correlation in hippocampal atrophy severity, according to neuroimaging studies using structural brain MRI. Elevations in CSF total Tau and P-Tau also appear to be associated with a quicker rate of hippocampal atrophy progression (Daniilidou et al., 2023).

9.3.18. CSF Biomarkers for the Differential Diagnosis Between Alzheimer's Disease and Other Dementias

The use of CSF biomarker analysis in the differential diagnosis of Alzheimer's disease (AD) and other dementias has grown. The best accuracy in differentiating between AD and other degenerative dementias is provided by the combined analysis of CSF biomarkers, as evidenced by data from multiple centers. P-Tau/Aβ42 in particular proved to be the most effective biomarker for distinguishing AD from semantic dementia and the behavioral variant of frontotemporal lobar degeneration, with specificity and sensitivity of 92.6 and 84.2, respectively, and 81.7 and 98.3, respectively. These results, which show a specificity of 96.6% in a group of patients with diagnostic confirmation either by genetics or by post-mortem examination, are consistent with earlier findings regarding the performance for the differential diagnosis between AD and frontotemporal lobar degeneration.

Additionally helpful in identifying patients with focal atypical presentations of AD are CSF biomarkers. Atypical focal forms of AD include non-amnestic focal cortical syndromes like posterior cortical atrophy (PCA), logopenic aphasia, and the frontal variant of AD, which show characteristic histological lesions of AD-type pathology at post-mortem examination. These differ from the typical amnestic profile "of the hippocampal type." For example, in nearly 60% of patients with primary progressive aphasia (PPA) and in over 80% of PCA cases at post-mortem examination, the retained diagnosis is AD-type pathology. It was noted that 60% of PCA patients (9/15) and 61.5% (16/26) of aphasic subjects had an AD biological profile, with both altered Tau/Aβ42 and P-Tau/Aβ42 ratios. These patient groups' biomarker assay results are consistent with the pathological studies. Additionally, in a group of PCA patients, a concordance between CSF markers and amyloid imaging with PiB was reported. Interestingly, two different brain perfusion profiles were found in a group of 34 PPA patients who underwent lumbar puncture and brain perfusion SPECT for CSF biomarkers. The PPA patients with an AD CSF profile displayed a perfusion pattern akin to that seen in logopenic aphasia, while the PPA patients without an AD CSF biomarker profile displayed a pattern of brain perfusion akin to that reported in semantic dementia. According to other research, logopenic aphasia is linked to significant PiB uptake, whereas semantic dementia and non-fluent aphasia do not show signs of amyloidosis on molecular imaging. This finding is consistent with the categorization of semantic dementia and non-fluent APP as language variants of frontotemporal lobar degeneration, and logopenic aphasia as a focal variant of AD. Patients with the so-called frontal variant of AD, a behavioral presentation resembling the behavioral variant of frontotemporal lobar degeneration, may also exhibit AD pathology. When combined, these findings provide credence to the use of CSF biomarkers in the diagnosis of AD pathology in patients presenting in an unusual way. CSF biomarkers help determine an underlying AD pathology in these patients because their positive results may reorient the diagnosis and, consequently, the therapeutics (Daniilidou et al., 2023).

A Closer Look

Tau Protein and Alzheimer's Disease

Tau is a tiny protein with a catchy moniker and a well-deserved reputation. This protein, which is mostly located in the brain, has several purposes in healthy brain cells. Tau is susceptible to environmental changes and genetic errors, just like the majority of proteins. These elements may render tau unable to perform its normal function, a condition linked to numerous brain disorders. The aberrant tau accumulates to form "tangles," which inflame and harm cells, exacerbating the symptoms of Alzheimer's disease. The majority of tau is present in neurons, which are the brain's messenger cells. Even the most basic tasks in our daily lives require communication between these cells. The unusual shape of neurons can be categorized into three sections: a long hallway, a messaging-sending end, and a messaging-receiving end. A superhighway system that moves critical molecules throughout the cell is located inside. This shuttle system needs to cross the neuron's lengthy axon, or hallway. The superhighway, or "skeleton" of the cell, is made up of microtubules, which resemble tubes. Tau helps these microtubules function at their best by stabilizing them. In the voids between neurons, tau also exists in smaller forms known as oligomers. When present in high doses, this can disrupt brain cell communication and cause disorientation. Decades before memory loss and other telltale signs of Alzheimer's disease manifest, there are elevated tau levels in the brain. In Alzheimer's disease, aberrant tau builds up and starts to cling to one another in structures known as neurofibrillary tangles. The cell's typical methods of getting rid of "trash" don't work well for these tangles. The accumulation impairs the microtubule superhighway, impairing the normal functioning of neurons.

The brainstem, which joins the brain and spinal cord, is where tau tangles first appear. They extend upward from the brainstem toward two crucial areas of the brain for memory. The brain's learning center is accessed through the entorhinal cortex, which is the first stop. Here are some of the brain cells that show some of the early signs of Alzheimer's disease damage. It then moves on to the hippocampus, which is the learning center. This is the process by which the brain forms a short-term memory and learns something new, like the rules of a board game. One of the many biological consequences of Alzheimer's disease that causes memory loss and other symptoms is the buildup of tangles in these areas. The degree and stage of the disease are correlated with the quantity of aberrant tau in the brain. Monitoring tau levels is a good way to spot cognitive decline early on and is a reliable predictor of it. Alzheimer's disease-related aberrant tau can be identified by two commercially available blood tests. These tests measure tau that has experienced hyperphosphorylation, a molecular alteration that results in abnormalities linked to Alzheimer's disease. To identify tau, specialized imaging techniques can also be employed. To visualize the brain, a doctor will first inject a brain tau-binding agent (also known as "tracers") into a vein. A positron emission tomography (PET) scan is used by medical professionals to visualize the tau by detecting a signal from the tracer. The amounts and locations of tau in the brain can then be seen by clinicians by examining the images obtained from these scans. Tau PET scans can offer a biomarker measurement that usefully shows the course of the disease. By 2020, the U.S. S. The first tau PET tracer (F-18 flortaucipir) was approved by the FDA. Tau PET scans are now a common component of Alzheimer's clinical trials as a potential biomarker of disease severity. One of the numerous ways Alzheimer's disease can damage brain cells and result in symptoms like memory loss is represented by this hallmark protein. Researchers are using this data to support earlier treatment and improved patient outcomes in the future by using it for early detection and diagnosis.

SUMMARY

- Alzheimer's disease is a neuropsychological ailment characterized by progressive degeneration of neurons, which results in dementia and mental impairment.
- Aβ is the main pathological hallmark of Alzheimer's disease, and CSF and PET biomarkers for Aβ pathology become abnormal decades before dementia symptom onset.
- The clinical value of these assays for quantification of plasma Aβ has been validated in different cohorts covering the complete continuum of Alzheimer's disease. The assays have also been compared with established Alzheimer's disease biomarkers (CSF $A\beta_{1-42}$ and Aβ-PET) and in relation to cognitive performance and cognitive decline (both baseline and longitudinal changes).
- GFAP is a major cytoskeletal constituent of astrocytes. In Alzheimer's disease, reactive astrocytosis has been implicated as a potential driver or effect of Alzheimer's disease pathological changes.
- Alzheimer's disease has a monogenetic determined cause in rare cases, with a mutation in either the PSEN1, PSEN2, or APP gene, or a multiplication of the APP gene, which also occurs in Down syndrome due to the chromosome 21 trisomy.
- Biomarker dynamics of pTau and NfL in individuals with genetically determined Alzheimer's disease are consistent with findings in people with sporadic Alzheimer's disease and provide insights into the timing of changes in these biomarkers.
- Alzheimer's disease participants were significantly older than subjective cognitive decline and mild cognitive impairment individuals ($P = 0.005$), whereas sex distribution did not differ between the three diagnostic groups ($P = 0.68$). In addition, MMSE score was lower in Alzheimer's disease compared with the other two groups after age adjustment ($P < 0.0001$).
- A biological marker of AD should detect with high accuracy a fundamental feature of AD's pathology early in the course of the disease. The core pathological hallmarks of the AD are the extracellular deposits of Aβ peptide and the intracellular accumulation of abnormally hyperphosphorylated tau protein.
- A multitude of studies has consistently demonstrated that AD patients exhibit a decrease in CSF $A\beta_{42}$ and an increase in CSF Tau and P-tau when compared with healthy controls. Data provided by these studies confirm that each of these biomarkers differentiates AD patients from age-matched controls with 80–90% sensitivity and specificity.
- The pathophysiological process of AD starts decades before the clinical onset of the disease, with a gradual loss of synapses, axons and neurons that progress before the appearance of the first cognitive symptoms, most often episodic memory impairment.

REFERENCES

1. Akterin, S., Cowburn, R. F., Miranda-Vizuete, A., et al. (2006). Involvement of glutaredoxin-1 and thioredoxin-1 in beta-amyloid toxicity and Alzheimer's disease. *Cell Death & Differentiation, 13*(9), 1454–1465. https://doi.org/10.1038/sj.cdd.4401811.

2. Arodin, L., Lamparter, H., Karlsson, H., et al. (2014). Alteration of thioredoxin and glutaredoxin in the progression of Alzheimer's disease. *Journal of Alzheimer's Disease, 39*(4), 787-797. https://doi.org/10.3233/JAD-131776.

3. Ballard, C., Gauthier, S., Corbett, A., Brayne, C., Aarsland, D., & Jones, E. (2011). Alzheimer's disease. *The Lancet, 377*(9770), 1019–1031. https://doi.org/10.1016/S0140-6736(10)61349-9.

4. Bateman, R. J., Xiong, C., Benzinger, T. L., et al. (2012). Clinical and biomarker changes in dominantly inherited Alzheimer's disease. *New England Journal of Medicine, 367*(9), 795–804. https://doi.org/10.1056/NEJMoa1202753.

5. Blennow, K., Hampel, H., Weiner, M., & Zetterberg, H. (2010). Cerebrospinal fluid and plasma biomarkers in Alzheimer's disease. *Nature Reviews Neurology, 6*(3), 131–144. https://doi.org/10.1038/nrneurol.2010.4.

6. Buerger, K., Ewers, M., Pirttilä, T., et al. (2006). CSF phosphorylated tau protein correlates with neocortical neurofibrillary pathology in Alzheimer's disease. *Brain, 129*(11), 3035–3041. https://doi.org/10.1093/brain/awl269.

7. Camporesi, E., Nilsson, J., Brinkmalm, A., et al. (2020). Fluid biomarkers for synaptic dysfunction and loss. *Biomarkers Insights, 15*, 1177271920950319. https://doi.org/10.1177/1177271920950319.

8. Cosarderelioglu, C., Nidadavolu, L. S., George, C. J., et al. (2020). Brain renin-angiotensin system at the intersect of physical and cognitive frailty. *Frontiers in Neuroscience, 14*, 586314. https://doi.org/10.3389/fnins.2020.586314.

9. Daniilidou, M., Eroli, F., Alanko, V., et al. (2023). Alzheimer's disease biomarker profiling in a memory clinic cohort without common comorbidities. *Brain Communications, 5*(5), fcad228. https://doi.org/10.1093/braincomms/fcad228.

10. De Meyer, S., Schaeverbeke, J. M., Verberk, I. M. W., et al. (2020). Comparison of ELISA- and SIMOA-based quantification of plasma Aβ ratios for early detection of cerebral amyloidosis. *Alzheimer's Research & Therapy, 12*, 162. https://doi.org/10.1186/s13195-020-00720-5.

11. Devi, G., & Scheltens, P. (2018). Heterogeneity of Alzheimer's disease: Consequence for drug trials? *Alzheimer's Research & Therapy, 10*(1), 122. https://doi.org/10.1186/s13195-018-0458-9.

12. Forgrave, L. M., Ma, M., Best, J. R., & DeMarco, M. L. (2019). The diagnostic performance of neurofilament light chain in CSF and blood for Alzheimer's disease, frontotemporal dementia, and amyotrophic lateral sclerosis: A systematic review and meta-analysis. *Alzheimer's & Dementia: Diagnosis, Assessment & Disease Monitoring, 11*, 730–743. https://doi.org/10.1016/j.dadm.2019.09.001.

13. Forlenza, O. V., Diniz, B. S., & Gattaz, W. F. (2010). Diagnosis and biomarkers of predementia in Alzheimer's disease. *BMC Medicine, 8*, 89. https://doi.org/10.1186/1741-7015-8-89.

14. Gerenu, G., Persson, T., Goikolea, J., et al. (2021). Thioredoxin-80 protects against amyloid-beta pathology through autophagic-lysosomal pathway regulation. *Molecular Psychiatry, 26*(4), 1410–1423. https://doi.org/10.1038/s41380-020-00980-6.

15. Gil-Bea, F., Akterin, S., Persson, T., et al. (2012). Thioredoxin-80 is a product of alpha-secretase cleavage that inhibits amyloid-beta aggregation and is decreased in Alzheimer's disease brain.

EMBO Molecular Medicine, 4(10), 1097–1111. https://doi.org/10.1002/emmm.201201380.

16. Grimmer, T., Riemenschneider, M., Forstl, H., et al. (2009). Beta amyloid in Alzheimer's disease: Increased deposition in brain is reflected in reduced concentration in cerebrospinal fluid. *Biological Psychiatry, 65*(10), 927–934. https://doi.org/10.1016/j.biopsych.2008.10.030.
17. Hansson, O. (2021). Biomarkers for neurodegenerative diseases. *Nature Medicine, 27*(6), 954–963. https://doi.org/10.1038/s41591-021-01368-y.
18. Herr, D. R., Chew, W. S., Satish, R. L., & Ong, W. Y. (2020). Pleiotropic roles of autotaxin in the nervous system present opportunities for the development of novel therapeutics for neurological diseases. *Molecular Neurobiology, 57*(1), 372–392. https://doi.org/10.1007/s12035-019-01747-5.
19. Jack, C. R. Jr, Bennett, D. A., Blennow, K., et al. (2018). NIA-AA Research Framework: Toward a biological definition of Alzheimer's disease. *Alzheimer's & Dementia, 14*(4), 535–562. https://doi.org/10.1016/j.jalz.2018.02.018.
20. Janelidze, S., Mattsson, N., Stomrud, E., et al. (2018). CSF biomarkers of neuroinflammation and cerebrovascular dysfunction in early Alzheimer's disease. *Neurology, 91*(9), e867–e877. https://doi.org/10.1212/WNL.0000000000006114.
21. Kellar, D., & Craft, S. (2020). Brain insulin resistance in Alzheimer's disease and related disorders: Mechanisms and therapeutic approaches. *The Lancet Neurology, 19*(9), 758–766. https://doi.org/10.1016/S1474-4422(20)30242-1.
22. Keshavan, A., Pannee, J., Karikari, T. K., et al. (2021). Population-based blood screening for preclinical Alzheimer's disease in a British birth cohort at age 70. *Brain, 144*(2), 434–449. https://doi.org/10.1093/brain/awaa426.
23. Lange, C., Storkebaum, E., de Almodóvar, C. R., Dewerchin, M., & Carmeliet, P. (2016). Vascular endothelial growth factor: A neurovascular target in neurological diseases. *Nature Reviews Neurology, 12*(8), 439–454. https://doi.org/10.1038/nrneurol.2016.88.
24. Li, W. W., Shen, Y. Y., Tian, D. Y., et al. (2019). Brain amyloid-β deposition and blood biomarkers in patients with clinically diagnosed Alzheimer's disease. *Journal of Alzheimer's Disease, 69*(1), 169–178. https://doi.org/10.3233/JAD-181209.
25. Lodeiro, M., Puerta, E., Ismail, M. A. M., et al. (2017). Aggregation of the inflammatory S100A8 precedes Aβ plaque formation in transgenic APP mice: Positive feedback for S100A8 and Aβ productions. *The Journals of Gerontology Series A: Biological Sciences and Medical Sciences, 72*(3), 319–328. https://doi.org/10.1093/gerona/glw122.
26. Loera-Valencia, R., Goikolea, J., Parrado-Fernandez, C., Merino-Serrais, P., & Maioli, S. (2019). Alterations in cholesterol metabolism as a risk factor for developing Alzheimer's disease: Potential novel targets for treatment. *Journal of Steroid Biochemistry and Molecular Biology, 190*, 104–114. https://doi.org/10.1016/j.jsbmb.2019.03.004.
27. Mateos, L., Ismail, M. A. M., Gil-Bea, F. J., et al. (2011). Upregulation of brain renin angiotensin system by 27-hydroxycholesterol in Alzheimer's disease. *Journal of Alzheimer's Disease, 24*(4), 669–679. https://doi.org/10.3233/JAD-2011-101938.
28. McLimans, K. E., & Willette, A. A. (2017). Autotaxin is related to metabolic dysfunction and predicts Alzheimer's disease outcomes. *Journal of Alzheimer's Disease, 56*(1), 403–413. https://doi.org/10.3233/JAD-160875.

29. Milà-Alomà, M., Brinkmalm, A., Ashton, N. J., et al. (2021). CSF synaptic biomarkers in the preclinical stage of Alzheimer's disease and their association with MRI and PET: A cross-sectional study. *Neurology, 97*(21), e2065–e2078. https://doi.org/10.1212/WNL.0000000000013086.

30. Murray, M. E., Graff-Radford, N. R., Ross, O. A., et al. (2011). Neuropathologically defined subtypes of Alzheimer's disease with distinct clinical characteristics: A retrospective study. *The Lancet Neurology, 10*(9), 785–796. https://doi.org/10.1016/S1474-4422(11)70156-9.

31. Nakamura, A., Kaneko, N., Villemagne, V. L., et al. (2018). High performance plasma amyloid-β biomarkers for Alzheimer's disease. *Nature, 554*(7691), 249–254. https://doi.org/10.1038/nature25456.

32. Nitsch, L., Schneider, L., Zimmermann, J., & Müller, M. (2021). Microglia-derived interleukin 23: A crucial cytokine in Alzheimer's disease? *Frontiers in Neurology, 12*, 639353. https://doi.org/10.3389/fneur.2021.639353.

33. Olsson, B., Lautner, R., Andreasson, U., et al. (2016). CSF and blood biomarkers for the diagnosis of Alzheimer's disease: A systematic review and meta-analysis. *The Lancet Neurology, 15*(7), 673–684. https://doi.org/10.1016/S1474-4422(16)00070-3.

34. Querfurth, H. W., & LaFerla, F. M. (2010). Alzheimer's disease. *New England Journal of Medicine, 362*, 329–344. https://doi.org/10.1056/NEJMra0909142.

35. Rosenberg, A., Solomon, A., Jelic, V., Hagman, G., Bogdanovic, N., & Kivipelto, M. (2019). Progression to dementia in memory clinic patients with mild cognitive impairment and normal β-amyloid. *Alzheimer's Research & Therapy, 11*(1), 99. https://doi.org/10.1186/s13195-019-0555-2.

36. Sarazin, M., Dorothee, G., de Souza, L. C., & Aucouturier, P. (2013). Immunotherapy in Alzheimer's disease: Do we have all the pieces of the puzzle? *Biological Psychiatry, 74*(5), 329–332. https://doi.org/10.1016/j.biopsych.2013.04.006.

37. Scheltens, P., De Strooper, B., Kivipelto, M., et al. (2021). Alzheimer's disease. *Lancet, 397*(10281), 1577–1590. https://doi.org/10.1016/S0140-6736(21)00278-8.

38. Schindler, S. E., Bollinger, J. G., Ovod, V., et al. (2019). High-precision plasma β-amyloid 42/40 predicts current and future brain amyloidosis. *Neurology, 93*(16), e1647–e1659. https://doi.org/10.1212/WNL.0000000000008081.

39. Strozyk, D., Blennow, K., White, L. R., & Launer, L. J. (2003). CSF Aβ42 levels correlate with amyloid-neuropathology in a population-based autopsy study. *Neurology, 60*(5), 652–656. https://doi.org/10.1212/01.WNL.0000046581.91536.0C.

40. Tapiola, T., Alafuzoff, I., Herukka, S. K., et al. (2009). Cerebrospinal fluid β-amyloid 42 and tau proteins as biomarkers of Alzheimer-type pathologic changes in the brain. *Archives of Neurology, 66*(3), 382–389. https://doi.org/10.1001/archneurol.2009.43.

41. Tapiola, T., Overmyer, M., Lehtovirta, M., et al. (1997). The level of cerebrospinal fluid tau correlates with neurofibrillary tangles in Alzheimer's disease. *Neuroreport, 8*(16), 3961–3963. https://doi.org/10.1097/00001756-199712220-00030.

42. Thijssen, E. H., Verberk, I. M. W., Vanbrabant, J., et al. (2021). Highly specific and ultrasensitive plasma test detects Abeta (1–42) and Abeta (1–40) in Alzheimer's disease. *Scientific Reports, 11*, 9736. https://doi.org/10.1038/s41598-021-89191-8.

43. Tolboom, N., van der Flier, W. M., Yaqub, M., et al. (2009). Relationship of cerebrospinal fluid markers to 11C-PiB and 18F-FDDNP binding. *Journal of Nuclear Medicine, 50*(9), 1464–1470. https://doi.org/10.2967/jnumed.109.064360

44. Vergallo, A., Mégret, L., Lista, S., et al. (2019). Plasma amyloid β 40/42 ratio predicts cerebral amyloidosis in cognitively normal individuals at risk for Alzheimer's disease. *Alzheimer's & Dementia, 15*(6), 764–775. https://doi.org/10.1016/j.jalz.2019.01.009.

45. Vermunt, L., Sikkes, S. A. M., van den Hout, A., et al. (2019). Duration of preclinical, prodromal, and dementia stages of Alzheimer's disease in relation to age, sex, and APOE genotype. *Alzheimer's & Dementia, 15*(7), 888–898. https://doi.org/10.1016/j.jalz.2019.03.004.

46. Wimo, A., Winblad, B., & Jonsson, L. (2010). The worldwide societal costs of dementia: Estimates for 2009. *Alzheimer's & Dementia, 6*(2), 98–103. https://doi.org/10.1016/j.jalz.2010.01.010.

Chapter

10

RISK ASSESSMENT AND PREVENTION OF ALZHEIMER'S DISEASE

Contents

Introduction 348
10.1. Risk Factors for Alzheimer's Disease 350
10.2. Fall Risk Assessment Among Older Adults with Mild Alzheimer's Disease 354
10.3. The Prevention of Alzheimer's Disease 358
10.4. Challenges For Alzheimer's Disease Therapy 365
Summary 376
References 377

INTRODUCTION

In medicine, the phrases "prevention" and "risk reduction" are frequently used synonymously to describe therapeutic approaches intended to postpone or stop the onset of an illness. Every term has different implications, some of which could suggest that a suggested intervention has different therapeutic effects. The terms used to describe interventions intended to maintain cognitive function and/or slow the progression of Alzheimer's disease (AD) are the subject of much discussion. Furthermore, when utilizing these terms, it's critical to distinguish between Alzheimer's disease prevention and Alzheimer's dementia prevention.

Growing interest has been shown in "preventative" interventions, which include co-morbid medical conditions that are linked to an increased risk of AD dementia, pharmacologic approaches that target disease pathology (such as anti-amyloid immunotherapies), and lifestyle changes (such as increased physical activity and improved nutrition). The interventions are intended to give patients an evidence-based plan in an attempt to slow down or stop the progression of the disease from preclinical (asymptomatic) AD to more advanced stages. Even though "prevention" may be the ultimate objective, there are a variety of "risk reduction" interventions that may be used in conjunction with a wide range of other strategies (e.g., removal of pathology, enhancement of cognitive reserve, focus on resilience).

The language surrounding pre-AD dementia interventions is particularly important because there is currently no cure for AD. Furthermore, although earlier research has established evidence-based standards for the various stages of AD, there are currently no established clinical consensus standards to direct doctors' practical application of these terms (Cummings et al., 2016; Ritchie et al., 2016; Winblad et al., 2016; Livingston et al., 2020).

Orientation and Directional Terms

Term	Definition	Illustration
Mendelian randomization	Mendelian randomization can be used to look at whether levels of a substance found naturally in a person's body is linked to disease. Measuring the levels themselves can be a problem because the levels can change in response to other factors that could be related to the disease, such as diet, smoking, or alcohol use.	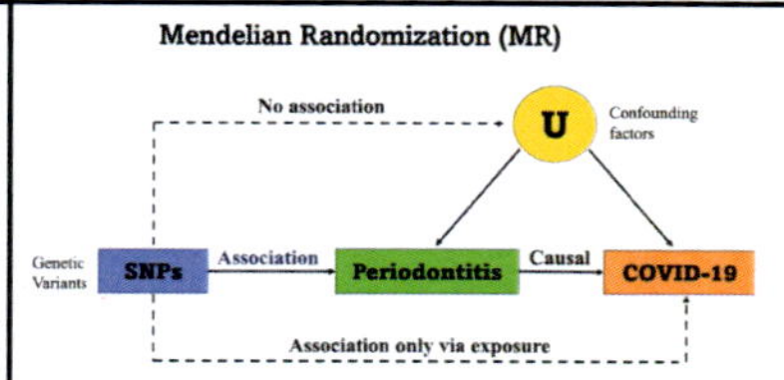
Dyslipidemia	Dyslipidemia is defined as having blood lipid levels that are too high or low. Blood lipids are fatty substances, such as triglycerides and cholesterol. Dyslipidemia may not always cause symptoms but it can lead to other conditions.	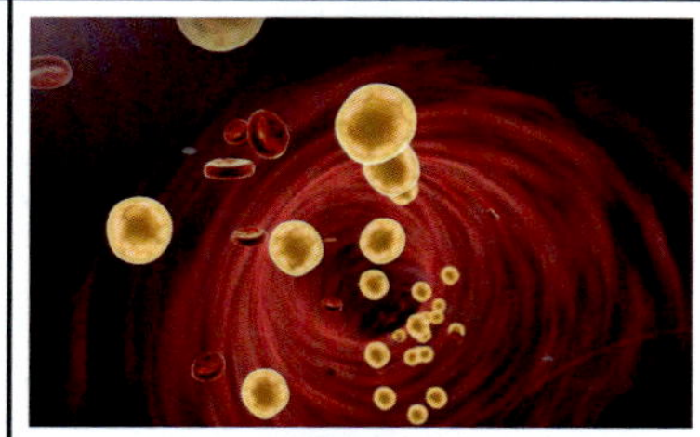
Blood lipids	Blood lipids are lipids in the blood, either free or bound to other molecules. They are mostly transported in a phospholipid capsule, and the type of protein embedded in this outer shell determines the fate of the particle and its influence on metabolism.	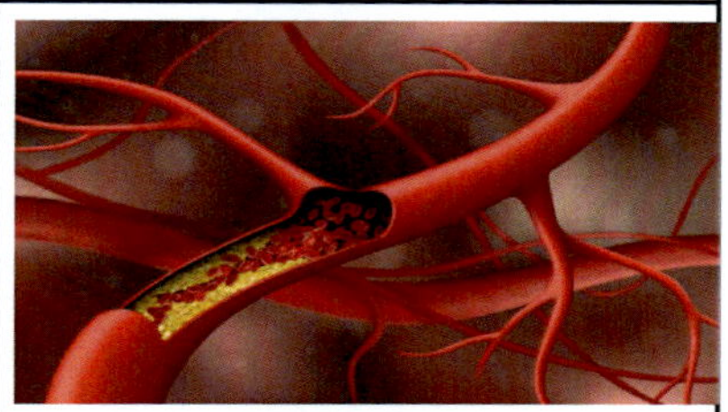
Body mass index	Body mass index is a value derived from the mass and height of a person. The BMI is defined as the body mass divided by the square of the body height, and is expressed in units of kg/m^2, resulting from mass in kilograms and height in meters.	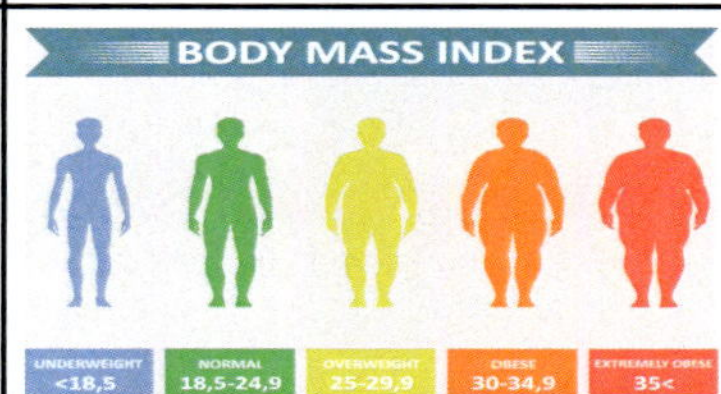
Hyperhomocysteinemia	Hyperhomocysteinemia refers to the condition where there is greater than 15 micromol/L of homocysteine in the blood. This condition is present in a wide range of diseases, and in many cases, it is an independent risk factor for more serious medical conditions	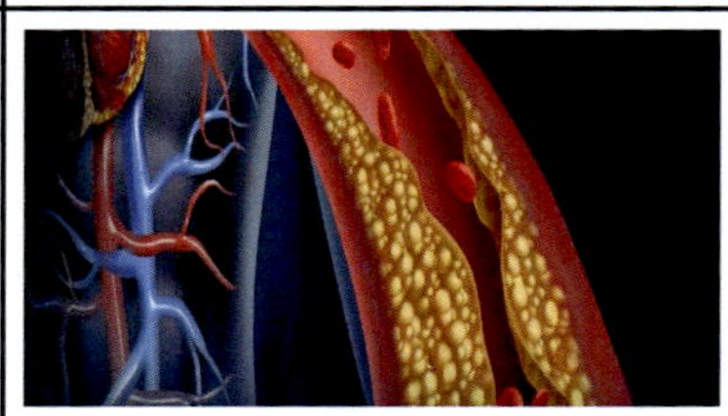
Catheter ablation	Catheter ablation is a procedure that uses radio-frequency energy or other sources to terminate or modify a faulty electrical pathway from sections of the heart of those who are prone to developing cardiac arrhythmias such as atrial fibrillation, atrial flutter and Wolff-Parkinson-White syndrome.	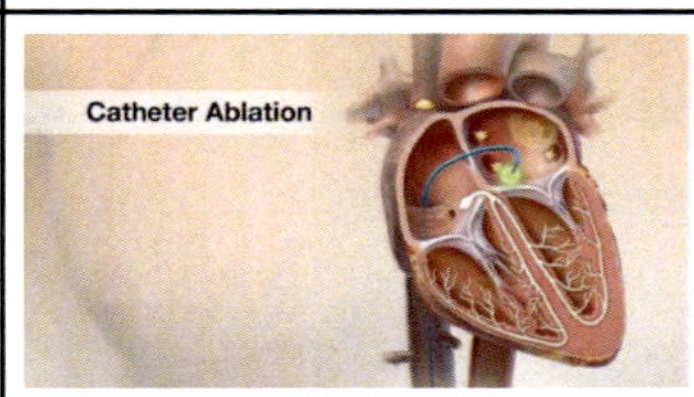

10.1. RISK FACTORS FOR ALZHEIMER'S DISEASE

Over the past few years, evidence from observational studies has accumulated and revealed several potentially modifiable risk factors. Some potentially workable recommendations regarding AD prevention are provided (Figure 10.1).

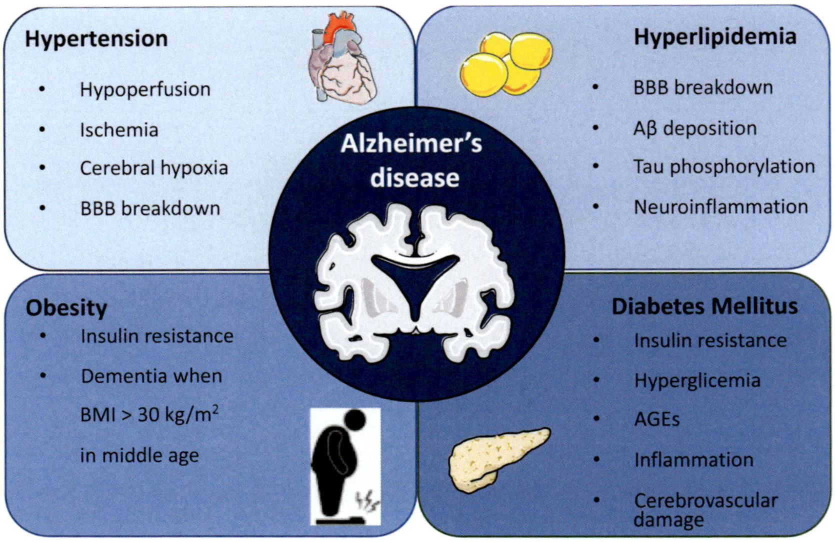

Figure 10.1. *Potential risk factors for Alzheimer's disease.*

Source: Ezkurdia A, Ramírez MJ, & Solas M, (2023). Metabolic syndrome as a risk factor for Alzheimer's disease: A focus on insulin resistance. International Journal of Molecular Sciences, 24(5), 4354. https://doi.org/10.3390/ijms24054354.

10.1.1. Psychosocial Factors

Researchers have looked into whether these psychosocial factors could have a particular impact on cognition in some prospective cohorts.

10.1.1.1. Educational Attainment

Lower education is associated with higher burden of vascular risk factors in mid-life and higher risk of dementia in late life. We aim to understand the causal mechanism through which vascular risk factors potentially mediate the relationship between education and dementia.

More education was associated with 8 to 44% lower risk of dementia compared to grade school-level education in a dose–response pattern, while the relationship between education and post-stroke dementia was not statistically significant. Up to 25% of the association between education and dementia was mediated through mid-life vascular risk factors, with a smaller percentage mediated for lower levels of education.

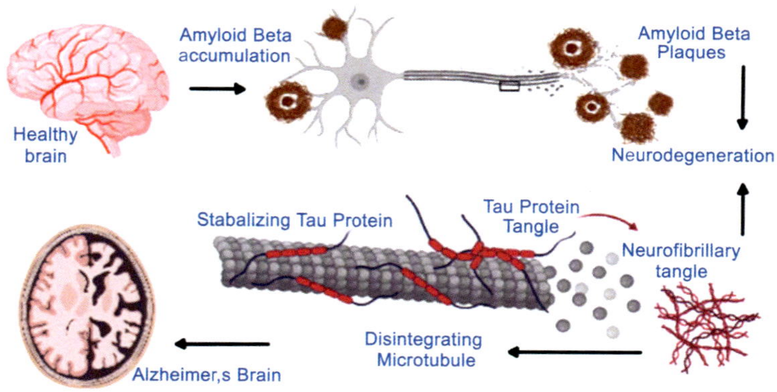

Figure 10.2. *Implications for preventing Alzheimer's disease and slowing its progression.*

Source: Abduljawad AA, Elawad MA, Elkhalifa MEM, Ahmed A, Hamdoon AAE, Salim LHM, Ashraf M, Ayaz M, Hassan SSu, & Bungau S, (2022). Alzheimer's disease as a major public health concern: Role of dietary saponins in mitigating neurodegenerative disorders and their underlying mechanisms. Molecules, 27(20):6804. https://doi.org/10.3390/molecules27206804.

10.1.1.2. Cognitive Activity and Bilingualism

According to the Swedish study, engaging in cognitive activities actively was associated with a 46% lower risk of AD. In particular, the Lothian cohort study found that playing more analog games was associated with a slower decline in memory and cognitive speed. This finding may have something to do with the strong connections between the superior frontal cortex and the hippocampus.

Cognitive advantage in bilingual dementia is the result of brain reserve and neural compensation due to the lifelong usage of two or more languages. Comparable cognitive performance was noted in bilinguals with dementia despite greater neuronal degeneration in the brain than in monolinguals with dementia. The modulation in functional connectivity in specific brain regions in bilingual older adults helps to cope with the pathology due to neurodegeneration. Only a few community studies have investigated the role of bilingualism on the prevalence, incidence, and progression of dementia and mild cognitive impairment (MCI). The risk of developing cognitive impairment was reduced with an increase in the number of languages spoken by older individuals. The potential advantage of bilingualism on late-life cognition and protection against age-related cognitive decline was found to be independent of childhood intelligence.[4] Further, the incidence and the risk of progression to MCI from healthy aging were lower in individuals who learned an additional language in early life.

10.1.1.3. Social Engagement

Social connections play an important role in maintaining cognitive function in dementia. Older adults with cognitive impairments such as dementia are at heightened risk of loneliness and depression. Often their cognitive difficulties are related not only to memory problems, but also to problems with interacting and engaging socially with others. As their condition worsens, social networks grow smaller for people living with dementia. We have co-designed a novel social skills intervention with people living with dementia or mild cognitive impairment.

10.1.1.4. Depression and Stress

It can be hard to know what is causing depression in dementia. For many people, the challenges of living with dementia can lead to feelings of deep sadness or hopelessness. In addition, the diseases that cause dementia may damage parts of the brain involved in emotions and behaviour.

Other factors that can contribute to depression include:

- a history of traumatic or upsetting events
- other health conditions or disabilities – particularly heart problems, breathing difficulties, chronic pain or hormonal problems
- side-effects of medications – including certain sleeping pills, steroids, beta-blockers and drugs used to treat Parkinson's disease
- not having enough meaningful things to do, social isolation or a lack of social support
- not getting enough good-quality sleep
- bereavement – this can make a person more vulnerable to depression, although grief itself is not normally thought of as a type of depression
- feeling stressed about issues such as money, relationships or the future
- drinking too much alcohol.

A person with dementia is much more likely to become depressed if they have had depression in the past – particularly if they've had it several times during their life.

Depression can increase problems with thinking and memory caused by dementia. It may also contribute to changes in behaviour, such as becoming more agitated or not wanting to eat.

For people in the later stage of dementia, symptoms of depression often include tearfulness and poor appetite.

10.1.2. Lifestyles

10.1.2.1. Physical Activity

In the Hisayama Study, higher daily physical activity participation was linked to a roughly half-decreased risk of AD. Furthermore, the cognitive advantages of consistent resistance training and choreographic intervention may postpone the neurodegenerative process, particularly in areas linked to dementia conversion. Additionally, aerobic exercise improved oral fluency and executive function, possibly as a result of its protective effects on hippocampal volume and neuronal health. A prospective study found improvements in cardiorespiratory function, specifically cerebral perfusion and memory ability, after a year of aerobic exercise training. More research is required to fully understand the neurotrophic effects of active exercise; in particular, the kind, intensity, duration, and timing of the exercise may have a greater impact on the prevention of AD. Reverse causality may be responsible for the association between active exercise and a lower risk of Alzheimer's disease (AD), as people in the preclinical stage of the disease tended to be less physically active than older, healthy individuals in the Whitehall II study. Physical activity, however, did not appear to have any neuroprotective effects on cognitive functioning. Whether reverse causality can account for the positive effects of exercise on cognition is still up for debate.

10.1.2.2. Sleep Disturbances

A higher accumulation of neurotoxic substances was observed in those with sleep disorders due to a decreased ability to clear metabolites, which was one of the risk factors for AD identified by insomnia and sleep disordered breathing. A 66% (95% confidence interval [CI] 1.03–2.68) higher risk of AD was seen in individuals with severe obstructive sleep apnea (≥30 vs. 9 hours) revealed a risk of AD that was more than twice as high, and the risk of AD after a habit of getting less sleep was 1.25 (95% CI 0.88–1.76). Furthermore, it showed a V-shaped relationship between daily sleep duration and cognitive decline and the ensuing risk for dementia. Both short duration (≤6 hours) and long duration (≥8 hours) had negative effects on cognitive function. Notably, individuals with inadequate or excessive nocturnal sleep duration tended to exhibit higher levels of amyloid deposition. Additionally, a Mendelian randomization study found a causal link between increased cortical thickness and duration of sleep. Additionally, there might be a reciprocal relationship between the pathology of AD and sleep dysregulation; while sleep disorders may promote the build-up of tau and Aβ, the increased tau and Aβ aggregation may aggravate the development of sleep disturbances. To better investigate the possible function of sleep dysregulation as a biomarker of AD and the possible reciprocal relationship, more extensive longitudinal studies are required. Maintaining cognitive function greatly depends on getting enough sleep, so patients experiencing sleep issues should see a doctor and start therapy as soon as possible.

10.1.2.3. Smoking

In a meta-analysis comprising 37 longitudinal studies, smoking was found to increase the risk of AD (RR 1.40, 95% CI 1.13–1.73). This risk was also significant among non-APOE ε4 carriers. Notably, the initiation of smoking was linked to a decrease in cortical thickness. The oxidative stress caused by smoking in the brain may promote the development of tau or amyloid pathology. On the other hand, never-smokers had an 18% lower risk of AD than lifetime smokers, suggesting that quitting smoking at an early age would have a greater positive impact on cognition.

10.1.2.4. Alcohol Consumption

There may be disagreement over the effects of alcohol consumption on cognitive function in many epidemiological findings. In Nord-Trøndelag Health, frequent alcohol users (≥5 times/two weeks) had a 47% increased risk of AD (95% CI 1.00–2.16) compared to non-drinkers drinkers who don't often (1–4 times). It was believed that this relationship, which was thought to be J-shaped, could protect against dementia if alcohol consumption was appropriate (<12 g/day), much like the relationship between coffee consumption and AD. Drinking too much alcohol on a daily basis is not advised because in heavy users, the extracellular cold-inducible RNA-binding protein (eCIRP) may mediate tau phosphorylation, which advances alcohol-induced AD.

A randomized trial verified the improvement in cognitive status following the addition of matured hop bitter acid from beer. In particular, wine's alcohol content seemed to be more strongly inversely correlated with dementia risk, and wine's antioxidant and polyphenolic contents demonstrated stronger neurodegenerative protective effects. To elucidate the underlying mechanism explaining the alcohol-related risk of AD, more primary studies are necessary.

A mendelian randomization study revealed the only known causal relationship between alcohol consumption and an earlier onset of AD. This finding suggested that moderate alcohol consumption may be detrimental to brain health but not helpful. Future research should clearly and completely define this relationship in order to account for potential confounding factors, particularly the survival bias.

10.1.2.5. Coffee and Tea

A proposed J-shaped relationship between coffee intake and AD found that consuming less than 1–2 cups per day, but not more than 3 cups per day, was associated with an 18% reduction in AD risk (RR 0.82, 95% CI 0.71–0.94, vs < 1 cup/day), with a greater effect observed in women. This gender trait, however, differed from tea consumption. Green tea's cognitive-protective benefits were more pronounced in males. Drinking coffee or green tea may contain certain neuroprotective ingredients like caffeine and L-theanine. Green tea's anti-amyloid properties, which primarily inhibit Aβ aggregation and reduce Aβ-induced oxidative stress, may also protect against AD. The public should be encouraged to drink green tea and coffee in moderation. Those who regularly drank green tea had lower levels of CSF total-tau protein, most likely as a result of improved aberrant tau metabolism. On the other hand, neither black tea nor oolong tea demonstrated any cognitive advantages among the elderly Han participants in the study.

10.1.2.6. Diets

The risk of AD was found to be inversely correlated with three dietary patterns: the Mediterranean diet (HR 0.46, 95% CI 0.26–0.79), the DASH diet (HR 0.61, 95% CI 0.38–0.97), and the MIND diet (HR 0.47, 95% CI 0.26–0.76). The protective effects of these dietary patterns on cognition may be attributed to enough mono- and polyunsaturated fats as well as anti-oxidant, anti-inflammatory, and anti-diabetic effects. More intriguingly, the Three-City study put forth the idea that a novel diet pattern—one that is more varied and rich in fresh fruits, vegetables, and seafood—might be especially advantageous to cognitive function. In particular, the gut mycobiome may be altered by ketogenic diets, lowering the risk of AD. Conversely, the HR for AD increased by 27% when higher glycemic load foods were consumed. Furthermore, increased consumption of fish (RR 0.93, 95% CI 0.90–0.95) and marine-derived dietary docosahexaenoic acid (RR 0.63, 95% CI 0.51–0.76) may reduce the risk of developing AD, according to a meta-analysis incorporating 21 cohort studies. Additionally, APOE ε4 carriers who regularly consume seafood have a lower burden of AD brain pathology, which is unaffected by higher brain mercury levels.

Individuals who consumed higher amounts of B vitamins in their early adult years, such as folate, niacin, vitamin B-6, and vitamin B-12, were probably going to develop better cognitive function later in life. Furthermore, women who carry the APOE 4 gene were more likely to benefit from vitamin C's potential cognitive benefits, whereas men who do not carry the APOE 4 gene may benefit from higher blood vitamin E levels. Increased consumption of flavonoids through diet may lower the incidence of AD by 38% (95% confidence interval [CI] 0–39–0–98). This reduction in risk is unrelated to other lifestyle factors or cardiovascular-related illnesses. In order to determine whether these links between the intake of micronutrients and cognition are causal, more Mendelian randomization studies as well as additional research are necessary to identify the plausible biologic explanations. It's important to appropriately consume specific vitamins and other micronutrients from regular meals (Cummings et al., 2016; Ritchie et al., 2016; Winblad et al., 2016; Livingston et al., 2020).

10.2. FALL RISK ASSESSMENT AMONG OLDER ADULTS WITH MILD ALZHEIMER'S DISEASE

Every year in the United States, about 30% of older adults (65 years of age and older) who live in communities fall, costing the country more than $20 billion in medical expenses. Injuries from falls rank as the fifth most common cause of death for older adults.

Research has focused on identifying fall risk and preventing falls and injuries in older adults who are cognitively intact. However, there is a lack of studies that address fall risk screening in older adults with Alzheimer's disease (AD). Individuals with AD are more likely to fall and sustain more serious injuries compared to those who are cognitively intact.

The annual incidence of falls in older adults with AD is between 60% to 80%, which is more than twice the rate of cognitively intact older adults of the same age. Furthermore, seniors with AD experience nearly three times as many fall-related fractures compared to those with normal cognition.

The measurement of physical mobility in individuals with AD in the advanced stages of the disorder has been the focus of research. The effects of mild AD on physical function are poorly understood in the early stages of the disease.

The exact mechanisms by which AD raises older adults' risk of falling are still being investigated. The following conditions have been proposed as potential causes of falls in this population: cognitive impairment; changes in balance and gait associated with AD; impaired reaction time; side effects of commonly prescribed medications (e.g., antidepressants, anxiolytics, and antipsychotics); and risky behavior, such as wandering.

For older adults with mild AD, finding a trustworthy fall assessment tool could be helpful in identifying fall risk early in this extremely vulnerable population. Furthermore, not many studies have looked at how factors like age, gender, education, gait assistance, cognitive ability, functional mobility, and fall risk interact with one another. Early detection of fall risk during a disease may help lower morbidity and mortality as well as fall-related expenses.

10.2.1. Physiological and Cognitive Implications in Alzheimer's Disease

There are currently 52.2 million Americans who suffer from Alzheimer's. It is a cytoskeleton-related degenerative illness of the brain that affects several different neural systems. Two of the main characteristics of this illness are extracellular deposits (plaques) of the protein β-amyloid and intraneuronal neurofibrillary tangles. For the previous 20 years, scientists believed that AD mostly impacted cognition in the early stages of the disease and spared motor function until later on. But new research is starting to cast doubt on this idea. Researchers are now seeing that changes in cognitive function linked to AD contribute to gait disturbances and increase fall risk in those with this disorder. Walking is now understood to be a cognitive process requiring higher-level control.

Functional mobility is impacted by a number of physiological and cognitive changes related to AD. Executive dysfunction and loss of attention control are thought to be widespread in AD. Cognitive control, which refers to the mental processes that direct behavior and thought in line with self-generated objectives or plans, is synonymous with executive function. Attention deficits may account for some of the functional decline associated with aging and dementia, as well as impede information processing in the brain on several levels. Evidence currently available indicates that attention is the first nonmemory domain affected by AD, preceding deficits in language and visuospatial functions, following an initial stage of amnesia. Attention deficits may be linked to difficulties with daily living activities, which can arise in patients with mild dementia as well. Furthermore, a person's incapacity to adjust to erratic sensory input may raise their risk of falling. Task complexity can lead to capacity overload and decreased performance.

Visuospatial disorientation, impaired sensori-motor processing, and trouble suppressing visual distraction are all linked to Alzheimer's disease. Chong et al. evaluated how well subjects with AD balanced on the Sensory Organization Test in comparison to subjects with Parkinson's disease and healthy age-matched individuals. The purpose of the Sensory Organization Test is to evaluate a subject's ability to remain balanced while standing in various combinations of normal, absent, and/or inconsistent vestibular, somatosensory, and visual conditions. Subjects must use the congruent signals while suppressing the incongruent ones in order to stay balanced. During testing, the subjects wore a harness that was suspended from the ceiling. Although the subjects were able to move freely, the harness kept them from making contact with the ground in the event of a total loss of balance. When a participant stepped or fell into the harness, it was considered a fall. The subjects with AD did not show improvement with repetitions and fell more frequently than those in the other 2 groups, despite having normal vestibular system function. Because they were unable to suppress inconsistent visual and somatosensory information, AD subjects frequently fell when vestibular information was necessary for orientation.

10.2.2. Age, Falls, and Alzheimer's Disease

As people age, they experience physical and cognitive changes that can increase the likelihood of falls, such as sensory, musculoskeletal, neurological, and metabolic changes. Those over 80 years old are at the highest risk for falling and sustaining injuries. However, it is not solely age that raises the risk of falls; multiple age-related health conditions can significantly increase this risk. Age is closely linked to Alzheimer's Disease (AD), with the National Institute on Aging identifying age as the most significant risk factor for AD. A study by Bassiony et al. found that falls in older adults with AD were more common in those of advanced age, even after considering other contributing factors.

10.2.3. The Effects of Education on Falls in Individuals with Alzheimer's Disease

A negative correlation was found by Ott et al. between dementia development and education. Furthermore, research has indicated that obtaining a higher degree may postpone the manifestation of AD symptoms. Researchers have hypothesized that older adults with AD who are more educated might possess greater neural reserve and neural networking, potentially delaying neurodegeneration in some way. Therefore, as AD worsens and some neurons die, other neurons may perform comparable functional tasks, lessening the symptoms of cognitive and functional impairment.

Bennett and colleagues found compelling evidence that a higher level of formal education offers a cognitive or neural reserve that can mitigate the negative impact of senile plaques on cognitive abilities. Their research indicated that education provides a cognitive edge, as individuals with more years of schooling tend to have better cognitive function throughout adulthood and, as a result, require more pathology to experience any significant cognitive decline.

10.2.4. Functional Mobility and Fall in Individuals with Alzheimer's Disease

Walking may be thought of as a "automatic" activity, but if the walking surface suddenly changes or if it requires multitasking—such as carrying an object or using an assistive device—it may require more attention and executive function. Changes in the primary sensory domains—vision, hearing, vestibular, somatosensory—are a normal part of aging. As a result, it might take more mental work to account for these systemic changes. The network that regulates locomotion may become disorganized as a result of progressive cognitive decline, as seen in AD patients. This can cause problems with gait timing, speed, and postural control.

According to O'Keeffe et al., patients with mild AD are not immune to gait abnormalities; in fact, the most common gait abnormality in these patients is a "cautious gait." A cautious gait is a way of walking that is connected to perceived or actual instability. This seems to be comparable to the fear of falling that some older adults have, and it could decondition them and increase their risk of falling. In healthy older adults, fear of falling has been demonstrated to alter both the temporal and spatial gait parameters.

Reduced stride length, wider strides, slower gait speeds, and longer double limb support times are a few examples of altered gait parameters. These kinds of gait abnormalities are more common in subjects who have experienced falls in the past than in subjects who have not. Numerous studies have found that variability in stride length causes instability and is a major factor in the higher incidence of falls observed in the adult population with mild to moderate AD.

When two tasks were attempted independently, people with AD performed like controls in studies on dual-task performance; however, when the tasks were attempted simultaneously, their performance declined disproportionately. One reason why people with AD fall has been found to be related to impaired dual-task performance when walking. For instance, Camicioli et al. examined the performance of a dual task in community-dwelling healthy young adults (mean age, 72 years), healthy older old adults (mean age, 86 years), and adults with probable AD (mean age, 74 years). Participants were instructed to recite various masculine names aloud while moving at a comfortable yet fast pace down a 15-foot hallway. Compared to the other 2 groups, the subjects with AD walked noticeably more slowly. There was no discernible difference in walking speed between the two groups without AD. The authors came to the conclusion that people with AD had a tendency to perform worse on dual tasks involving gait, which was consistent with a higher risk of falls and injuries than what was seen in the other elder groups.

It has been demonstrated that gait speed is a significant predictor of disability. Furthermore, in older people without dementia, gait speed is associated with executive and cognitive function. A 0.6 m/s or slower gait has been linked to a higher risk of falls in older adults who are cognitively intact. Seniors with AD are more likely to fall because they typically walk even more slowly than adults without AD. In fact, studies have shown that older persons with AD who have slow gait speeds are more likely to fall. Additionally, research has demonstrated that the gait patterns (i.e., step length) of older adults with AD differed from those of older adults who are cognitively intact but of a similar age. According to Wang et al., gait slowing and poor balance in older adults may even be early indicators of AD (Cummings et al., 2016; Ritchie et al., 2016; Winblad et al., 2016; Livingston et al., 2020).

10.2.5. The Effects of Gait Aid Usage on Falls in Individuals with Alzheimer's Disease

Walking aids and canes are examples of assistive technology that can help with gait and improve balance control because they offer both somatosensory feedback and mechanical benefits. In addition to boosting self-assurance and a sense of security, gait aids can help older adults become more active and independent. However, some studies show a strong correlation between the use of gait aids and falls and injuries. Using gait devices comes with demands on the attentional, neuromotor, musculoskeletal, physiologic, and metabolic systems. There are also a number of possible ways in which these demands could negatively impact balance control. Fall risk may also be increased by improper device prescription, insufficient user education, or the use of non-prescribed devices.

According to some experts, using a gait aid could just be a sign of balance issues, a decline in functioning, or a higher risk of falling. Some have contended that using a gait device might actually raise your risk of falling because it can make you trip or impair your ability to maintain your balance. When participating in activities that compete for available attentional and cognitive resources, older adults in particular seem to experience a reduction in postural stability (dual task performance).

According to Carter et al., older adults who were living in the community and were cognitively intact and used a gait aid had a 3–4 times higher risk of falling than those who did not. According to Murray et al.'s study of elderly people living in the community, 80% of participants who had experienced a fall in the previous 12 months used a gait aid.

It is crucial to determine whether gait aids are linked to falls in this population of older adults with mild AD because of the distinct cognitive and functional deficits that these individuals experience. When using a gait aid, older adults with mild AD may have attention deficits, impaired dual task performance, and visuospatial skills that significantly impact gait performance. These factors can make safe mobility even more difficult. To find out if gait aids and fall risk in AD patients are related, more research is required (Cummings et al., 2016; Ritchie et al., 2016; Winblad et al., 2016; Livingston et al., 2020).

10.3. THE PREVENTION OF ALZHEIMER'S DISEASE

Alzheimer's disease (AD) affects more than 5 million Americans and is very expensive for families, patients, and the community. According to Alzheimer's Association projections, over 16 million cases of AD will occur in the US and over 60 million cases worldwide by the year 2050 if nothing is done. Only five symptomatic drugs—four of which are still on the market—have successfully completed Phase III clinical trials and reached their endpoints in the previous 25 years. Since 2003, problems with safety and/or efficacy have caused every symptomatic and disease-modifying medication to fail in Phase II/III trials. This prompted the National Alzheimer's Plan Act to propose the audacious goal of creating a disease-modifying therapy (DMT) by 2025. This target date is linked to two significant ideas. First, only drugs that have started Phase II trials will be able to meet the 2025 deadline for DMTs to reach the market. Second, the 16 million Americans expected to have AD in 2050 would drop to 5.7 million cases if a DMT were available by 2025, saving the country $367 billion. A concentrated effort is being made to start preventive measures in asymptomatic individuals in addition to efforts to develop a DMT for people with symptomatic AD. These initiatives align with the 2025 target goal as well. Nonetheless, the question of whether AD can be avoided is crucial. Numerous risk factors have been identified to date, including those that are non-modifiable (such as age, sex, and genetics) and modifiable (such as exposures, lifestyle, and social habits). The role of biomarkers in defining the pathologic cascade has been made clearer by recent revisions to the clinical criteria for AD and mild cognitive impairment (MCI). Additionally, the addition of research criteria for presymptomatic disease paves the way for improved modeling of the preclinical and prodromal stages of the disease. It is now feasible to investigate underlying pathologic alterations in amyloid, tau, dopamine transport, inflammation, signaling pathways, and eventually alpha-synuclein and TDP-43 in symptomatic, prodromal, and presymptomatic individuals thanks to efforts to develop and validate fluid and imaging biomarkers. Developments in epigenetic, genetic, and "omic" (such as proteomics, lipidomics, and metabolomics) techniques will make it possible to model modifications in transcription, translation, and post-translation. Moreover, neurodegenerative diseases are being treated with precision medicine techniques that have shown promise in oncology. Thus, the framework for starting preventative efforts is in place (Table 10.1).

Table 10.1. The Effects of Diets and Life Situations Negatively Influencing the Alzheimer's Disease

Authors	**Type of Diet/ Life Situation**	**Study Design**	**Study Population**	**Results**
Lee et al.	Obesity	Pilot study	10 obese patients before and after weight loss intervention	Changes in adipocyte APP expression correlated with changes in plasma Aβ40 levels ($R = 0.74$, $p = 0.01$).
Ye et al.	Malnutrition	Longitudinal study	747 patients with aMCI	The underweight group had a higher risk of probable Alzheimer's disease dementia (pADD), and the decreased-BMI (HR: 2.29, 95% CI: 1.41–3.72) groups were at increased risk of progression to pADD.
Hanson et al.	Malnutrition	Prospective cohort	256 nursing home residents with advanced dementia and feeding problems	Significant mortality risk in patients with feeding problems
Laitinen et al.	High-fat diet	Population-based study	1449 patients with 117 who had dementia	Moderate intake of polyunsaturated fats in mid-life decreased the risk of dementia even after adjustment for demographic variables, especially among the ApoE epsilon4 carriers.
Ruan et al.	High-fat diet	Meta-analysis of cohort studies	8630 participants and 633 cases	A higher dietary saturated fat intake was significantly associated with increased risks of 39% and 105% for AD and dementia.

Jacka et al.	Western diet	Longitudinal study	255 persons from the Personality and Total Health Through Life Study	Higher consumption of an unhealthy "Western" dietary pattern was associated with smaller left hippocampal volume.
Gibson et al.	Western diet	Observational study	23 women with polycystic ovary syndrome from 25 to 45 years old	Greater intakes of saturated and trans fats, and higher saturated-to-unsaturated fat ratio (Sat:UFA) were associated with more errors in the visuospatial task and poorer word recall and recognition.

Source: Doroszkiewicz J, Mroczko J, Rutkowski P, & Mroczko B, (2023). Molecular aspects of a diet as a new pathway in the prevention and treatment of Alzheimer's disease. International Journal of Molecular Sciences 24(13), 10751. https://doi.org/10.3390/ijms241310751.

With earlier identification of at-risk individuals, increased opportunities for quicker and earlier diagnoses, improved at-risk patient stratification, higher enrollment in randomized clinical trials (RCTs) by lowering screen failure rates, and ultimately more effective treatments, these efforts have a great deal of potential for both pharmaceutical and non-pharmacological approaches. Although AD will be the main topic of this chapter, the concepts covered here apply to other neurodegenerative disorders as well (e.g., Parkinson's disease, Lewy body dementia, vascular dementia). Preventing or just postponing the onset of dementia could drastically alter the course of the illness, assuming that curing AD remains a significant unmet challenge (Cummings et al., 2016; Ritchie et al., 2016; Winblad et al., 2016; Livingston et al., 2020).

10.3.1. Pharmacologic Approaches to Prevention

Numerous studies on prevention are being conducted for both autosomal dominant and sporadic forms of AD. The Anti-Amyloid Treatment in Asymptomatic Alzheimer's (A4) study is one such project that is looking for people 65 to 86 years old who have normal cognitive function but positive AD biomarkers (amyloid deposition by PET scan). For a duration of three years, these individuals receive treatment with an anti-amyloid monoclonal antibody. People with normal cognitive function who have two copies of the ApoE e4 allele, which puts them at high risk of Alzheimer's disease (AD), will be the subject of a study by the Alzheimer's Prevention Initiative (API). These patients receive treatment with an alternative anti-amyloid monoclonal antibody for a period of two years. People 65 to 83 years old with normal cognitive function who have a polymorphism in the TOMM40 gene linked to an increased risk of AD will be recruited for the TOMMORROW Study. Patients are treated with the anti-diabetes medication pioglitazone for five years. Parallel to these trials in sporadic cases with elevated risk, monoclonal antibody-based trials, such as the Dominantly Inherited Alzheimer's Network – Treatment Unit (DIAN-TU) and API, are being conducted in people with autosomal dominant forms of AD. One special benefit of the trials in familial AD is the predictable age of onset, which increases the likelihood of detecting any DMT effect. Whether the findings of these trials apply to the far more prevalent sporadic forms, where risk factors other than genetics may predominate, is a potential drawback. Prodromal studies, which are similar to prevention trials, are numerous and primarily concentrate on people who have motor cortex injuries. Many of these trials are still awaiting results, but at least one Phase II study produced encouraging findings. Aducanumab immunotherapy against the amyloid protein showed significant improvements in cognitive and functional measures over a 54-week period, in addition to changes in CSF amyloid in a dose-dependent manner. These results lend credence to the theory that there might be a window of opportunity within which these agents should be used to maximize the chances of success.

10.3.2. Lifestyle Modification Interventions

10.3.2.1. Modifiable Lifestyle Factors

Numerous factors that can be changed to reduce the risk and prevent AD have been identified through observational research. Numerous studies have shown that diabetes, hypertension, kidney failure, alcohol and tobacco use, high cholesterol, coronary heart disease, depression, sedentary lifestyle, low cognitive activity, and diet are important risk factors. Together, these variables are responsible for more than half of the AD-attributable risk. Diet is the hardest of these to control because it depends so much on one's ability to pay for and obtain fresh food. A 19% increased risk of dementia was linked to a 1-point increase in Lifestyle for Brain Health (LIBRA) scores, which are modifiable risk factors, in a 16-year observational study involving 949 participants. Crossword puzzles, card games, computer use, arts and crafts, lifelong learning, group discussions, and music were found to have a protective effect (odds ratio=0.58) in a meta-analysis of 19 studies on cognitive leisure activities. Furthermore, physical activity can lower the risk by 20–65%, depending on the kind and level of intensity, through a variety of mechanisms such as decreased risk of vascular disease, enhanced respiratory function, increased stimulation of trophic factors, and decreased inflammation and oxidative stress. An increase in the risk of dementia in later life was shown by an objective measurement of midlife vascular risk factors. Work-related stress raised the odds of MCI (odds ratio=1.38), dementia (odds ratio=1.53), and AD (odds ratio=1.55) in a study involving 2,000 people aged 71–78 years.

The aforementioned studies, along with numerous others, converge on a short list of risk factors that appear to be crucial in the development or prevention of AD and related disorders, despite variations in study ages, countries of origin, culture, and language. Because of this consistency, several dementia prevention initiatives have been put into place to change these risk factors, the majority of which are not directly related to the deposition of tau or amyloid.

10.3.2.2. Ongoing Prevention Initiatives

The European Prevention of AD (EPAD) initiative is recruiting now to investigate whether pathophysiological changes that occur decades before dementia onset are amplified by changes in early- and mid-life risk factors for AD. The Innovative Midlife Intervention for Dementia Deterrence (In-MINDD) trial enrolled 600 people to take part in an online education program while taking into account 11 risk factors that have been identified and account for 50% of the attributable risk, such as diabetes, hypertension, and renal disease. The FINGER study, which is enrolling 1260 people in an educational intervention that consists of modules on diet, exercise, cognitive training, and vascular risk reduction, is currently the largest initiative. For global cognition, executive function, and processing speed, overall between-group differences reached statistical significance, but not for episodic memory. These findings imply that, despite a tiny effect size, changing one's lifestyle may have some positive effects on cognitive function.

10.3.3. Precision Medicine Approaches to Prevention

Although it is the single biggest risk factor for AD, getting older is not a given. According to the most accurate estimates, there is a 42% chance of developing AD at age 85. Naturally, this indicates that even in cases where amyloid is found in the brain, 58% of elderly people do not experience dementia. Although the causes are unknown, a number of risk factors, both modifiable and non-modifiable, may contribute to the explanation. It is possible to prevent up to 30% of AD cases by modifying risk factors and making behavioral adjustments to lessen the impact of non-modifiable risk factors. The question of whether the available evidence is enough to launch preventive programs is still being debated because: (a) it can be challenging to establish a causal relationship from observational studies; and (b) it can be challenging to combine data from several RCTs because of variations in study design, measurements, and expected results. The cornerstone of disease prevention and brain health may be a well-balanced, healthy lifestyle; however, individual risk factors (vascular, lifestyle, and psychosocial) may act independently and compound the effects of one another. Consequently, a prevention program must be multimodal and customized to target specific risks.

These specifications provide many design and analytical difficulties. Time-to-event analytic techniques are widely used in prevention RCTs to show a DMT effect. When expected treatment effects are known to be constant over time, such designs are ideal; however, in the case of dementia prevention, this is unknown. Therefore, time-to-event techniques like hazard ratios might not be the most effective way to model effects, especially if the intervention's detectable signal manifests itself as a late effect. Because AD is highly variable in terms of risk factors, age at onset, presentation, progression, and pathology burden, large sample sizes (tens of thousands to thousands) must be followed for extended periods (years to decades) when designing a study to treat individuals as a homogenous population. This significantly raises study expenses, staff workloads, and participant workloads. RCT design will continue to be difficult because of the lack of reliable biomarkers that indicate the beginning and progression of disease rather than just the existence of pathology. The following are some of the obstacles that preventive studies face: a lack of standardization in study design, definitions, and outcomes; a lack of understanding of the true relationship between dementia risk factors and the impact of risk reduction; the complexity of the life course on dementia risk factors; challenges in converting RCT findings into practical applications; social and cultural barriers to implementation; a lack of research capacity to enroll large research cohorts for extended periods; and the widespread social stigma associated with AD.

Using precision medicine designs from oncology trials to customize interventions to a patient's genotype and phenotypic expression would be an alternative strategy, as effective preventive strategies are still elusive despite significant advances in our understanding of the biology and pathophysiology of AD. Trial-ready cohorts can be more effectively targeted with pharmaceutical and non-pharmacological interventions (made to ameliorate particular pathologic mechanisms based on specific biomarkers and patient characteristics) with improved patient classification and phenotyping. Subsequent studies could be designed to ascertain safety and efficacy faster (i.e., "fast to fail") by shifting from generalized methods to patient-specific, precision treatments.

Rethinking trial design for preventative measures and switching to more "N-of-1" designs would also be necessary for this. N-of-

1 trials use the same study designs and statistical methods as RCTs, but they focus only on the individual patient as the unit of observation in order to examine the effectiveness and/or negative effects of an intervention. They are also guided by objective, data-driven criteria. Since each patient's risk and molecular profile for AD are unique, classifying people into single entities (placebo vs. treatment-arm) might combine "super-responders" and "non-responders," meaning that treatment effects that are only noticeable in post-hoc analyzes would be eliminated. It may be preferable to compare the time-to-disease progression of a single patient using a novel therapeutic approach to the same patient's time-to-disease progression for the treatment paradigm that came right before. Due to recruitment delays and difficulties in extrapolating significant p-values from large treatment groups to the care of a single patient, which is the ultimate goal of clinical practice, N-of-1 trials may be less constrained by risks to the generalizability of large RCTs. 50 of the 57 completed N-of-1 trials in the meta-analyzes of 70 N-of-1 trials offered conclusive clinical or statistical answers, and 39% of those trials led doctors to modify their treatment plans. According to the findings of another meta-analysis, which looked at 108 trials with 2154 participants, 54% of the participants had their subsequent treatment decisions altered. Some requirements must be satisfied in order to establish the platform for these trials. Patients need to have detailed phenotyping, including genetic, biomarker, clinical, psychological, cognitive, and functional characteristics. In an ideal world, these patients would consent to an autopsy to confirm diagnosis and treatment effects on brain pathology, as well as to being followed up on over time and having their samples banked for later analysis. Both within- and between-subject comparisons as well as alternative time-series analyzes may be advantageous from a statistical perspective. Last but not least, when an expensive intervention—like an off-label treatment involving a pricey medication—is planned, the cost of care must be carefully considered (Table 10.2).

Table 10.2. Possible Mechanisms of the Effects of Physical Activity and Exercise Interventions on Cognitive Decline and Dementia Prevention

Possible Mechanisms	
1.	Improvement in cardiovascular factors (e.g., diabetes, hypertension, hyperlipidemia, and obesity)
2.	Increased neurotrophic factor expression (e.g., BDNF, IGF-1, and VEGF)
3	Increased amyloid-β turnover
4	Increased cerebral blood flow
5	Decreased inflammatory responses (e.g., CRP, IL-6, and TNF-α)

Abbreviation: BDNF, brain-derived neurotrophic factor; CRP, C-reactive protein; IGF-1, insulin-like growth factor 1; IL-6, interleukin-6; TNF-α, tumor necrosis factor-alpha; VEGF, vascular endothelial growth factor.

Source: Yamasaki T, (2023). Preventive strategies for cognitive decline and dementia: Benefits of aerobic physical activity, especially open-skill exercise. Brain Sciences, 13(3), 521. https://doi.org/10.3390/brainsci13030521.

10.3.4. Example of a Personalized Medicine Approach to Dementia Prevention

We are creating N-of-1 trials to personalized dementia prevention using an evidence base derived from a thorough literature review and the outcomes of an NIH-funded project to conduct dementia screening in multicultural communities, as an example of how this may be applied practically. To increase acceptance of dementia screening and better understand the effects of co-morbid disease on cognitive performance, broader medical screening for diabetes, hypertension, vascular risk factors, obesity, mobility, physical performance, frailty, and depression was added to the cognitive impairment screening process as part of a "Healthy Body, Healthy Mind" approach. This cross-sectional study produced new findings connecting cognitive performance to sarcopenia and mobility while also validating many findings of observational studies about the relationship between cognitive performance and diabetes, hypertension, obesity, vascular risk factors, and depression. These combined results were used in a prospective manner to create N-of-1 trials.

For instance, a 68-year-old woman with a college degree reported subjective memory complaints (such as losing car keys, forgetting conversations, and becoming defensive when discussing memory problems) that she had been experiencing for a year, but she was still able to function independently in her daily activities. Her pertinent past medical history is noteworthy in terms of her high cholesterol and blood pressure. Her physical examination revealed mild hypertension (132/92), but her peripheral vascular and cardiac exams were normal (Figure 10.3).

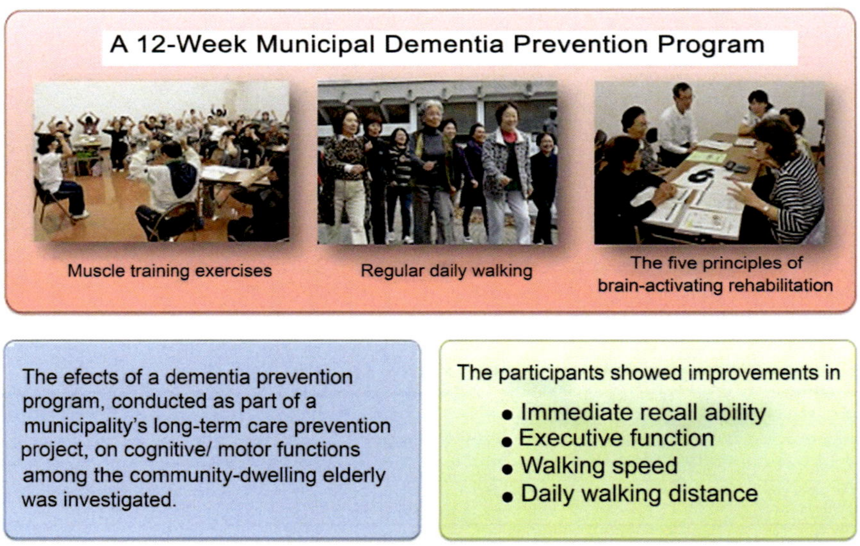
A 12-Week Municipal Dementia Prevention Program
Muscle training exercises
Regular daily walking
The five principles of brain-activating rehabilitation
The efects of a dementia prevention program, conducted as part of a municipality's long-term care prevention project, on cognitive/ motor functions among the community-dwelling elderly was investigated.
The participants showed improvements in
• Immediate recall ability
• Executive function
• Walking speed
• Daily walking distance

Figure 10.3. *Model of a dementia prevention initiative.*

Source: Kamegaya T, & Yamaguchi H, (2016). Long-term-care prevention team of Isesaki city community general support center. Effects of a 12-week municipal dementia prevention program on cognitive/motor functions among the community-dwelling elderly. Geriatrics, 1(3), 18. https://doi.org/10.3390/geriatrics1030018.

Neurologic findings of note include mild postural instability, diminished vibration sensation in the lower extremities, and mild symmetric weakness. Cognitive testing revealed working memory and executive dysfunction, global deficits (Montreal Cognitive Assessment score 19/30), and episodic memory deficits on list learning that vanished with cued recognition. Low lean muscle mass, at-risk nutritional status, moderate daily physical activity, mild deficits in physical functionality (Short Physical Performance Battery score 7/12), and mild frailty (Fried Frailty Phenotype Score 3/5) were all found during physical and functional testing. The results of the gait and balance test showed postural sway with closed eyes, slowed gait speed (1.07 m/s), and noticeable slowing (22.9%) during a dual-task challenge (walking while talking). Blood-based biomarkers showed evidence of insulin resistance (higher fasting glucose, hemoglobin A1c, and estimated average glucose), an abnormal lipid profile (elevated total, LDL- and non-HDL cholesterol; elevated LDL and small LDL particles; and reduced HDL particles); and elevated inflammatory markers (hs-CRP and myeloperoxidase). Quantitative MRI showed confluent white matter hyperintensities with frontal lobe predominance, but normal lateral ventricle volume and hippocampal size. Auditory event-related potentials showed normal amplitudes and latencies at all other peaks, including the P50 peak associated with amyloid deposition, but delayed median reaction times and reduced amplitude at the N200 peak (linked to impaired attention and executive function) and left-right asymmetry with frontal predominance (linked to vascular injury). This comprehensive phenotypic assessment yielded useful results in the following areas: biomarker testing (lipid profile, inflammation, insulin resistance, ApoE4 genotype suggesting poor response to statins), MRI (preserved hippocampal and cortical volume, extensive white matter disease), EEG (executive dysfunction and evidence of vascular injury), physical testing (sarcopenia, at-risk nutritional status, poor physical functionality, and early frailty), and gait testing (slowed gait speed, impaired dual tasks, and postural instability with eyes closed). These findings supported a diagnosis of vascular cognitive impairment.

A personalized treatment plan was then developed focusing on:

- dietary counseling (MIND diet, high protein snacks, glycemic control);
- physical therapy for gait, balance, strengthening, and conditioning;
- referral to a personal trainer for aerobic, resistance, and flexibility training;
- mindfulness (yoga, meditation) for stress reduction;
- cognitive exercise focusing on problem-solving skills;
- omega-3 supplementation and possible resin therapy for cholesterol-lowering;
- improved blood pressure monitoring; and
- initiation of a baby aspirin to improve blood flow.

But if successful, such a trial could lower long-term healthcare costs, improve patient-centered outcomes, improve the precision of future treatment decisions, and give a direct estimate of the effects of each individual treatment (Cummings et al., 2016; Ritchie et al., 2016; Winblad et al., 2016; Livingston et al., 2020).

10.4. CHALLENGES FOR ALZHEIMER'S DISEASE THERAPY

Longer lifespans have led to a sharp increase in the prevalence of age-related illnesses, such as dementia. The most common cause of dementia, accounting for 60–80% of cases, is Alzheimer's disease (AD). According to epidemiological studies, AD will become even more prevalent by the middle of the century, posing a serious threat to both individual and societal well-being. AD mainly affects people in their later years; its prevalence doubles approximately every five years after the age of 65, impacting about 47 million people globally. It is anticipated that during the next 20 years, this number will rise. Dementia is expected to cost the world $1 trillion by 2018 after being valued at about $818 billion in 2010. This is made even more striking by the fact that approximately 60% of dementia patients reside in low- and middle-income nations.

AD is a multifaceted illness. Genetic mutations cause a rare (<0.5 percent) familial form of AD, whose symptoms manifest earlier, usually between the ages of 30 and 50. The majority of sporadic cases of AD affect people over 60. Furthermore, the incidence of AD varies significantly between men and women. Given that women account for almost two thirds of AD patients, it is intriguing to consider the possibility that there are biological mechanisms explaining why women experience a higher incidence of AD cases. These mechanisms need further research.

The primary feature of AD is progressive cognitive impairment. But as the illness worsens, additional crippling non-cognitive symptoms appear, such as decreased appetite and sleep, as well as neuropsychiatric changes (e.g., depression and apathy). Furthermore, an increasing body of epidemiological research has confirmed a connection between metabolic disorders and AD. Since AD is thought to be a memory disorder, research on the pathophysiology of AD has mostly focused on how memory and cognitive decline occur, with other symptoms and co-morbidities largely disregarded. It follows that the lack of accurate and trustworthy biomarkers for early disease diagnosis is not surprising. Although definitive diagnosis has primarily been established by post-mortem examination, it is now generally acknowledged that pathophysiological alterations start to occur in a preclinical or presymptomatic stage decades before the onset of cognitive symptoms. Furthermore, a change in the way AD is viewed as a pathological entity has been sparked by the addition of novel biomarkers to diagnostic criteria. This has increased the understanding that AD is a complex process that progresses along a continuum rather than a disease with distinct clinical stages. When neuropsychological, fluid, and imaging biomarkers are combined, relatively accurate diagnosis and prompt therapies are expected to be attained.

Even medications with successful preclinical evaluation have not been able to reverse or slow down the progression of AD in large-scale clinical trials, despite the fact that advances in animal and clinical research over the past few decades have improved our understanding of the pathophysiological course of AD. These limitations might result from the fact that, since the amyloid cascade theory has been the focal point of therapeutic prospection, clinical trials have mostly concentrated on anti-amyloid strategies. Such unsatisfactory results also point to potential issues with adapting treatments from rodent model species for human use. This translational impedance is a result of animal model studies and their inadequate control over sex differences. As a result, promising treatments that are effective in one species of animal—typically male rodents—often do not translate to human trials where female participants predominate (often 2:1 female: male in large trials). Furthermore, the specifics of the mechanism involving central and peripheral derangements remain unclear, despite the widespread recognition of the neuropathological features of AD. Owing to the intricate pathology of AD, it is now thought that medications that target several molecular pathways and disease-modifying therapies may be able to provide more effective treatment. It is imperative that these take into account gender differences, as was recently observed (Cummings et al., 2016; Ritchie et al., 2016; Winblad et al., 2016; Livingston et al., 2020).

10.4.1. Molecular Pathogenesis of AD

10.4.1.1. Tau Phosphorylation, Amyloid Deposition, and A Oligomers

The two most characteristic abnormalities found in the memory-related brain regions of Alzheimer's disease patients are extracellular amyloid plaques and intracellular neurofibrillary tangles (NFTs). Tau protein that has been aberrantly phosphorylated and aggregated makes up the majority of NFTs, which weaken microtubules and jeopardize axonal transport. Tangles have been demonstrated to cause neuronal loss and defects in spatial memory, suggesting a connection between tau pathology and cognitive deficits in early AD. While it was previously believed that pathological changes in tau were caused by Aβ deposition, it is also possible that tau and Aβ act in tandem to intensify each other's harmful effects and start the pathogenic processes related to AD. Additionally, recent research has implicated soluble, diffusible tau oligomers as significant synaptotoxic mediators and potential causes of the distinct spread of tau pathology throughout the brain.

According to the amyloid cascade theory, a key factor in AD is the build-up of the amyloid-β peptide (Aβ) in the brain, which is caused by the β- and γ-secretase enzymes cleaving the APP one after the other. Due to conformational changes leading to a high β-sheet content, soluble Aβ is more likely to aggregate into polymeric forms such as larger insoluble fibrils and soluble oligomers. In the brains of AD patients, these fibrils eventually deposit into extracellular amyloid plaques.

The peptidases neprilysin, an insulin-degrading enzyme, and endothelin-converting enzyme physiologically break down Aβ. Furthermore, Aβ can be removed by transit to peripheral circulation via a variety of routes, such as the glymphatic-lymphatic pathways, arachnoid villi, interstitial fluid bulk flow, and blood-brain barrier. Furthermore, perivascular macrophages, astrocytes, and microglia can phagocytose and degrade Aβ aggregates. Thus, inefficient clearing systems may cause an imbalance between the brain's production and clearance of Aβ, which could lead to neurodegeneration and subsequent neuronal dysfunction.

However, an increasing amount of data suggests that plaque deposition is not the only cause of the impairments seen in AD. Conversely, the idea that Aβ oligomers (AβOs) are the primary toxins causing synapse dysfunction and cognitive deficits in AD has garnered significant attention to advance our knowledge of the disease's mechanisms. Plaques are believed to function as a reservoir from which soluble oligomers diffuse or as a means of sequestering them until they attain a physiological plateau.

Several studies have shown that AβOs build up in the brains and cerebrospinal fluid (CSF) of AD patients. They are also linked to synapses in the brains of patients exhibiting clinical signs of dementia, which lends clinical significance to their involvement in AD. According to these studies, memory loss may result from synapse-associated AβOs promoting harmful alterations in synapse composition and structure. This increasing amount of data supports an earlier theory that suggests that synapse loss and failure in AD contribute to cognitive decline in addition to the extracellular and intracellular buildup of tau.

The precise mechanisms by which AβOs cause toxicity are still unknown, even after extensive research. Aβ aggregates' binding to different receptors may impair important neuronal processes. But more work needs to be done to fully understand the underlying signaling pathways and the precise nature of the receptors they bind to.

It has been discovered that AβOs attach to receptors on the cell surface, leading to the activation of various harmful signaling pathways. These pathways include calcium signaling, oxidative stress, disruptions in receptors related to plasticity, and an increase in glutamate release from pre-synaptic terminals. AβOs also contribute to tau hyperphosphorylation, hindered axonal transport, and inhibit long-term potentiation (LTP) and memory function.

10.4.1.2. Inflammatory Markers in the Brain

The pathophysiology of AD seems to involve robust interactions with the brain's immune mechanisms. In the brains of mice and nonhuman primates, AβOs cause aberrant reactivity of microglia and astrocytes. More research has revealed that disruptions in peripheral immune cells and microglia may be important factors in AD-related neurodegeneration and synapse loss. These findings are consistent with growing data that suggests inflammation plays a critical role in the pathophysiology of the disease, since the brain, CSF, and plasma of AD patients have been found to contain higher levels of inflammatory markers like TNF-α, IL-1β, IL-6, and other cytokines.

Reactive microglia's increased pro-inflammatory signaling causes aberrant synaptic pruning, lowers Aβ clearance, triggers tau and Aβ pathologies, and impairs synapse function. Crucially, memory impairments and depressed-like conduct in AD mice seem to be fueled by TNF-α-dependent pathways, suggesting that inflammation plays a causal role in harmful processes associated with AD.

10.4.1.3. Unfolded Protein Response and Defective Proteostasis

Neuronal stress is reported to be induced by pro-inflammatory pathways triggered by AβOs, particularly via TNF-α, which likely leads to defective proteostasis. Additionally, it has been shown recently that AβOs promotes the phosphorylation of eIF2α. eIF2α is a hub in the brain that maintains neuronal integrity in both health and disease and regulates learning and memory that is dependent on protein synthesis. However, eIF2α attenuates the start of global protein synthesis when it is phosphorylated.

The main molecular pathways causing synapse and memory failure in AD models have been identified as aberrant eIF2α phosphorylation and inhibition of protein synthesis. According to this theory, in mouse models of AD, deletion of eIF2α kinases such as PKR, PERK, or GCN2 restores memory and synapse function.

An abnormal build-up of misfolded proteins within the endoplasmic reticulum sets off a series of signaling branches known as the unfolded protein response (UPR), which aims to reestablish cellular normalcy. On the other hand, prolonged UPR signaling may impair neuronal functions and cause neurodegeneration. Recent research has provided strong evidence that the brains of AD mice exhibit elevated UPR markers, and that memory impairments in AD mice are caused, at the very least, by the UPR branches IRE-1a and PERK. Moreover, AβO-induced memory deficits in mice are mitigated by the chemical chaperone 4-phenylbutyrate, demonstrating the involvement of UPR in mediating neurotoxicity in AD. Thus, the core of synaptic and memory failure in AD may consist of misfolded protein accumulation, brain immune response activation, and impaired proteostasis (Cummings et al., 2016; Ritchie et al., 2016; Winblad et al., 2016; Livingston et al., 2020).

10.4.2. Novel Pathophysiological Mechanisms in AD

Recent scientific developments have increased our understanding of the cellular and molecular components of AD. However, AD is still primarily idiopathic, and there are currently no effective treatments to slow the disease's progression. It is not surprising that the great majority of studies focus on mechanisms linked to cognitive decline, since AD is primarily associated with memory loss. As a result, much less is known about the mechanisms underlying AD's main comorbidities as well as how AD affects brain regions that are not directly related to memory.

The effects of Aβ on the hippocampus and cortex, which are known to be centrally involved in the formation, consolidation, and recall of new episodic memories, have been the subject of numerous studies. Early research, however, suggested that AD may also impact brain areas unrelated to learning and memory. Notably, AD patients show notable non-cognitive deficits like sleep-wake disturbances and neuroendocrine changes linked to hypothalamic dysfunction.

10.4.2.1. Impaired Hypothalamic Function

There have been reports of disturbances in the hypothalamic nuclei in both AD patients and animal models. Sleep disturbances can be partially explained by impairments in the function of the hypothalamus, as it is the organ responsible for controlling the circadian rhythm. Nevertheless, research examining whether hypothalamic defects mediate sleep disturbances in AD is still necessary, even though preliminary findings have already illuminated how sleep becomes dysregulated in AD.

Peripheral metabolism dysregulation and its aftermath are primarily caused by dysregulation of hypothalamic functions. For example, impaired proteostasis and hypothalamic inflammation are important pathogenic events in the development of peripheral insulin resistance in metabolic disorders. However, very few research have looked into hypothalamic dysfunction in AD to date.

Early postmortem investigations revealed neurodegeneration with pronounced dendritic retraction in early AD, as well as Aβ deposits in the hypothalamic nuclei of AD patients. Furthermore, AβO-injected mice and non-human primates showed signs of insulin resistance, inflammation, and hypothalamic endoplasmic reticulum stress. AβO-induced hypothalamic dysfunction linked to the development of persistent peripheral glucose intolerance was further shown in human patients and multiple transgenic mouse models of AD.

10.4.2.2. Defective Glucose Metabolism and Insulin Signaling

Changes in peripheral metabolism, characterized by elevated blood sugar and insulin levels—two hallmarks of type 2 diabetes (T2D)—have been found to positively correlate with the emergence of AD-like brain pathology in humans. On the other hand, AD has been linked to a higher risk of T2D, indicating that there may be a two-way relationship between AD and T2D. Reduction of cerebral glucose metabolism in the forebrain, which includes parts of the temporal and occipital lobes as well as the posterior parietal lobe, is positively correlated with the progression of AD. An important factor that could be responsible for AD's impaired glucose metabolism is a malfunction in the insulin signaling pathways. Lower insulin levels as well as decreased insulin receptor (IR) expression and sensitivity are seen in AD brains. Furthermore, post-mortem brain tissue and animal models of AD have been shown to have impairments in the downstream machinery of insulin signaling. According to recent research, AβOs are the toxins that are linked to impaired hippocampal insulin signaling because they block downstream hippocampal insulin signaling by promoting the internalization and cellular redistribution of insulin receptors. A plethora of data has demonstrated new molecular similarities between AD and T2D.

It is still unclear how exactly impaired glucose metabolism and insulin signaling relate to the pathogenesis of AD at the molecular level. However, a growing body of research indicates that inflammation plays a key role in the relationship between AD and metabolic disorders, such as type 2 diabetes. One important aspect of the pathophysiology of metabolic disorders is the overproduction of pro-inflammatory cytokines, particularly TNF-α. Notably, peripheral metabolic dysregulation and impaired neuronal insulin signaling in AD have both been linked to brain inflammation in recent times.

10.4.2.3. Disturbances in Monoamine Signaling and Mood

Growing research points to the possibility that brain inflammation and microglial activation are additional causes of mood disorders, including depressive behaviors. Apathy and/or depression have been identified as risk factors for AD and have been reported to occur frequently in AD patients.

The mechanisms linking depression and AD at the molecular and cellular levels have only recently started to be established, although clinical and epidemiological studies have shown a strong correlation between these disorders. Recent research demonstrates that AβOs cause memory deficits and depressive-like behavior in mice, and they also correlate with lower brain serotonin levels, which is similar to what is seen in transgenic mice models of AD. These findings provide clues about the mechanistic relationship between memory and mood disturbances in AD. Following microglial activation, reduced serotonin levels may be associated with increased levels and activity of indolamine 2,3-dioxygenase (IDO). It's interesting to note that AD patients had higher quinolinic acid levels, lower plasma tryptophan levels, and higher IDO immunoreactivity in microglia. These results raise the possibility that AβO-induced brain inflammation may be a common factor in cognitive and mood alterations in AD since inflammation is known to play a significant role in depression.

Reduced levels of dopamine and its receptors, as well as other dopaminergic system alterations, have also been documented in AD patients and experimental models. These changes are frequently connected to both cognitive and non-cognitive symptoms of the disease. In a transgenic mouse model of AD, it has recently been demonstrated that inflammation and apoptosis occur in the ventral tegmental area, leading to selective degeneration of the dopaminergic nuclei before senile plaque deposition, tangles, or any indication of neuronal loss in cortical and hippocampal regions.

Dopaminergic degeneration in the ventral tegmental area may play a major role in the impairments in hippocampus-dependent memory and reward circuits because dopaminergic neurons from this area not only influence hippocampal synaptic plasticity but also target the cerebral cortex and the nucleus accumbens. These results may offer a compelling explanation for recent observations in AD patients showing a correlation between early non-cognitive symptoms like depression and apathy and the clinical diagnosis of dementia. All things considered, these new findings point to a possible connection between the non-cognitive and cognitive symptoms of AD patients and inflammation as the cause of synaptic failure in the monoaminergic systems (Cummings et al., 2016; Ritchie et al., 2016; Winblad et al., 2016; Livingston et al., 2020).

10.4.3. Challenges for AD Therapy

Over the past three decades, there has been extensive research into the mechanisms underlying AD pathogenesis, but little progress has been made in developing effective treatments or preventative or curative measures. Given the sharp increase in AD cases, society will face significant economic and social challenges if a treatment regimen is not discovered in the coming years. It is also noteworthy that the global burden of AD would be greatly reduced by advancements in therapeutic approaches that even slightly delay the onset or progression of the disease.

In light of the recent conceptual paradigm shift in the field, AD is now understood to be a complex process that progresses along a continuum rather than just having discrete and defined clinical stages. It is currently understood that pathophysiological alterations start many years before clinical signs of AD appear, thanks to the developing field of biomarker research. For instance, it has been demonstrated that alterations in CSF tau levels occur approximately 15 years before the onset of clinical AD, whereas CSF Aβ42 levels may decline as early as 20 years before symptoms appear.

AD ranges from profoundly impaired to clinically asymptomatic. These limits are difficult to draw, though, because the line separating preclinical AD from healthy aging is not clearly defined in our current knowledge. Since early detection biomarkers have emerged as a key area of study, it is likely that this unanswered question will be addressed in the future.

Given that women make up nearly two-thirds of AD patients and represent the majority of those affected, gender differences should also be considered as a biological variable in the pathogenesis of AD. Women may have longer lifespans than men, which could contribute to the higher frequency of AD in this population. Nevertheless, even after accounting for women's longer lifespans than men's, the risk of late-onset AD remains higher in them. There is still much to learn about the biological basis of women's higher risk of AD.

However, it is now acknowledged that the disruption of multiple estrogen-regulated systems that occurs during the transition from perimenopause to menopause affects various domains of cognitive function. In fact, new preclinical research suggests that a change in the brain's bioenergetics system at the onset of menopause may act as an early trigger for a higher risk of AD in the brains of women. These biological factors could contribute to a mechanism that triggers AD by increasing fatty acid catabolism, Aβ deposition, and impairing synaptic plasticity. Therefore, it is plausible that the disparities in metabolism between men and women could account for some of the underwhelming results observed in clinical trials. Therefore, the research community should fully support recommendations to include both male and female animals in preclinical research.

Although the amyloid cascade theory has dominated research for the past 20 years, the last 10 years have seen a shift toward the development of disease-modifying drugs, which may be necessary to create strategies that disrupt the underlying disease processes.

Combination pharmacotherapy may also offer advantages for AD treatment. This approach has demonstrated efficacy in treating a number of illnesses, such as cancer, HIV/AIDS, cardiovascular disease, and tuberculosis. It may also improve the effectiveness of medications that are ineffective when taken alone but have synergistic or additive effects when used in combination.

Strategies aimed at repurposing already marketed drugs become an intriguing option to expedite drug discovery in AD, given the well-known high failure rates in drug development targeting the central nervous system. Repurposing such compounds could expedite drug development since metabolic derangements appear to be central to AD and numerous medications for metabolic disease have already received human use approval. This is due to the possibility of quicker progress in preclinical toxicology, human safety, tolerability, and pharmacokinetic evaluations. The molecular pathophysiology of sporadic AD appears to be largely driven by impaired brain insulin signaling or brain insulin resistance. Therefore, drugs that have already been approved for the treatment of diabetes mellitus, such as insulin and medications that increase insulin sensitivity, could be developed more quickly for the treatment of AD if they target brain insulin signaling through their administration. It is important to remember that anti-diabetic medications like liraglutide, exenatide, and insulin have already been put to the test in ongoing clinical trials.

A vicious cycle of neuronal damage, proinflammatory factor release, and microglial activation is supported by neuroinflammation, particularly in its early stages. Furthermore, there is a possibility that TNF-α-induced inflammatory processes are coordinated between the brain and the peripheral, suggesting a connection between peripheral metabolic dysregulation and AD. Findings showing altered AD risk is linked to gene variants for immune receptors, including TREM2, which further supports the critical role of neuroinflammation in AD.

There is a good deal of evidence to suggest that inflammation in AD may be a target for therapeutic intervention. Even though lifetime use of NSAIDs has been linked to a lower risk of developing AD, trials involving anti-inflammatory substances, such as TNFα signaling inhibitors, minocycline, peroxisome proliferator-activated receptor-γ (PPAR-γ) activators, and non-steroidal anti-inflammatory drugs (NSAIDs), have not yet produced encouraging results.

Results from the evaluation of additional therapeutic approaches involving intravenous immunoglobulins and/or monoclonal antibodies are still pending. Anti-inflammatory medications target general neuroinflammatory components in AD rather than specific neuroinflammatory components, which may account for some of these ambiguous results. Therefore, to fully grasp the potential of targeting inflammation in neurodegeneration, it will be imperative to identify specific modulators of inflammation during the early stages of the disease (Cummings et al., 2016; Ritchie et al., 2016; Winblad et al., 2016; Livingston et al., 2020).

A Closer Look

Non-Modifiable Risk Factors of AD

The most significant known non-modifiable risk factors for AD and dementia are age, gender, ethnicity, and genetic composition. The most prevalent type of AD, known as sporadic Alzheimer's disease, is primarily caused by these risk factors; it is not inherited and is therefore non-familial in nature. The confluence of environmental elements and lifestyle traits (a.k.a. lifestyle medications) impact the state of risk.

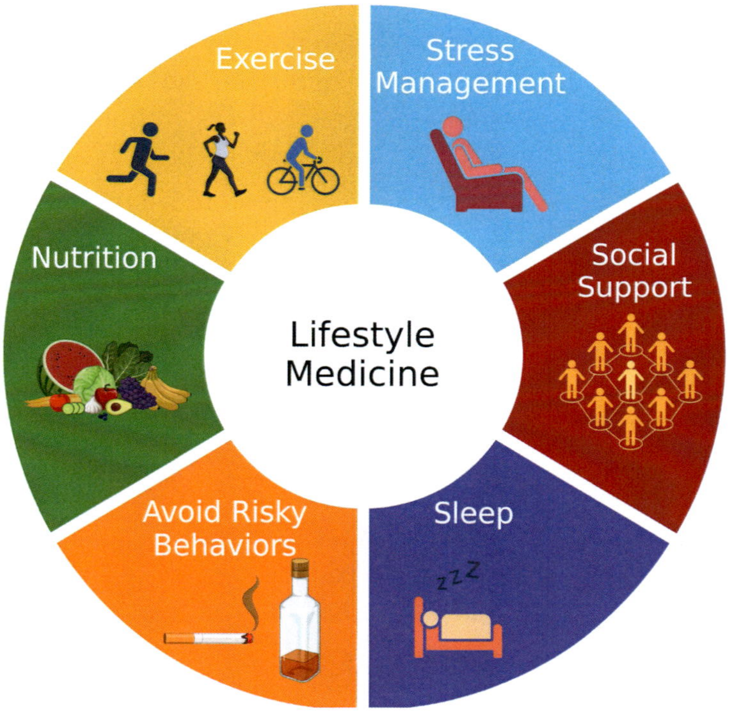

Arora S, Santiago JA, Bernstein M, & Potashkin JA. (2023) Diet and lifestyle impact the development and progression of Alzheimer's dementia. Front. Nutr., 10, 1213223. doi: 10.3389/fnut.2023.1213223.

- **Genetics:** Less than 5% of AD cases are hereditary and result from familial AD. It is caused by particular gene mutations or alterations. Three well-established genes—two presenilin genes (PSEN1 and PSEN2) and an amyloid precursor protein (APP) gene—have been connected to the onset of familial AD. Merely 50% of familial cases can be attributed to these three genes combined, indicating the possible involvement of additional genes that have not yet been identified. Furthermore, the pathology and clinical characteristics differ based on the mutation. There is a 50% chance that children of parents with these genes will inherit AD. There are at least 21 susceptibility genes known to raise the possibility of sporadic Alzheimer's disease. APOE, CLU, CR1, BIN1, PICALM, CD33, ABCA7, CD2AP, EPHA1, MS4, and TREM2, for example, are associated. It is important to note that the related genes are mainly grouped into three pathways: endosomal vesicle cycling, immune system and inflammatory response, and cholesterol and lipid metabolism. A person's lifetime susceptibility to developing AD is influenced by both lifestyle choices and environmental factors. However, the susceptibility gene APOE4 is thought to have the biggest impact on a person's likelihood of getting sporadic AD. Testing for APOE4 genetically is a contentious topic.

- **Aging:** A recognized risk factor for late-onset AD (LOAD) is age. AD affects almost one-third of adults over 85. People typically live longer thanks to medical advancements. As a result, there are more seniors in the population overall, and dementia incidence rises at the same time. Increased atrophy in particular brain regions that develop more quickly in AD patients compared to normal aging phenomena is one known difference between normal aging and AD, though the cause of this difference is still unknown. Even though AD and aging are distinct conditions, they both exhibit aberrant stem cell activity, inflammation, and proteostasis at the molecular and cellular levels. To fill in the knowledge gaps about AD and dementia, there is a greater need to comprehend the process of normal aging.
- **Gender:** AD is not limited to being more common in women than in men. Furthermore, there are gender differences in the clinical symptoms, rates of brain atrophy (which progress even faster in ApoE4 carriers), and responses to pharmaceutical therapy. The implications of ApoE4 in females are more severe than in males, and the primary cause of this bias remains poorly understood. Men have a 10% chance of developing AD at 45, while women have a 20% risk, according to the Alzheimer's Association. The higher incidence of AD in women may be partially explained by the fact that women outlive men and by the low level of education attained by women in their 20s. It is also assumed that the ApoE4 genotype in females interacts with estrogen to modify the risk in females. Cardiovascular and cerebrovascular risk factors are similar, if not higher in women, after menopause or age 60. Certain medical conditions, like depression and sleep disorders, are more prevalent in women and have been linked to an increased risk of AD.
- **Race:** There exists variation in the prevalence of AD across various racial groups. After the age of 65, 10.3% of white people, 12.2% of Hispanic/Latinos, and 13.8% of black/African Americans have been diagnosed with AD. This discrepancy is thought to be caused by lifestyle choices, medical disorders like diabetes and cardiovascular disease, and socioeconomic status. African Americans and Hispanics (Mexican-Americans or Caribbean-Americans) have higher rates of diabetes and cardiovascular diseases. The discrimination that African Americans and Hispanics experience is also characterized by lower levels of education and higher rates of poverty. The widespread misdiagnosis of African Americans is another significant problem. Compared to non-Hispanic Whites, African Americans and Hispanics have a two- and one-point-five-fold increased risk of developing AD, respectively. There appears to be little genetic variation in the prevalence of AD among different racial and ethnic groups. There is a strong correlation between APOE4 and ABCA7 and late-

onset AD (LOAD) in African-American individuals. Certain mutations in the ABCA7 gene have also been linked to an increased risk of AD in populations with European ancestry and those living in the Arctic. It has been determined that the CLU gene poses a risk to Caucasian people, particularly in relation to the transition from the MCI state to AD. The TREM2 variant is probably not linked to AD in the East Asian population, but it is in the Caucasian population.

- **Post-Traumatic Stress Disorder:** Post-traumatic stress disorder (PTSD) is one of the psychosocial determinants that raises the risk of AD, although there is a dearth of information regarding these factors. Epigenetics and chronic low-grade neuro-inflammation are two of the suggested mechanisms. The anterior cingulate, prefrontal, and hippocampal regions—all of which are anatomical structures implicated in AD pathology—are altered in PTSD patients. Serum glial fibrillary/serum glial fibrillary acidic protein, tumor necrosis factor-alpha, interleukin, MMP2 and MMP9, and brain-derived neurotrophic factor (BDF) and nerve growth factor-beta (NGFβ), which are markers of brain damage, were found to be higher in PTSD veterans compared to healthy veterans in a case-control study. These are potential early biomarkers for nervous system damage diseases like PTSD before the clinical onset because they would not be visible on brain scans like magnetic resonance imaging. These biomarkers may indicate the early pathogenesis that eventually leads to AD, as PTSD is a risk factor for AD. Alternatively, to help with treatment, these biomarkers can be utilized to identify the cause of AD. These biomarkers are particularly helpful because, according to certain studies, there is very little chance that a patient with PTSD will test positive for amyloid.

SUMMARY

- The terms "prevention" and "risk reduction" often are used interchangeably in medicine when referring to clinical interventions that aim to delay or prevent the onset of a disease.
- Evidence from observational studies has accumulated during the past few years and shown several potentially modifiable risk factors, concerning AD prevention some potential feasible suggestions are provided.
- Frequent social contact with friends was related to a modest decrease in dementia risk, owing to the creation of cognitive reserve at the early stage via regular healthy social engagement.
- Evidence supporting the higher risk of affecting with AD among diabetics [relative risks (RR) 1.43, 95% CI 1.25–1.62] was based on 24 longitudinal studies.
- Consistent pieces of evidence have proposed a higher risk of developing AD among middle-aged patients with raised body mass index (BMI) whereas overweight or obesity in late-life might have protective effects on cognition.
- A meta-analysis incorporating 5 prospective studies found a linear dose-response relationship between blood homocysteine (Hcy) levels and risk of AD (HR 1.15, 95% CI 1.04–1.26, per 5 μmol/L increment).
- Sleep disturbances (insomnia and sleep disordered breathing) were risk factors for AD, and those with sleep disorders were more likely to experience more accumulation of neurotoxic substances as a result of the decreased metabolite clearance ability.
- Persons in early adulthood taking more B vitamins including niacin, folate, vitamin B-6, and vitamin B-12 were likely to acquire better cognitive performance in late life.
- Approximately 30% of community-living older adults (≥65 years of age) in the United States fall each year, resulting in medical costs of more than $20 billion per year. Fall-related injuries are the fifth leading cause of death in older adults.
- Numerous tests and intervention programs have been researched to identify fall risk and to reduce falls and injuries in cognitively intact older adults.
- Normal aging inevitably brings physical and cognitive changes that may contribute to the risk of falls, including sensory, musculoskeletal, neurological, and metabolic changes.
- Assistive devices, such as canes and walkers, used to aid gait can improve balance control by providing mechanical advantages as well as somatosensory feedback.
- Many prevention studies are ongoing in both sporadic and autosomal dominant forms of AD. One such study is the Anti-Amyloid Treatment in Asymptomatic Alzheimer's (A4) recruiting individuals aged 65–86 with normal cognitive function but positive AD biomarkers (amyloid deposition by PET scan).
- The most distinctive features present in memory-associated brain regions of AD patients are the intracellular neurofibrillary tangles (NFTs) and the extracellular amyloid plaques.

- The amyloid cascade hypothesis suggests that brain accumulation of the amyloid-β peptide (Aβ), produced by sequential cleavage of the amyloid precursor protein (APP) by the β- and γ-secretase enzymes, is a central event in AD.
- Alterations in the dopaminergic system have also been reported in AD patients and experimental models, including reduced levels of dopamine and its receptors, and are commonly linked to cognitive and non-cognitive symptoms of the disease.
- Despite intensive investigation of mechanisms of pathogenesis in AD during the past three decades, little has been achieved in terms of effective treatments or approaches to prevent or cure it.

REFERENCES

1. Albert, M. S., DeKosky, S. T., Dickson, D., et al. (2011). The diagnosis of mild cognitive impairment due to Alzheimer's disease: Recommendations from the national institute on aging-Alzheimer's association workgroups on diagnostic guidelines for Alzheimer's disease. *Alzheimer's & Dementia, 7*, 270–279. https://doi.org/10.1016/j.jalz.2011.03.008.
2. Alcolea, D., Carmona-Iragui, M., Suárez-Calvet, M., et al. (2014). Relationship between β-secretase, inflammation and core cerebrospinal fluid biomarkers for Alzheimer's disease. *Journal of Alzheimer's Disease, 42*(s3), 157–167. https://doi.org/10.3233/JAD-132570.
3. Anker, J. N., Hall, W. P., Lambert, M. P., et al. (2009). Detection and identification of bioanalytes with high resolution LSPR spectroscopy and MALDI mass spectrometry. *Journal of Physical Chemistry C, 113*(14), 5891–5894. https://doi.org/10.1021/jp811687s.
4. Appleby, B. S., & Cummings, J. L. (2013). Discovering new treatments for Alzheimer's disease by repurposing approved medications. *Current Topics in Medicinal Chemistry, 13*(18), 2306–2327. https://doi.org/10.2174/15680266113136660257.
5. Bartels, C., Wagner, M., Wolfsgruber, S., Ehrenreich, H., & Schneider, A. (2018). Impact of SSRI therapy on risk of conversion from mild cognitive impairment to Alzheimer's dementia in individuals with previous depression. *The American Journal of Psychiatry, 175*(3), 232–241. https://doi.org/10.1176/appi.ajp.2017.17020147.
6. Chan, K. Y., Wang, W., Wu, J. J., et al. (2013). Epidemiology of Alzheimer's disease and other forms of dementia in China, 1990–2010: A systematic review and analysis. *The Lancet, 381*(9882), 2016–2023. https://doi.org/10.1016/S0140-6736(13)60221-4.
7. Cummings, J., Aisen, P. S., DuBois, B., et al. (2016). Drug development in Alzheimer's disease: The path to 2025. *Alzheimer's Research & Therapy, 8*, 39. https://doi.org/10.1186/s13195-016-0207-9.
8. Diniz, B. S., Butters, M. A., Albert, S. M., Dew, M. A., & Reynolds, C. F. (2013). Late-life depression and risk of vascular dementia and Alzheimer's disease: Systematic review and meta-analysis of community-based cohort studies. *The British Journal of Psychiatry, 202*, 329–335. https://doi.org/10.1192/bjp.bp.112.118307.
9. Estanga, A., Ecay-Torres, M., Ibañez, A., et al. (2017). Beneficial effect of bilingualism on Alzheimer's disease CSF biomarkers and cognition. *Neurobiology of Aging, 50*, 144–151. https://doi.org/10.1016/j.neurobiolaging.2016.11.004.

10. Fancourt, D., Steptoe, A., & Cadar, D. (2020). Community engagement and dementia risk: Time-to-event analyses from a national cohort study. *Journal of Epidemiology and Community Health, 74*(1), 71–77. https://doi.org/10.1136/jech-2019-212777.

11. Global, regional, and national burden of Alzheimer's disease and other dementias, 1990-2016: A systematic analysis for the Global Burden of Disease Study 2016. (2019). *The Lancet. Neurology, 18*(1), 88–106. https://doi.org/10.1016/S1474-4422(18)30403-4.

12. Grady, C. L., Luk, G., Craik, F. I. M., & Bialystok, E. (2015). Brain network activity in monolingual and bilingual older adults. *Neuropsychologia, 66*, 170–181. https://doi.org/10.1016/j.neuropsychologia.2014.11.021.

13. Hanson, L.C.; Ersek, M.; Lin, F.C.; Carey, T.S. Outcomes of Feeding Problems in Advanced Dementia in a Nursing Home Population. J. Am. Geriatr. Soc. 2013, 61, 1692–1697.

14. Jacka, F.N.; Cherbuin, N.; Anstey, K.J.; Sachdev, P.; Butterworth, P. Western Diet Is Associated with a Smaller Hippocampus: A Longitudinal Investigation. BMC Med. 2015, 13, 215.

15. Laitinen, M.H.; Ngandu, T.; Rovio, S.; Helkala, E.L.; Uusitalo, U.; Viitanen, M.; Nissinen, A.; Tuomilehto, J.; Soininen, H.; Kivipelto, M. Fat Intake at Midlife and Risk of Dementia and Alzheimer's Disease: A Population-Based Study. Dement. Geriatr. Cogn. Disord. 2006, 22, 99–107.

16. Lee, Y.H.; Martin, J.M.; Maple, R.L.; Tharp, W.G.; Pratley, R.E. Plasma Amyloid-Beta Peptide Levels Correlate with Adipocyte Amyloid Precursor Protein Gene Expression in Obese Individuals. Neuroendocrinology 2009, 90, 383–390

17. Leigh Gibson, E.; Barr, S.; Jeanes, Y.M. Habitual Fat Intake Predicts Memory Function in Younger Women. Front. Hum. Neurosci. 2013, 7, 838.

18. Livingston, G., Huntley, J., Sommerlad, A., et al. (2020). Dementia prevention, intervention, and care: 2020 report of the Lancet Commission. *The Lancet, 396*(10248), 413–446. https://doi.org/10.1016/S0140-6736(20)30367-6.

19. Matyas, N., Keser Aschenberger, F., Wagner, G., et al. (2019). Continuing education for the prevention of mild cognitive impairment and Alzheimer's-type dementia: A systematic review and overview of systematic reviews. *BMJ Open, 9*(10), e027719. https://doi.org/10.1136/bmjopen-2018-027719.

20. McKhann, G. M., Knopman, D. S., Chertkow, H., et al. (2011). The diagnosis of dementia due to Alzheimer's disease: Recommendations from the National Institute on Aging-Alzheimer's Association workgroups on diagnostic guidelines for Alzheimer's disease. *Alzheimer's & Dementia, 7*, 263–269. https://doi.org/10.1016/j.jalz.2011.03.005.

21. Norton, S., Matthews, F. E., Barnes, D. E., Yaffe, K., & Brayne, C. (2014). Potential for primary prevention of Alzheimer's disease: An analysis of population-based data. *The Lancet. Neurology, 13*(8), 788–794. https://doi.org/10.1016/S1474-4422(14)70136-X.

22. O'Donnell, C. A., Browne, S., Pierce, M., et al. (2015). Reducing dementia risk by targeting modifiable risk factors in mid-life: Study protocol for the Innovative Midlife Intervention for Dementia Deterrence (In-MINDD) randomized controlled feasibility trial. *Pilot and Feasibility Studies, 1*, 40. https://doi.org/10.1186/s40814-015-0033-5.

23. Ohara, T., Hata, J., Yoshida, D., et al. (2017). Trends in dementia prevalence, incidence, and survival rate in a Japanese community. *Neurology, 88*(20), 1925–1932. https://doi.org/10.1212/WNL.0000000000003962.

24. Ritchie, C. W., Molinuevo, J. L., Truyen, L., et al. (2016). European Prevention of Alzheimer's Dementia (EPAD) Consortium. Development of interventions for the secondary prevention of Alzheimer's dementia: The European prevention of Alzheimer's dementia (EPAD) project. *The Lancet Psychiatry, 3*, 179–186. https://doi.org/10.1016/S2215-0366(15)00454-X.

25. Ruan, Y.; Tang, J.; Guo, X.; Li, K.; Li, D. Dietary Fat Intake and Risk of Alzheimer's Disease and Dementia: A Meta-Analysis of Cohort Studies. Curr. Alzheimer Res. 2018, 15, 869–876.

26. Setiawan, E., Attwells, S., Wilson, A. A., et al. (2018). Association of translocator protein total distribution volume with duration of untreated major depressive disorder: A cross-sectional study. *The Lancet. Psychiatry, 5*(4), 339–347. https://doi.org/10.1016/S2215-0366(18)30048-8.

27. Sindi, S., Calov, E., Fokkens, J., et al. (2015). The CAIDE Dementia Risk Score App: The development of an evidence-based mobile application to predict the risk of dementia. *Alzheimer's & Dementia: Diagnosis, Assessment & Disease Monitoring, 1*, 328–333. https://doi.org/10.1016/j.dadm.2015.07.004.

28. Singh-Manoux, A., Dugravot, A., Fournier, A., et al. (2017). Trajectories of depressive symptoms before diagnosis of dementia: A 28-year follow-up study. *JAMA Psychiatry, 74*(7), 712–718. https://doi.org/10.1001/jamapsychiatry.2017.0660.

29. Sperling, R. A., Aisen, P. S., Beckett, L. A., et al. (2011). Toward defining the preclinical stages of Alzheimer's disease: Recommendations from the national institute on aging-Alzheimer's association workgroups on diagnostic guidelines for Alzheimer's disease. *Alzheimer's & Dementia, 7*, 280–292. https://doi.org/10.1016/j.jalz.2011.05.001.

30. Suo, C., Singh, M. F., Gates, N., et al. (2016). Therapeutically relevant structural and functional mechanisms triggered by physical and cognitive exercise. *Molecular Psychiatry, 21*(11), 1633–1642. https://doi.org/10.1038/mp.2016.19.

31. Wada, M., Noda, Y., Shinagawa, S., et al. (2018). Effect of education on Alzheimer's disease-related neuroimaging biomarkers in healthy controls, and participants with mild cognitive impairment and Alzheimer's disease: A cross-sectional study. *Journal of Alzheimer's Disease, 63*(3), 861–869. https://doi.org/10.3233/JAD-171121.

32. Winblad, B., Amouyel, P., Andrieu, S., et al. (2016). Defeating Alzheimer's disease and other dementias: A priority for European science and society. *The Lancet. Neurology, 15*(5), 455–532. https://doi.org/10.1016/S1474-4422(16)00062-4.

33. Yates, L. A., Ziser, S., Spector, A., et al. (2016). Cognitive leisure activities and future risk of cognitive impairment and dementia: Systematic review and meta-analysis. *International Psychogeriatrics, 28*, 1791–1806. https://doi.org/10.1017/S1041610216001151.

34. Ye, B.S.; Jang, E.Y.; Kim, S.Y.; Kim, E.J.; Park, S.A.; Lee, Y.; Hong, C.H.; Choi, S.H.; Yoon, B.; Yoon, S.J.; et al. Unstable Body Mass Index and Progression to Probable Alzheimer's Disease Dementia in Patients with Amnestic Mild Cognitive Impairment. J. Alzheimers Dis. 2016, 49, 483–491.

35. Zheng, Y., Wu, Q., Su, F., et al. (2018). The protective effect of Cantonese/Mandarin bilingualism on the onset of Alzheimer's disease. *Dementia and Geriatric Cognitive Disorders, 45*(5–6), 210–219. https://doi.org/10.1159/000487587.

INDEX

A

Active Immunization 211
Adrenaline (AduhelmTM) 207
Aducanumab 202, 207, 208, 217
Advance directive 283
Aging Demographics and Memory Study (ADAMS) 80
Agitation 201, 209, 211, 221
Air pollution 134
Alcohol 233, 235
Alleles of apolipoprotein E (APOE) 7
Alzheimer's disease (AD) 1, 3, 8, 11, 25, 26, 34
Alzheimer's Disease and Related Disorders Association (ADRDA) 53
Amantadine 209
Amyloid angiopathy 25, 26
Amyloid beta 6, 7, 8, 9, 12, 25, 26, 27, 28, 29, 34, 35
Amyloid hypothesis 209
Amyloid precursor protein (APP) 11, 26, 30, 108, 136, 145
Amyloid-related imaging abnormalities (ARIA) 164
Anticholinergics 155
Antihistamines 155
Anti-inflammation 217
Antioxidants 120
Anti-tau interventions 217
Anxiety 41, 49, 59, 60, 63, 64, 66
Apolipoprotein E (APOE) gene 108, 145
Apolipoprotein E ε4 (APOE ε4) 116
Association memory (AM) 257
Atrial fibrillation 117, 130
Autopsy 124
Autosomal-dominant Alzheimer's disease (ADAD) 327
Avagacestat 210
Aβ accumulation 130
Aβ antibodies 202
Aβ hypothesis 141
Aβ-induced oxidative stress 133

B

BACE Inhibitors 209
Balanced diet 279
Behavioral and psychological symptoms of dementia (BPSD) 250
Benzodiazepines 155
Bepineuzumab 202, 219
Beta-amyloid plaques 5, 32
Beta-Secretase Enzyme 202
Bilingualism 127
Billing records 78
Biological factors 116
Biomarkers 6, 13, 18, 21
Black and Hispanic populations 94
Blood-Based Biomarkers (BBBMs) 165
Blood lipids 129

Blood Pressure 117
Bloodstream 116
Blood tests 40
Body mass index (BMI) 118
Brain atrophy 5, 6, 11
Brain tumors 40
Brain vascularization 140
Budipine 209

C

Cache County Study 114
Caffeine 233, 235
Cardiovascular Disease 117
Care 269, 271, 274, 279, 291, 292, 293, 294, 295, 296, 298, 299, 300, 301, 304, 305, 306, 308
Caregiving 24
Central nervous system (CNS) 199
Cerebrospinal fluid (CSF) 6
Cerebrospinal fluid (CSF) biomarkers 150
Cerebrovascular Disease 118, 135, 136
Chelation therapy 211, 224
Chicago Health and Aging Project (CHAP) 73
Cholesterol 116, 119, 129, 139
Cholinesterase inhibitors 19, 20, 33, 199, 201, 217
Chronic disease 85
Clinical Laboratory Improvement Amendments (CLIA) 313
Clinical psychologists 169
Cognitive ability 87, 96
Cognitive skills 16
Cognitive stimulation therapy (CST) 248
Cognitive training 237, 238, 246, 247, 248, 249, 250, 256, 257
Cohorts 90
Communication gap 62
Community 110, 114, 115, 128, 140, 146
Compassionate allowances 299
Computed tomography (CT) 152, 167
Computerized Tomography (CT) 17
Confusion 49, 52
Cornell Scale for Depression in Dementia (CSDD) 251
Corticobasal syndrome (CBS) 157, 159
COVID-19 pandemic 63
Cramping 201
C-reactive protein 123, 140
Cross-Cultural Studies 82
Cytokines 25, 27, 28
Cytoskeleton 198

D

Deep brain stimulation (DBS) 254, 261, 262
Defective Proteostasis 368
Delphi Consensus Study 79, 80, 84
Dementia 37, 38, 40, 41, 42, 43, 46, 47, 48, 49, 50, 51, 52, 54, 55, 56, 57, 58, 65, 67, 68, 69
Demographics 74, 91
Demographic transition 108, 110
Demyelination 12
Department of Veterans Affairs 300
Depression 40, 41, 42, 44, 59, 60, 67
Developing nations 110, 112, 113, 115, 131
Dextrometorphan 209
Diabetes 108, 118, 119, 123, 129, 134, 135, 136, 137
Diabetes Mellitus 118, 135
Dietary fats 139
Diets 133
Diffuse plaques 26
Disability 115, 124
Disease-modifying therapies (DMTs) 157
Disorientation 49
Dizziness 201, 209, 221
Docosahexaenoic acid (DHA) 259
Doll Therapy 243
Dominantly Inherited Alzheimer's Network – Treatment Unit (DIAN-TU) 360
Do Not Resuscitate (DNR) Form 275
Dressing 278
Drugs 235, 253
Durable Power of Attorney for Finances 275
Durable Power of Attorney for Health Care 275
Dyslipidemia 119, 135
Dystrophic neurites 71

E

Efficacy 200, 213, 214, 215, 216
Eicosapentaenoic acid (EPA) 259
Elan vital 245

Electrocardiogram (ECG) 201
Elenbecestat (E2609) 210
Emesis 209
end-stage dementia 50
Enzyme-Assisted Derivatization for Sterol Analysis 326
Ervin Böhm's Psychobiographic Model 245
European Prevention of AD (EPAD) 361
Excitotoxicity 199, 205, 207, 218
Exercise 140
Exercise programs 230
Exhaustion 201
Extremely-low-frequency electromagnetic fields (ELF-EMF) 123

F

Family caregivers 59, 60
Fatigue 209
Fish products 235
Fluorodeoxyglucose (FDG) 17
Food and Drug Administration (FDA) 207
Free radicals 7, 138
Frontal variant of AD 339
Frontotemporal dementia (FTD) 43, 163
Functional magnetic resonance imaging (fMRI) 156
Functional MRI (fMRI) 328

G

Galantamine 197, 208, 222
Gamma-Secretase Enzyme 202
Gastrointestinal distress 201
GEDOC memory clinic subcohort 324
Gene alterations 7
Genetic mutations 111, 115, 145
Genetic predisposition 116, 145
Genetic risk factors 1, 7, 8, 10
Gentle deception 62
Geriatricians 153, 169
Geriatric Psychiatrists 153
Gingko biloba 235
Glial fibrillary acidic protein (GFAP) 165, 313
Glutamate 197, 199, 205, 207, 208, 209, 218, 222, 226
Grooming 278

H

Hallucinations 209
Hamilton Depression Rating Scale (HDRS) 251
Harmonized Cognitive Assessment Protocol (HCAP) 73
Headaches 209
Health and Retirement Study (HRS) 73
Healthy lifestyle 121
Hearing loss 131
Heart failure 117
Hemorrhagic infarcts 118, 146
Hippocampus 351, 369, 370
HIV/AIDS 93
Hormone Replacement Therapy 123
Huntington's disease 40
Hyperhomocysteinemia 131
Hypertension 117, 118, 119, 129, 134, 135, 136, 137
Hypoperfusion 111, 130, 135, 136
Hypothyroidism 155, 167

I

Immune cells 27
Immunization 202, 210
Immunofluorescence Staining 326, 335
Incontinence 282, 283
Indianapolis-Ibadan Dementia Project 83
Inflammation 123
Insomnia 155
Instrumental activities of daily living (IADLs) 49
insulin receptor (IR) 370
Intermittent theta burst stimulation (iTBS) 254, 262
Interval censoring 87
Intraneuronal neurofibrillary tangles 71
Intravenous (IV) infusion medication 207
Ischemic cortical infarcts 118, 146

K

Ketamine 209
Kufs disease 40

L

Lewy body dementia (LBD) 43
Lewy body disease 40
Lifelong environmental exposures 116
Liver metabolic rates 314
Living Trust 275
Living Will 275
Low-dose aspirin 133

M

Macushield 259
Magnetic Resonance Imaging (MRI) 17
Marginalization 92, 94
MCI-converters 338
Medicaid 293, 294, 295, 297, 298, 299, 300
Medical history 149, 169, 170
Medicare 292, 293, 294, 295, 297, 298, 299
Medications 133
Memantine 201, 205, 207, 208, 209, 227, 228
Memantine uncompetitively 201
Memory 41, 42, 43, 46, 51, 52, 62
Memory Impairment Screen 46
Memory loss 111
metabolic disorders 366, 369, 370
Metabolic Syndrome 119
Microglia 5, 11, 25, 27, 28
Microhemorrhages 207, 210, 211
Mild Cognitive Impairment 15
Mild cognitive impairment (MCI) 13
Mini-Mental State Examination (MMSE) 89, 150, 183, 184
Mixed dementia 43
Moderate cognitive decline 49
Montreal Cognitive Assessment (MoCA) 150
Mortality 110, 115, 125, 131, 146
multi-infarct dementia 43
Multi-target directed ligands (MTDL) 212

N

National Council on Aging (NCOA) 300
National Institute of Neurological and Communicative Disorders and Stroke (NINCDS) 53
National Institute on Aging – Alzheimer's Association (NIA-AA) 75
National Institutes of Health (NIH) 233
Neurocognitive disorder (NCD) 40
Neurofibrillary tangles 1, 6, 10, 12, 17, 25, 26, 32
Neurofibrillary tangles (NFTs) 198
Neurofilament light chain (NfL) 165
Neurogenesis 130, 140
Neuroinflammation 126, 127, 129, 134, 135, 136
Neurologists 153, 154, 169
Neurons 130
Neuron-to-neuron communication 5
Neuroprotection interventions 217
Neuropsychiatric Inventory (NPI) 251
Neuropsychiatric symptoms 41, 67
Neuropsychologists 153, 169
Nicotine 138, 233, 235
Nilvadipine 219
N-methyl-D-aspartate (NMDA) receptor 19, 199
Nonsteroidal anti-inflammatory drugs (NSAIDs) 133
Normal activities of daily living (ADLs) 49
N-terminal fragment of tau (NT1) 316

O

Obesity 118, 130, 135
Omega-3 fatty acids 235
Overconsumption 119
Overweight 118
Oxidative stress 353, 354, 361, 368

P

Parkinson's disease 40, 43
Parkinson's disease dementia (PDD) 43
Passive Immunization 210
Peptic ulcer disease 201
peripheral metabolism 369
Phagocytes 138
Phagocytosis 207
Pharmacotoxic psychosis 209
Physical activity 2
Physical environment 94
Placebo effects 260

Plasma 161, 162, 165, 168, 174, 178, 179, 180, 181, 188, 191, 193
Pollution 134, 136
polyunsaturated fatty acids (PUFAs) 120
Population aging 81, 99
Positron emission tomography (PET) 6, 26
Posterior cortical atrophy (PCA) 157, 159
Pre-Dementia 47
Pressure ulcers 304
Primary Care Physician (PCP) 169
probable AD dementia 56, 57, 58
Program of All-Inclusive Care for the Elderly (PACE) 299
Psychological variables 116

R

Race 85, 93, 94, 101, 102, 104
Radiologists 169
Randomized controlled trials (RCTs) 87
Rapid eye movement (REM) 43
Reactive astrocytosis 316
Reliability 87, 89
Reminiscence Therapy 239
Repetitive transcranial magnetic stimulation (rTMS) 254, 262
Restless legs syndrome 233
Restless leg syndrome 155
Retrogenesis 12

S

Score Composite 219
Sedatives 155
Semagacestat 202, 210
Semantic variant primary progressive aphasia (svPPA) 158, 159
Senile plaques 25, 26
Sensory Organization Test 356
severe dementia 48, 49, 52
Sexual and gender minority (SGM) groups 92
Simulated presence therapy (SPT) 24
Sleep apnea 155, 233
Slow waves 233
Smoking 110, 120, 135, 137
Snoezelen 24
Snoezelen therapy 231, 238, 239, 262
Social connections 351
Social Security Administration Programs 299
Social Security Disability Insurance (SSDI) 299
Social workers 170
Socioeconomic diversity 95
Socioeconomic status 85
Solanezumab 202
standard deviations (SD) 324
State Health Insurance Assistance Program (SHIP) 299
Stroke 154, 179
Structural MRI 328
Subjective cognitive decline 78, 79
Substrate presentation 30
Sundown syndrome 49
Supplemental Security Income (SSI) programs 299
Susceptibility gene 116
Swedish Kungsholmen Project 115
Synapses 3, 5, 25, 28, 34
Synucleinopathies 40

T

Tau 198, 203, 204, 217, 218, 227
Tauopathies 39, 40
Tau tangles 4, 5, 6
Thyroid dysfunction 150
Trade-offs 91
Tranquilizers 235
Transcranial direct current stimulation (tDCS) 254, 262
Transcranial pulse stimulation (TPS) 254, 262
Trustee 275
Ttraumatic brain injury (TBI) 130, 131
Type II Diabetes 137

U

umibecestat (CNP520) 210
Unfolded protein response (UPR) 368
U.S. Census Bureau 73

V

Validation 239, 240, 241, 242, 243
Validity 87, 88, 91
Vascular brain lesions 111
Vascular dementia 95
Vascular disease 40, 199
Vasculopathies 118, 135, 146
Vitamin deficiencies 150

W

Wandering 49, 66
Will 275

MIX
Papier | Fördert gute Waldnutzung
FSC® C083411

Kolibri 360 GmbH
Ferdinand-Jühlke-Straße 7
99095 Erfurt, Deutschland
produktsicherheit@kolibri360.de